jamie's kitchen

'There's only one Jamie Oliver. Great to watch. Great to cook'
Delia Smith

'If he can rescue 12 aimless drifters and imbue them with passion, excitement and pride, then it can be done in schools all over Britain' *Daily Mail*

'This is simply brilliant cooking, and Jamie's recipes are a joy'
Nigel Slater

'Acquire the book: it's irresistible' *Daily Telegraph*

'This beautifully illustrated book will inspire even the most jaded of cooks' *Daily Mirror*

'The design and photography are clear and luscious and the recipes are the kind you want to try and really can make at home' *Time Out*

'First class ... accessible easy meals to impress your friends with but which won't take for ever to make' *Guardian*

'He has created a foolproof repertoire of simple, feisty and delicious recipes which combine bold flavours with fresh ingredients. At the same time he avoids culinary jargon and any complicated time-consuming processes ... unpretentious, charismatic, streetwise and passionate about food'
Food and Wine Magazine

'Great, fabulous. There are some really hot tips and some scrumptious recipes that really hit the spot' *Spectator*

'The food is simply explained and superbly presented, and it makes you want to cook every dish' *Daily Express*

'Twelve-year-olds will like it . . . women will like it . . . men will like it . . . Problem solved' *The Times*

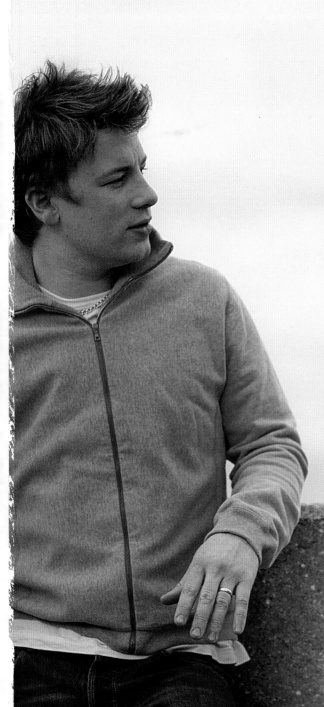

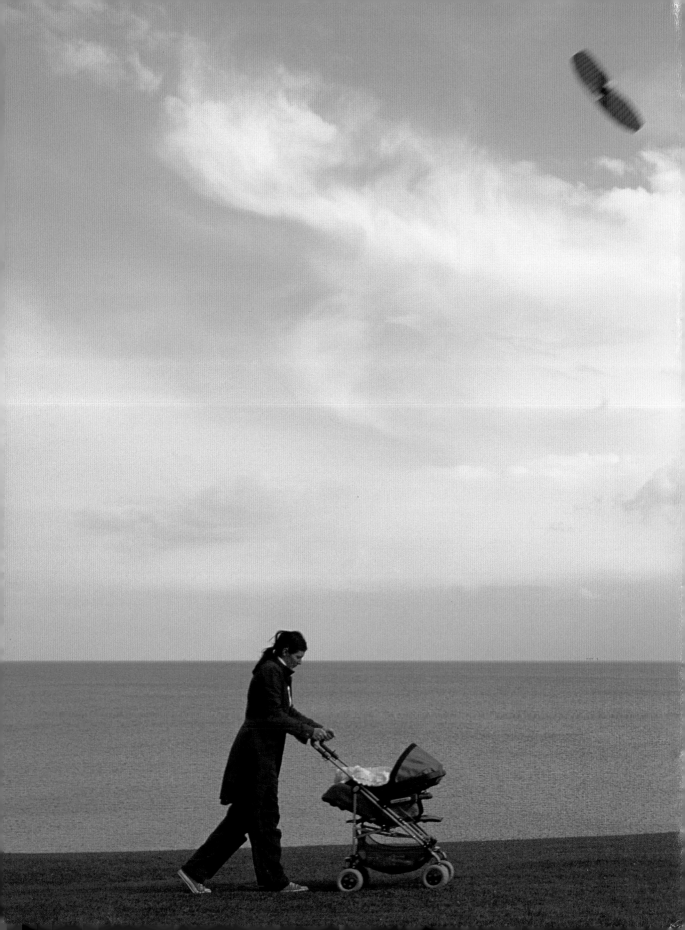

jamie's kitchen
jamie oliver

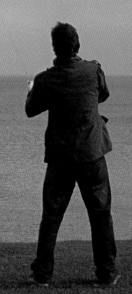

PENGUIN BOOKS

PENGUIN BOOKS

Published by the Penguin Group

Penguin Books Ltd, 80 Strand, London WC2R 0RL, England

Penguin Group (USA) Inc., 375 Hudson Street, New York, New York 10014, USA

Penguin Group (Canada), 90 Eglinton Avenue East, Suite 700, Toronto, Ontario, Canada M4P 2Y3
(a division of Pearson Penguin Canada Inc.)

Penguin Ireland, 25 St Stephen's Green, Dublin 2, Ireland (a division of Penguin Books Ltd)

Penguin Group (Australia), 250 Camberwell Road, Camberwell, Victoria 3124, Australia
(a division of Pearson Australia Group Pty Ltd)

Penguin Books India Pvt Ltd, 11 Community Centre, Panchsheel Park, New Delhi – 110 017, India

Penguin Group (NZ), 67 Apollo Drive, Rosedale, North Shore 0632, New Zealand
(a division of Pearson New Zealand Ltd)

Penguin Books (South Africa) (Pty) Ltd, 24 Sturdee Avenue, Rosebank, Johannesburg 2196, South Africa

Penguin Books Ltd, Registered Offices: 80 Strand, London WC2R 0RL, England

www.penguin.com

First published by Michael Joseph 2002
Published in Penguin Books 2004
Reissued in Penguin Books 2010

Copyright © Jamie Oliver, 2002
Food and reportage photography copyright © David Loftus, 2002
Photographs on pages 9, 12 and 323 copyright © Harry Borden, 2002

ISBN: 978-0-141-04299-2

jamieoliver.com

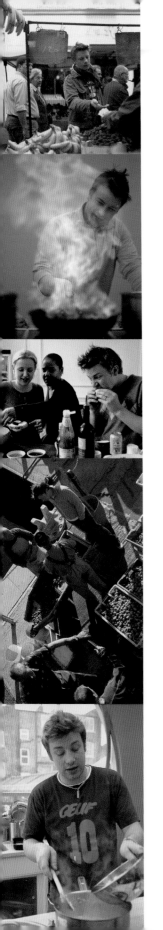

contents

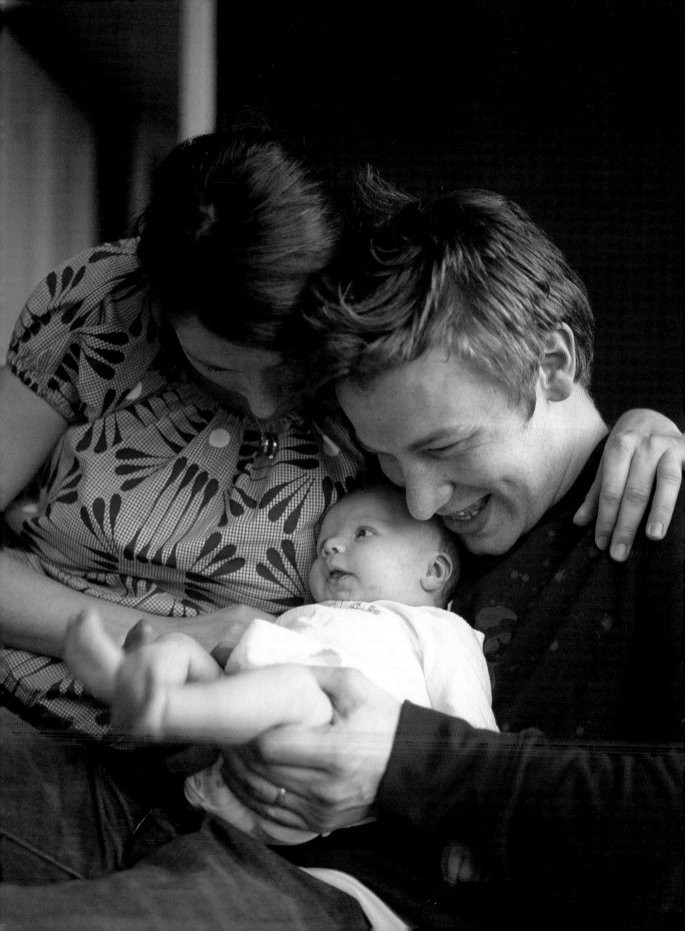

To my two great girls:

Lovely Jools, the best thing that ever happened to me, and little Poppy, the best thing that I've ever made.

Love Dad

X

WHAT A YEAR IT'S BEEN. Over the past 12 months I've really learnt a lot about myself and have gained so much from new experiences, especially from the birth of my daughter. Poppy has given me a massive wake-up call! Some things never change though – I am still absolutely passionate about food. Not just eating but the whole cooking thing, hunting down great produce and especially making up recipes. When I've found a new dish or tried out a new technique in cooking, I get the same feeling as when I first learnt how to ride a bike. I may never have been the best bike rider, but I always enjoyed it, even when I fell off or crashed. I want you to have the same attitude towards your cooking.

This year has been really exciting for me, because an idea has finally become a reality. Let me tell you about Jamie's Kitchen. About seven years ago, when I'd just started working at the River Café, I was having a cup of tea with a friend, Kirsty. At the time she was working with problem children – aggressive and bad-tempered, they weren't fitting into their school or home environments very well – and she was explaining to me that the main thing was to inspire and empower them and to give them some hands-on responsibility. She said that cooking classes had been going really well with them, because they could feel, smell and create things and above all it was fun. Plus they could eat what they'd made! Having not been the brightest banana in the bunch myself, I realized that my biggest weapon in life was the determination, enthusiasm, hands-on and 'actions speak louder than words' approach my father taught me, and I wanted to get this across to others, especially those interested in food. Having had five really great years I felt it was about time to give a little back and help inspire others. So that's where Jamie's Kitchen came from.

All my ideas got whittled down to one main one – to train a team of unemployed kids with an interest and passion for food and to open a new first-class restaurant in London to be run by them. The restaurant will be a charity, with all profits used to send the kids on scholarships to work with the best chefs around the world – Britain, Italy, France, Australia, Japan. Just look at the difference that the Roux brothers, Marco Pierre White and Gordon Ramsay have made in such a short period of time. They are all incredible chefs and we should aspire to be as good as they are. Together they have broken the mould for British food and now their protégés are continuing in their footsteps and cooking to a brilliantly high standard.

The aim of this book is the same as my TV programme's. It's not a clinical or overly serious 'learn to cook' book. It's more about giving you an honest and easy approach

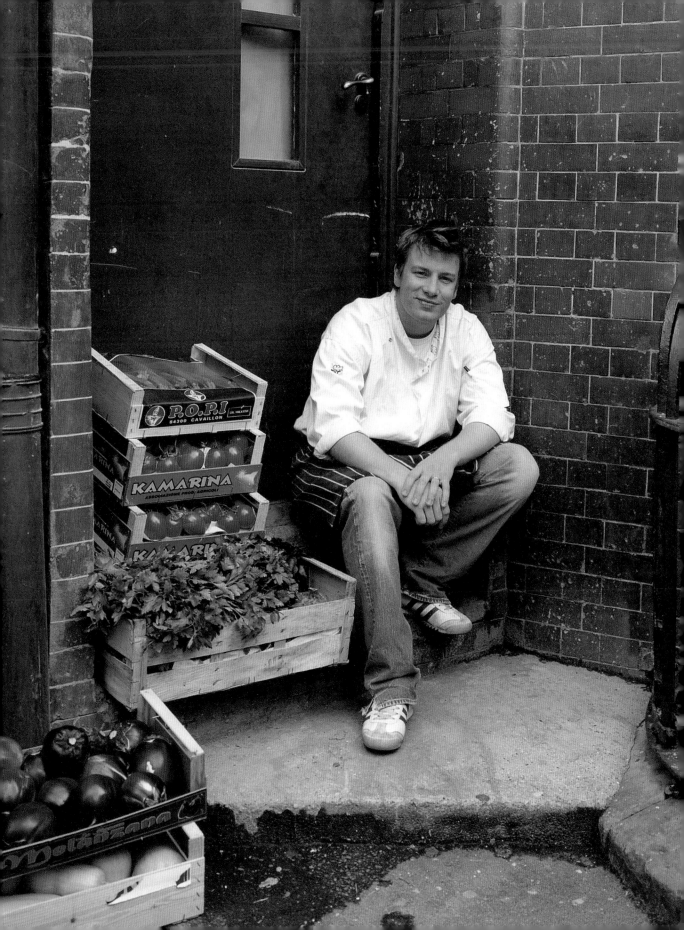

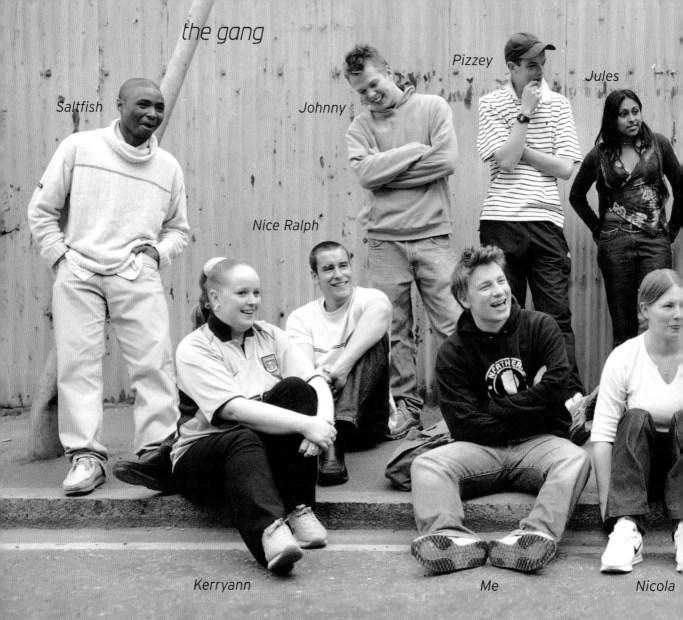

the gang

Saltfish

Johnny

Pizzey

Jules

Nice Ralph

Kerryann

Me

Nicola

to cooking from my point of view. With this book, you too can get stuck in along with the kids who are training as chefs. So far they've been brilliant – getting stuck into their training and displaying a real thirst for knowledge. But it hasn't all been plain sailing as they are 15 very different individuals. I'm pleased with how well they've been doing though, and I really hope they enjoy the training and the whole experience. If they can come out the other end as fully trained, passionate chefs, I'll be a happy man.

Recently I've travelled all over the world and have met some great people. I honestly can't tell you what a real sense of happiness and achievement I feel when I get everyone from kids, to OAPs, to students, to builders, to city boys, talking to me

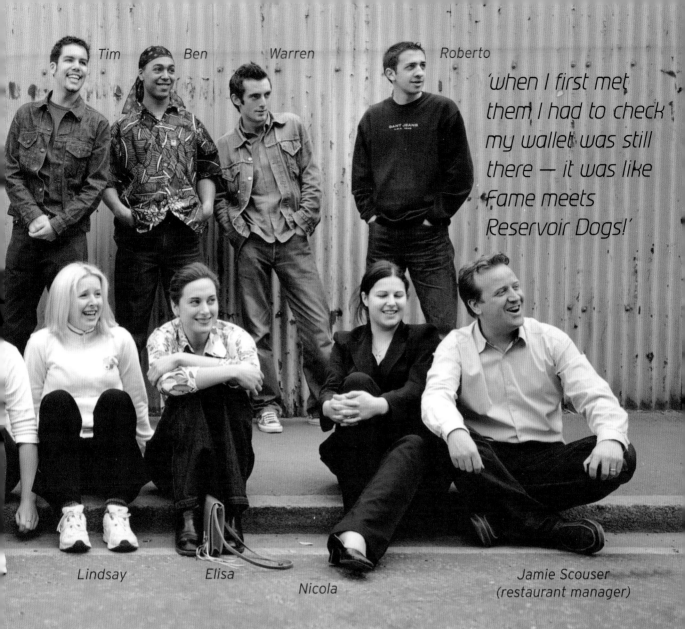

Tim Ben Warren Roberto

'when I first met them I had to check my wallet was still there — it was like fame meets Reservoir Dogs!'

Lindsay Elisa Nicola Jamie Scouser (restaurant manager)

about the recipes they've cooked from my books. It's an unbelievable feeling, but the best thing of all for me is when someone says they adapted a recipe as they preferred a nice cod steak to a bit of mullet, or 'I hate pears so I did it with peaches' or 'I turned that ravioli into a tortellini.' For me it doesn't get much better than that, because it makes me feel I've given you guys confidence in your own cooking. Just remember, it's not about being a professional chef, weighed down with facts and figures and techniques.

I'd like you to have a go on your own and think of me as a mate who's on hand to give you a bit of extra guidance. I want to give your cooking a kickstart, so be creative, give it your best shot and, as always, have a laugh.

Love Jamie O
xxx

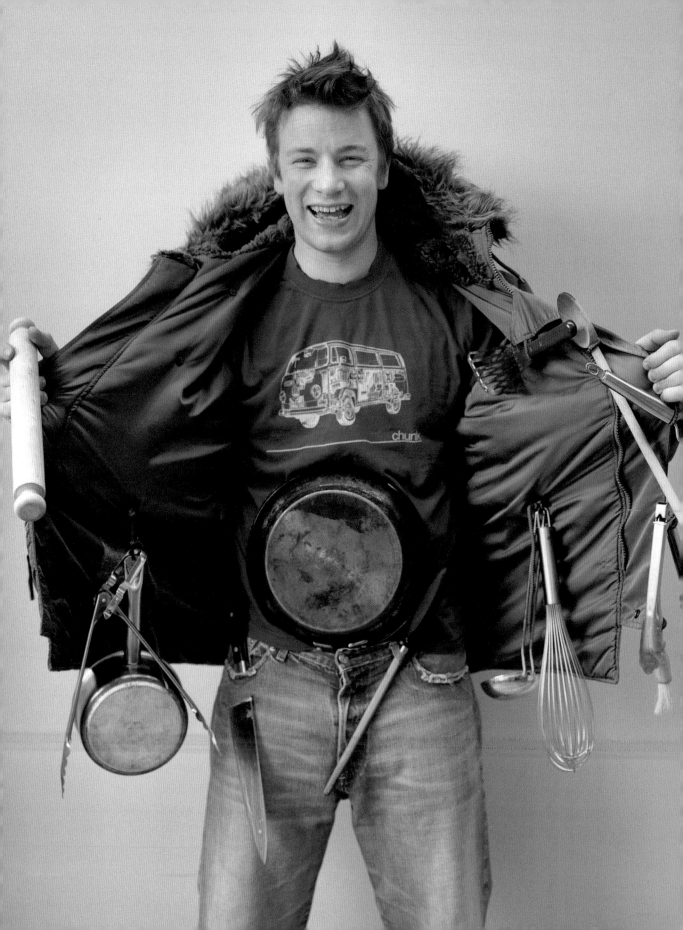

getting yourself kitted out

When shopping for kitchen equipment, you'll find that most cookshops and department stores have all these high-tech pans with glass lids, glass bottoms, removable handles and so on, but most of the time they're actually not very good. Just try to get yourself a minimal amount of decent sturdy kitchen equipment. Have a look in some professional kitchen shops – you'll be surprised to find that they don't charge over-the-top prices as they have to stock no-nonsense inexpensive equipment.

Here are a few of the things I couldn't live without:
* large non-stick frying pan
* large porcelain or stainless steel casserole
* some heavy, thick-bottomed saucepans – large, medium and small
* a couple of metal tongs
* wooden spoons
* thick, sturdy wooden chopping board – spend a bit more and it should last you a lot longer
* small plastic chopping board, for fish – small enough to fit in the dishwasher
* olive oil drizzlers
* medium large stone pestle and mortar – from all good stores and supermarkets
* Magimix food processor – these save time and are a good investment
* knives: 30cm/12 inch cook's knife, paring knife and bread knife to get you started – Victorinox, Gustav or Henkels are good makes
* stainless steel fish slice, slotted spoon, ladle and whisk – don't use plastic ones
* speed peeler – cheap as chips and really handy
* 2 or 3 good sturdy roasting trays – the thicker the better so they won't kink in the oven
* salad spinner – good ones only last a year, so buy yourself a cheap one
* electric scales
* a couple of sieves, fine and coarse
* measuring jug
* string
* 4-sided metal grater
* rolling pin
* cake tins
* wine rack

shopping tips

Some people think shopping for food is a bit of a hassle, but, to be honest, if you shop well for the best seasonal ingredients that's half the battle won. Here are some tips to help you get the best out of your shopping.

* Always keep your basic commodities stocked up so you're never short of herbs and spices. Check out my website at www.jamieoliver.com for a list of 'Cupboard Stuff'.
* If you are unhappy with anything you buy, make sure you take it back because if you don't complain the shop will never know and learn from their mistakes. If the supermarkets haven't got what you want on their shelves, you can ask them to stock it on a trial basis. Things like vanilla pods, semolina flour, good olive oils and vinegars should be there, so kick up a fuss if they're not and then blame it on me!
* There aren't many places you visit 2 or 3 times a week like clockwork, so make a point of getting to know your manager and let him know when displays of fresh goods look shabby. I do this all the time and it does make a difference.
* Don't just look, but smell and touch as well. Get to know your ingredients!
* The best beef is the darker meat which has been hung for longer as opposed to the bright red stuff. Look for meat that has hung for anything from 16 to 26 days, depending on the age and breed of the animal. The meat should be well-marbled with fat.
* Any really fresh fish will never ever smell – look for clear eyes, shiny scales and red gills. And always trust your instincts. If you can't get to the fish because it's behind a counter, have a look at the way it's been presented. If the tuna has been badly or unevenly cut, or if the cod is broken open as it has been dumped in a pile, or if the scallops are sitting in a puddle of fish juice or defrosted ice, then you know that the people behind the counter are not very knowledgeable or passionate about what they do. If, however, everything is neatly portioned and arranged and nothing's sitting in murky water, then the chances are you are in safe hands.
* If you don't know what to buy, ask the butcher or fishmonger what they are going to eat tonight or what they would buy from the selection, or if they've got anything else that's not on display. Sometimes the really fresh fish is sitting out the back waiting for the old fish to be sold before it gets offered to the customers.
* When at the butchers or fishmongers ask them to fillet and debone what you've bought – it's good to watch them do it.
* Try and buy regional produce from your own area or at least from your own country.
* Try and buy in season. Let the seasons dictate to you what to cook.
* Think about using the delivery service that local shops offer over the internet. It's a great way to get heavy and bulky objects home – with this out of the way you can enjoy walking round the shops a bit more.

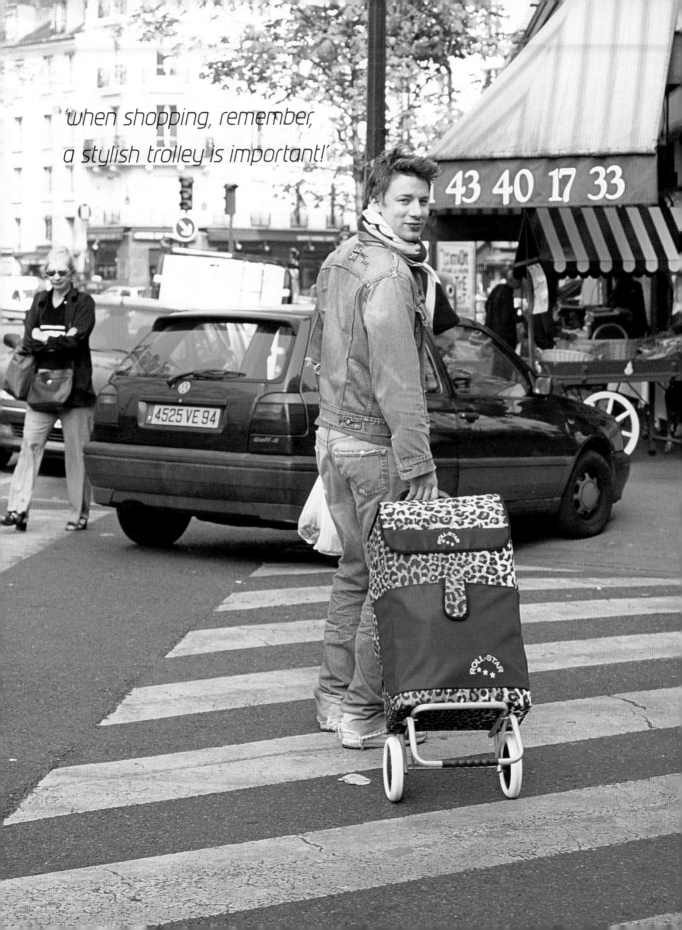

'when shopping, remember, a stylish trolley is important!'

now it's your turn

You may have wondered sometimes where a chef gets his inspiration from, so I thought I'd try to give you a sense of the things I enjoy. I think my style of light, fresh and colourful food has been shaped by the kind of person I am and the things I do, even though some of these may have nothing to do with food.

I'm quite an impulsive person and enjoy my friends, family and lifestyle as much as I do cooking. I often find that these things have an influence on my recipes, along with things like the clothes I wear, the music I listen to and stuff like that. My style of cooking is not intense and in-your-face as I'm not an uptight kind of person, so my food doesn't reflect that. I suppose what I'm trying to say is that it's important to put your own stamp on things. When you buy a house or rent a flat you decorate it in your own style; when you go to a wedding you might not want to wear a tie or hat; when you make a steak sandwich you might want to drink a really over-the-top glass of French claret with it. Life is full of rules and regulations, dos and don'ts and contradictions, but I like to be slightly odd, a bit naughty, a bit edgy and (hopefully!) a bit funky. It's the same in cooking.

I do love food – I'm obsessed by it. I think about breakfast in the evening and dinner at breakfast. I often daydream about family dinners ten days in advance. You can't always plan ahead, though – for instance, it's no good setting your heart on a particular sea bass recipe, just because you want to eat sea bass that day. It could be that it's been rough at sea and the fish will have been hanging round since the weekend and starting to smell. Better to ask the fishmonger what's fresh, use your nose, use your eyes, give the fish a feel and then decide what to buy. Certainly the most effortless way to be

inspired is simply to go for a walk down the market and see what's in season. It goes a bit like this: English asparagus has come in, the peas are sweet and bursting in your mouth, the mint in the herb box is growing like the clappers and strangling the rosemary, leafy Sicilian lemons are about – bloody hell, this is great – I know for a fact that I've got some extra virgin olive oil stashed in the back of a dark cupboard at home, some great Arborio risotto rice, some tagliatelle or spaghetti even, I've got fresh organic eggs which are double-yolkers and golden and I've got a couple of those goose eggs from Mr Turnip down at Borough Market. I could make a frittata with some Pecorino and Parmesan, or maybe some goat's cheese. My mouth's beginning to water; right, I'll buy those peas mate and I'll have that asparagus. I'll eat some of these peas raw while I'm waiting to pay.

It really is all about twists and turns and putting new tyres on old wheels. Sometimes I've thought I've invented something new and have found out that it's already been done slightly differently by someone else, but it doesn't stop me and it shouldn't stop you really taking cooking by the horns and making it a part of your life that you enjoy. Trust me, you'll love it. As far as I'm concerned, anyone who says they hate cooking or food just doesn't know that they like it yet.

Very often when I'm inventing new dishes I'll draw them before attempting to cook them for the first time. It helps me to see things visually, so try out whatever helps you – it's a bit like writing a shopping list or drawing up plans for a garden. Here's a funny little montage of things that inspire me – designs, feelings, people, experiences – things I feel I relate to and that make me happy. You're bound to have your own list, and everyone's will be different.

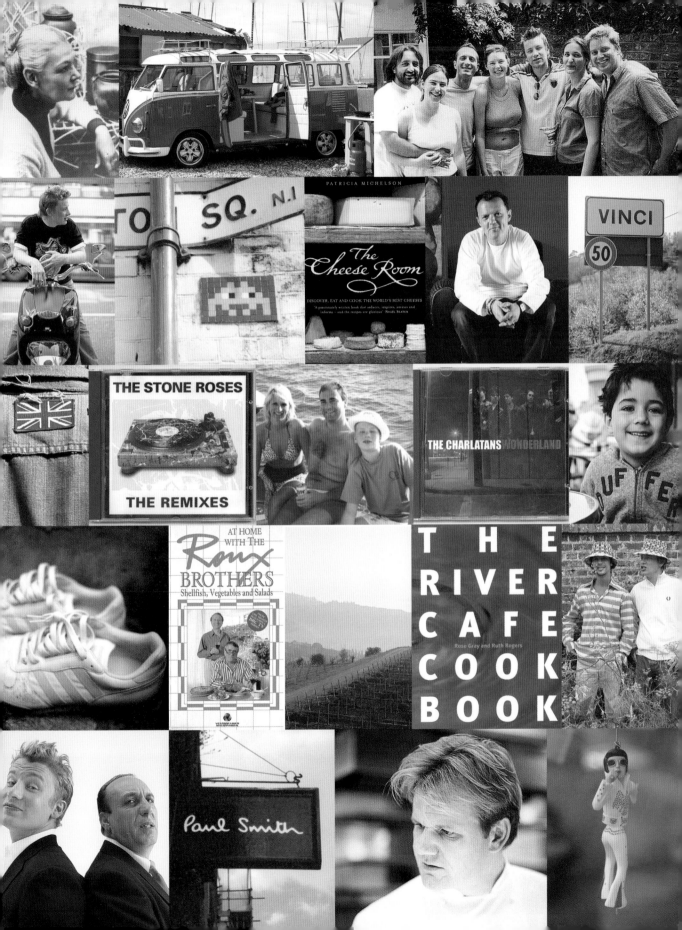

CRACKING SALADS

Unlike the other chapters in this book, this one doesn't generally concern itself with a particular method of cooking. There are still many easy skills that are needed for making great salads. I hope you get lots of inspiration from this chapter. It's all down to your sense of taste, having a good combination and keeping it as fresh as possible.

purple potato salad

I like to use a mixture of new potatoes and purple potatoes in this salad, but if you can't find any purple ones then just use all new potatoes instead. But try to hunt them down – they're great!

Make the dressing by mixing together the olive oil, lemon juice and crème fraîche or fromage frais. Cook the potatoes in plenty of boiling salted water for around 20 minutes until tender, and drain well. When the potatoes are cool enough to handle, rub off the skins with a knife and slice into bite-size pieces. Mix with the dressing, then add the radishes and herbs and season well to taste.

SERVES 6

6 tablespoons extra virgin olive oil

juice of 1-2 lemons, to taste

255g/9oz crème fraîche or fromage frais

500g/1lb 2oz baby new potatoes

500g/1lb 2oz purple potatoes

sea salt and freshly ground black pepper

1 bunch of radishes, finely sliced

1 handful of fresh mint leaves, chopped

1 handful of chives, chopped

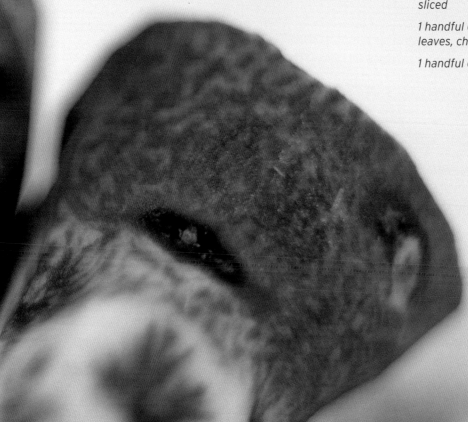

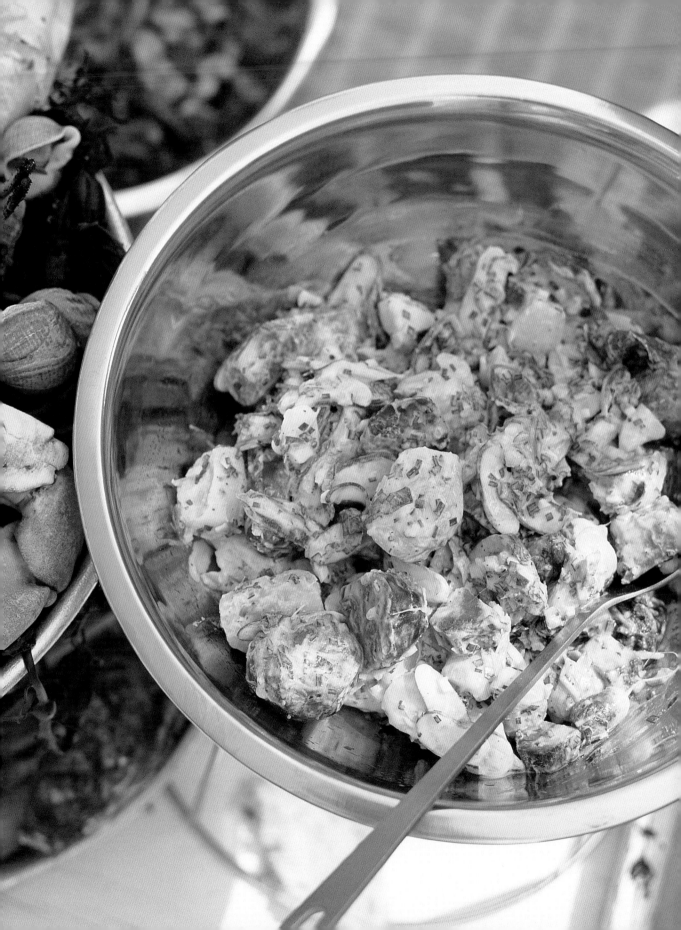

my new best salad

This salad is one of the best things that's happened to me this year. Really tasty, really clean and fresh. I haven't yet given it to anyone who didn't absolutely love it. The recipe uses tarragon instead of any other salad leaf. This is quite shocking for me, as I've always been scared of tarragon! It's a potent herb, but used aggressively and strongly like it is here it really works well. With the sweetness of the grapes and the saltiness of the goat's cheese, it's fantastic. If you can't get hold of enough tarragon, feel free to bulk the salad out with some rocket. This will be fine - but tarragon on its own is so amazing, you must try it some time.

The first job is to put the finely sliced shallots and vinegar together in a dish, making sure that the shallots are all covered by the vinegar. If the shallot slices are nice and thin they will need only about 10–15 minutes in the vinegar for the desired effect. They will be just like crunchy pickled onions when they're done.

Keep all the ingredients in the fridge until your guests are around the table. Crack open a bottle of crisp white wine for them, then get started. Throw the tarragon leaves into a bowl, add the grapes, the shallots with only 5 tablespoons of their vinegar, and the olive oil. Toss this all together, taste it and add a little seasoning if it's needed. Go easy on the salt though, as the cheese will be quite salty. Use some tongs to pick up the salad and divide it between 4 plates. Grate or crumble the goat's cheese on top of each salad and drizzle over any leftover dressing. You'll love it!

SERVES 4

2 banana shallots, or 6 normal-sized ones, peeled and very finely sliced

a good vinegar (champagne, white wine or sherry vinegar)

4 large handfuls of fresh tarragon, leaves picked

1 small bunch of seedless red grapes, halved

1 small bunch of seedless green grapes, halved

6 tablespoons extra virgin olive oil

sea salt and freshly ground black pepper

200g/7oz good goat's cheese or hard salted ricotta

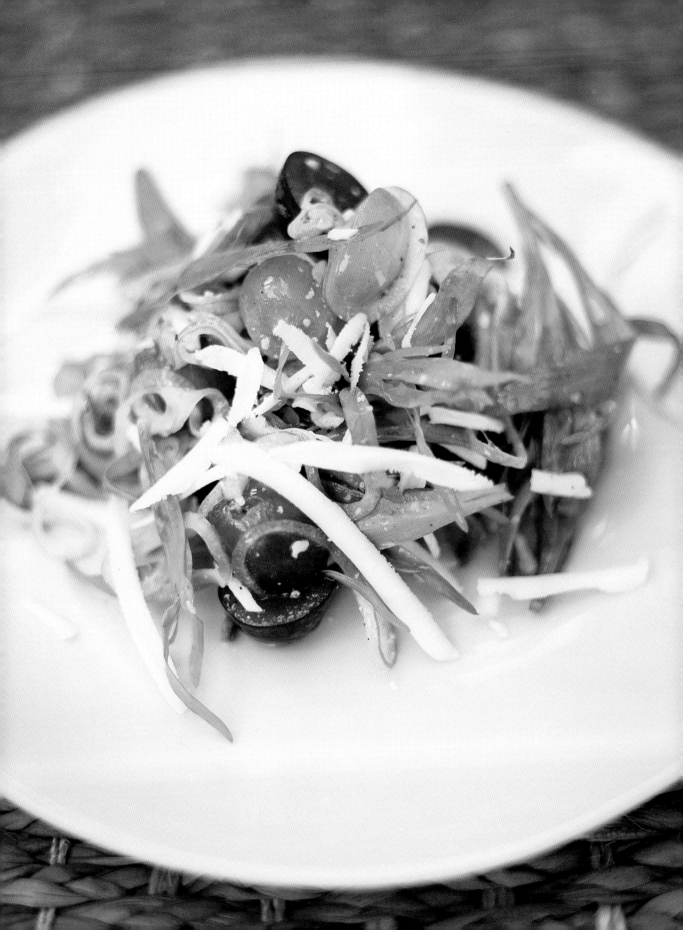

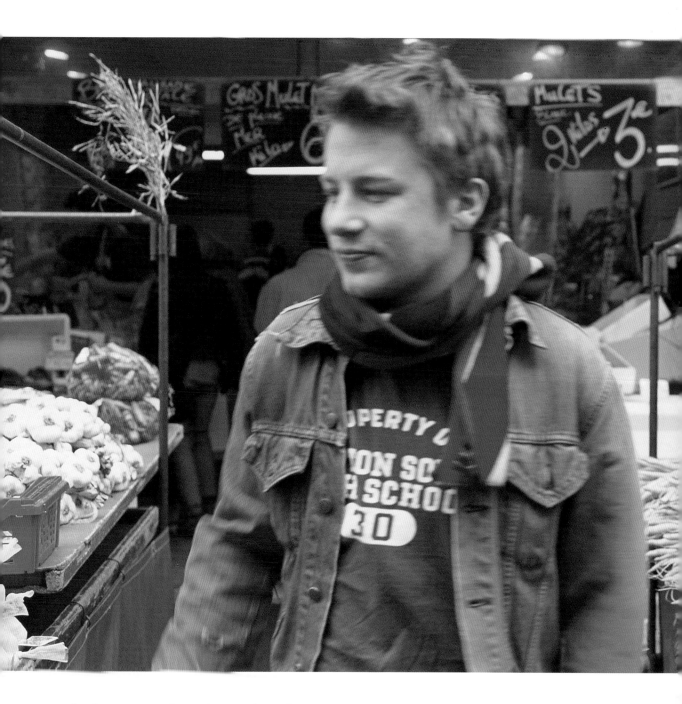

'when you're shopping keep your eyes peeled. get stuck
in, pick stuff up, grope it, smell it. trust your instincts ...
if it's good, buy it!'

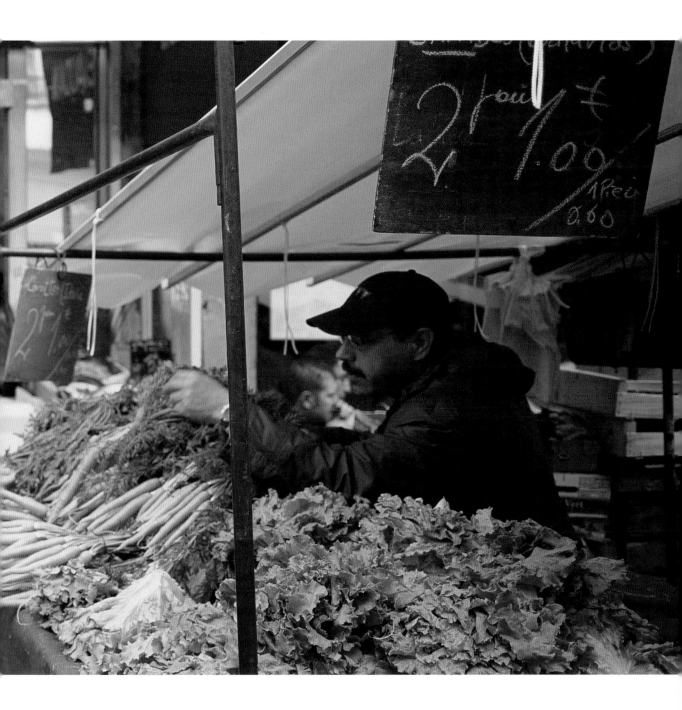

broad bean and crispy pancetta salad with a pea, pecorino and mint dressing

Even though this salad's really simple and really tasty, it's also quite a brave dish because it hasn't got lots of leaves everywhere – just some beautiful ingredients put together with a little common sense. It's one of those combos that makes the back of your mouth juice up when you think about it. Ideally use young peas and broad beans when they're in season. If they're a little older then take the skins off the beans, and if the peas are large it doesn't really matter as you'll be mushing them up anyway.

Bring a pot to the boil, half-filled with water, but with no salt as this makes broad beans and peas toughen. Add your garlic and allow the water to boil for a couple of minutes before adding the broad beans. Cook for around 3–5 minutes, depending on how young the beans are. Simply taste one to check. If you feel the skins are a little tough, which they can be sometimes, let them cool a little and then you can peel them very quickly by pinching and squeezing the bean out. Throw the skins away, and keep the garlic clove to one side. Place your pancetta on a baking tray, with the almonds spread out next to it. Place in a hot oven at 250°C/475°F/gas 9 – keeping an eye on the almonds to make sure they don't colour too much. You should be able to crisp up the pancetta at the same time as toasting the almonds, but simply remove one or the other if it is getting too far ahead.

To make the dressing, put your raw podded peas and the soft, boiled garlic clove into a pestle and mortar or a Magimix and bash or blitz until smooth. Add the cheese and most of the mint and stir or pulse to make a smooth paste. You want to turn this into a thick dressing, so add the olive oil and 4-5 tablespoons of lemon juice, to your preference. Season to taste – it should have an amazing flavour of sweet peas, twangy lemon, fragrant mint and a softness and roundness from the cheese. A balance is good, but you should also trust your own personal judgement – I generally like mine to be a bit more lemony, to cut through the smokiness of the pancetta.

Mix the dressing with the broad beans and sprinkle this over 4 plates. Crumble the pancetta over, followed by a sprinkling of the almonds, which can be crushed or bashed up a little. Tear a little mint over the top with a little shaved Parmesan if you like.

SERVES 4

1 clove of garlic, peeled and left whole

300g/10 1/2oz podded broad beans

8 slices of pancetta or smoked streaky bacon

1 handful of whole blanched almonds

150g/5 1/2oz podded fresh peas

70g/2 1/2oz Pecorino or Parmesan cheese, or a mixture of both, grated

1 handful of fresh mint, leaves picked

8 tablespoons extra virgin olive oil

juice of 1–2 lemons

sea salt and freshly ground black pepper

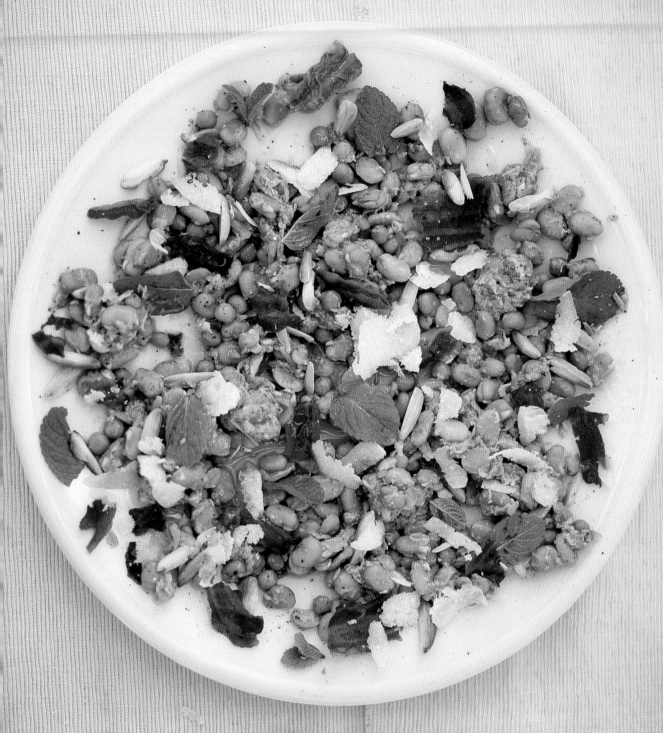

Try this: Fry the pancetta and just as it starts to get crispy add some sliced garlic to the pan, along with a handful of small shrimps or prawns and then the almonds. Carry on as before.

And this: Mush everything up and smear on some bruschetta or crostini or even some melba toast for a lovely snack.

Or this: Simply spoon over some steamed fish.

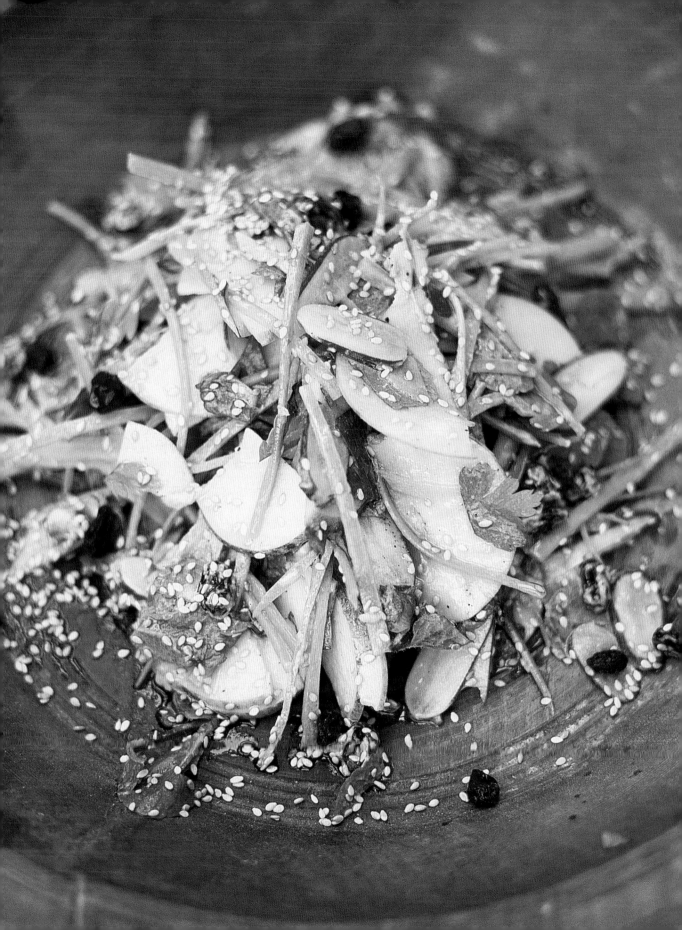

moorish crunch salad

This is a lovely little Moorish salad which gets the old tastebuds going – but more to the point, it's refreshingly crunchy and is right at home as a nice side salad or with a barbecue. You know, sometimes you haven't got salad leaves in your fridge, but you will probably have a couple of carrots and apples, and by getting on the Moorish vibe and using mint and tahini (a paste made out of sesame seeds which you can find in most supermarkets), I've pulled together this little combo. The reason I've stated that you should slice some ingredients and have matchsticks for others is because this really adds to the crunch. You can always use the coarse side of a grater for speed (see page 30).

First of all, finely slice your carrots into matchstick-sized batons (see page 266). Finely slice your radishes – you can leave a little of the tops on if you like. Quarter your apples, remove the cores and finely slice. Add all these to a bowl with the rest of the ingredients, apart from the sesame seeds. Toss together, carefully checking the seasoning, and serve with the sesame seeds sprinkled over the top. Eat straight away.

Try this: Turn it into a warm salad by adding some pan-seared chicken, prawns or scallops which have been dusted with a little paprika.

And this: Make it more of a snack by frying some halloumi cheese until golden with some chopped fresh chilli and crumbling this over the top.

Or this: Grill some pitta bread and serve stuffed with the Crunch Salad. Crumble in some feta cheese too. Lovely.

SERVES 4

300g/10 1/2oz carrots, peeled

150g/5 1/2oz radishes

2 crunchy eating apples

1 small handful of raisins or sultanas

1 handful of fresh parsley, roughly chopped

1 handful of fresh mint, roughly chopped

4 tablespoons sherry or red wine vinegar

8 tablespoons olive oil

1 tablespoon tahini

sea salt and freshly ground black pepper

2 tablespoons sesame seeds, toasted in the oven

GRATING AND PEELING

It sounds really basic, but graters and peelers can be used for so much more than just peeling carrots or potatoes and grating cheese. Here are a few ways that I use them to save time when preparing stuff.

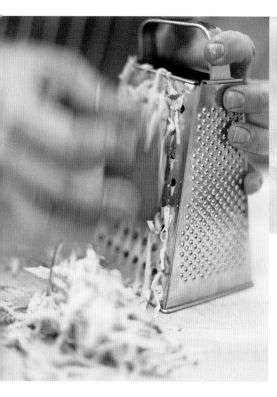

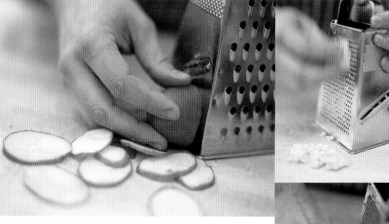

Grating potatoes for potato cakes or stovies (see page 220).

Slicing potatoes and loads of other things really quickly.

Grated ginger is much tastier than sliced or chopped.

Grating chocolate is a superb way to finish off desserts.

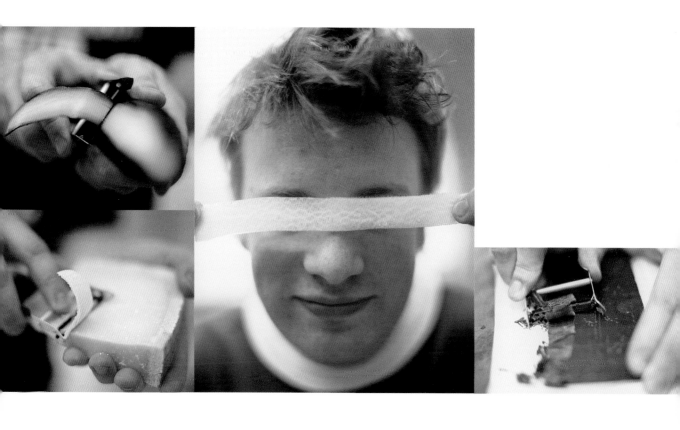

Thin slivers of cucumber, or any vegetable, are really crunchy and great for salads and veg dishes.

A simple way to do Parmesan shavings, to finish off dishes at the table.

Peelers are fast, efficient and can give you slices which are almost translucent and really fresh and crunchy – great for salads and stir-frying and loads more.

Shaving chocolate for desserts.

ribbon celeriac salad

Inspiration for this came from me being so bored with traditional celeriac rémoulade, which is an old-fashioned French salad kind of similar to this but using grated celeriac, mustard and mayonnaise. It's really handy to have a good peeler for this recipe (see page 31). I tend to use capers in vinegar for this dish and it works really well.

Once you've peeled the celeriac, chuck away the skin and then carry on peeling around it, giving you long ribbons. If they break every now and again it doesn't matter. Continue until you reach the fluffy tasteless inner core, which you should throw away. Remove and discard the chunky stalks from the parsley, then finely slice the thinner stalks and roughly chop the leaves.

Put your celeriac and parsley into a large bowl and mix together with all the other ingredients. Season to taste, adding a little more vinegar if need be, then serve straight away.

Try this: Put some of this salad on a plate, then cover it completely with some smoked salmon and plenty of ground black pepper.

Or this: Roast a nice chicken. Allow it to cool and serve with this salad.

SERVES 4

1 celeriac, peeled

1 bunch of fresh flat-leaf parsley

2 anchovies, finely chopped

2 heaped tablespoons good capers, finely chopped

2 heaped tablespoons small sweet and sour gherkins, finely chopped

5 tablespoons crème fraîche

1 heaped tablespoon Dijon mustard

3 tablespoons extra virgin olive oil

2–3 tablespoons sherry, red or white wine vinegar

sea salt and freshly ground black pepper

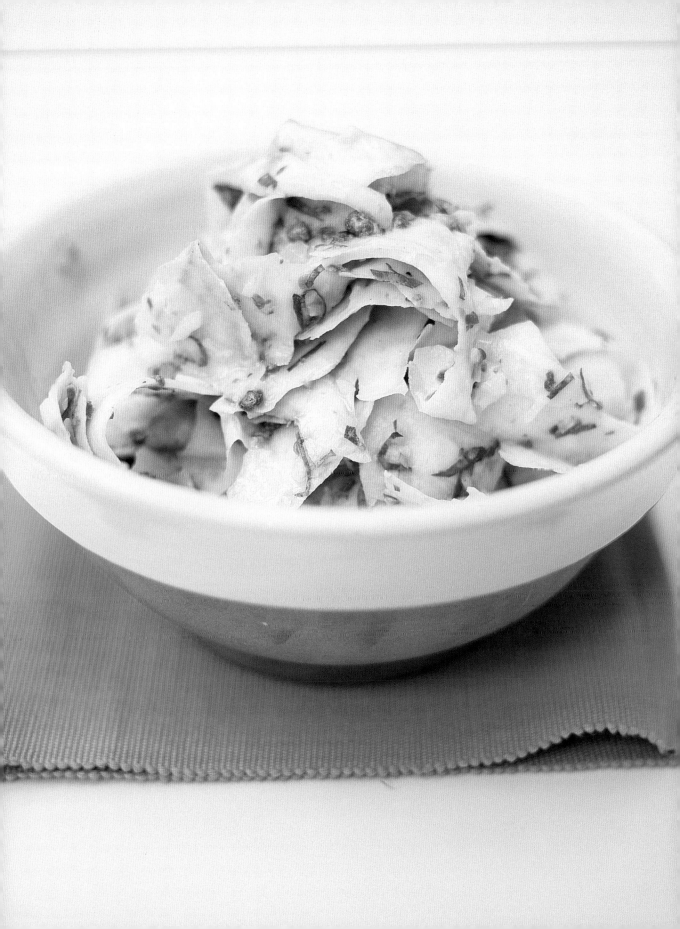

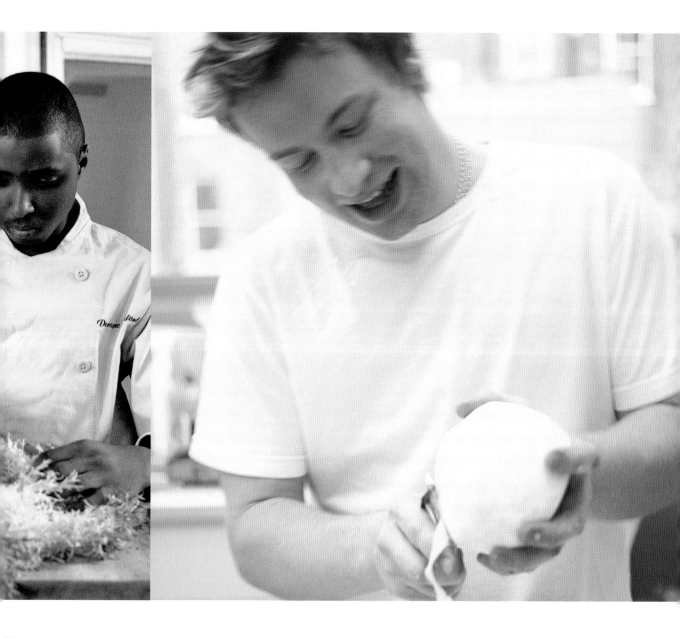

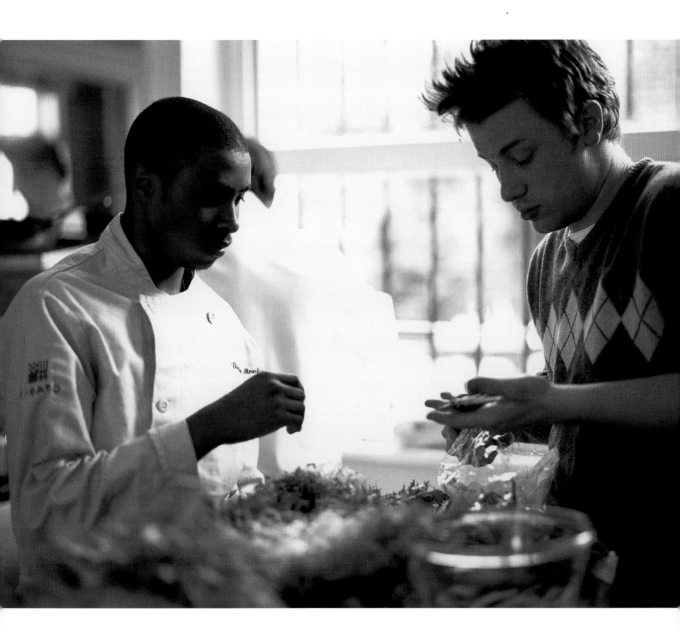

lamb's lettuce and lychee salad with lucky squid and chilli jam

As you know, I love the use of fruit in salads, and I've always wanted to do something with lychees as they are so fresh and fragrant. I thought that, coming from Asia, they'd be fantastic incorporated into a salad with my mate John Torode's Lucky Squid and Chilli Jam. Thanks for the inspiration, mate. If you haven't got time to make the chilli jam, then you can always wok-fry the squid with just the lime zest and a bit of fresh chilli. My mum's a bit of a pleb and uses tinned lychees, but they seem to work for her.

First you need to make your chilli jam, so blitz up all the jam ingredients roughly in a food processor, apart from the sugar and the fish sauce. Put the mixture in a wok or a pan and cook gently, stirring regularly, for about 20 minutes on a slow simmer. Put back into the food processor and blitz again until very, very smooth. Return the mixture to the pan, add the sugar, and simmer slowly again for half an hour, stirring regularly and making sure it doesn't catch. Season with fish sauce. Allow to cool, and keep in the fridge until you need it. It will keep for at least a couple of weeks. It's fantastic used in any stir-frying or salads.

Get your fishmonger to clean the squid and ask him to lightly score the inside in a criss-cross fashion. Finely slice your lime zest. Get a wok or pan really hot and add a lug of olive oil. Season the squid and lay it in the wok, sprinkling the lime zest on top. Give it a good shake about. It normally only takes about 2 minutes to cook, and should curl up at the edges. Remove from the heat, slice the squid up, add back to the pan with the chilli jam and stir around until it coats the squid completely. Add the lime juice and 4 tablespoons of olive oil. Lightly dress your lamb's lettuce and lychees with a little olive oil. Scatter your squid over the leaves and then sprinkle everything with chilli. Spoon over a little of the juice from the wok. A fantastic combination.

SERVES 4

4 medium-sized squid, cleaned

zest and juice of 2 limes

extra virgin olive oil

sea salt and freshly ground black pepper

4 handfuls of lamb's lettuce

455g/1lb lychees, peeled and deseeded

2 fresh chillies, finely chopped

for the sweet chilli jam

4 fresh red chillies,

1 red onion, peeled and halved

10 cloves of garlic, peeled

100g/3½oz fresh ginger, peeled

2 handfuls of fresh coriander

2 sticks of lemongrass, peeled and roughly chopped

1 tablespoon dried shrimps

150ml/5½fl oz sunflower oil

40g/1½oz palm sugar

fish sauce, to taste

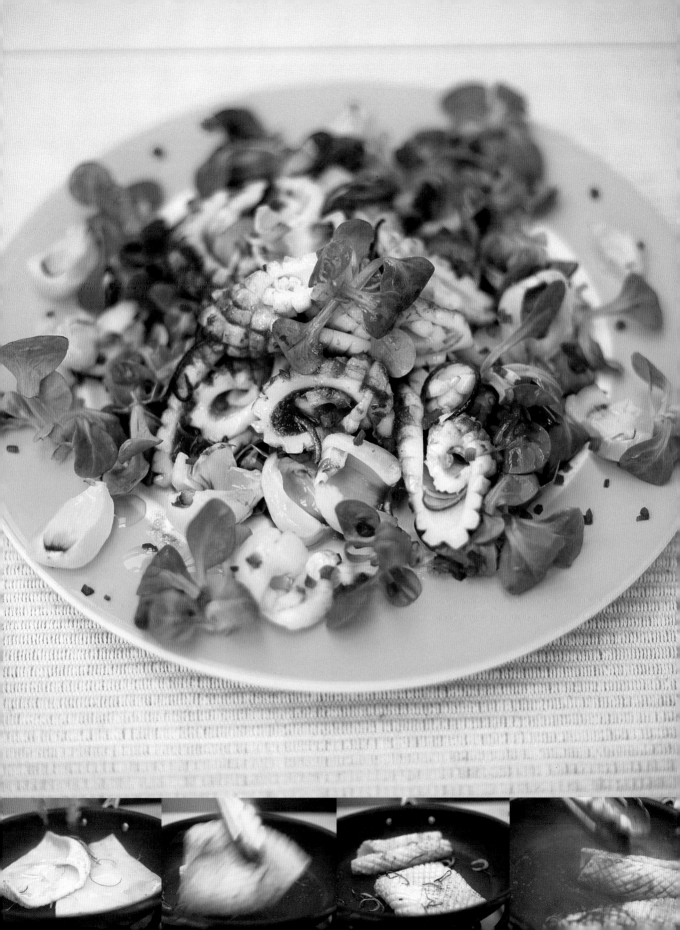

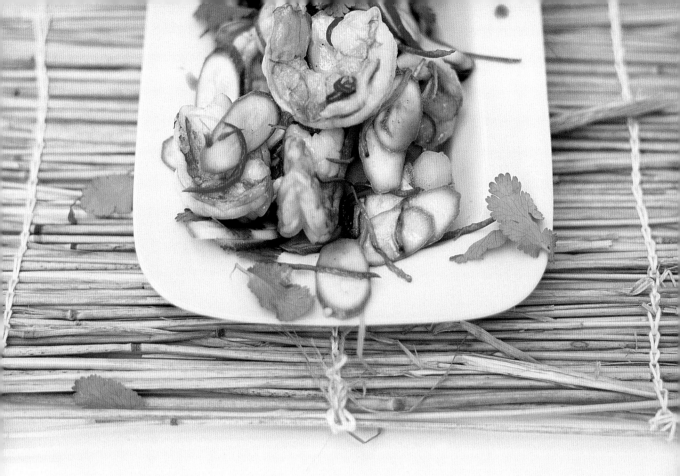

stir-fried warm salad of prawns and baby courgettes

I love the crunch of the raw baby courgettes you can easily get hold of these days. The zing of lime and ginger and the sweetness of the charred prawns are amazing.

First of all, run a sharp knife down the back of the prawns and remove the little vein. This will make the prawns look nicer and taste better, as they will take on more flavour. Get a wok or pan very hot while you very finely slice your baby courgettes at an angle. Place these in a bowl and have all your ingredients ready to go, which is really important when you're stir-frying. To your hot pan, add the oil, prawns, lime zest and ginger. Stir fry for around 2 minutes, until the prawns are lightly golden. Remove from the heat, and allow to cool for 30 seconds before adding your courgettes, lime juice, chilli and herbs. You can increase or decrease the quantity of chilli to your own taste. I prefer to use lots! Season with soy sauce and toss well, then serve on a plate. Eat straight away, while the courgettes are still nice and crunchy.

SERVES 4

20 medium to large prawns, peeled

10 baby courgettes

6 tablespoons sunflower or nut oil

zest and juice of 2 limes

1 heaped tablespoon grated fresh ginger

2 fresh red chillies, deseeded and finely chopped

1 small handful of mixed fresh coriander and mint

2 tablespoons soy sauce

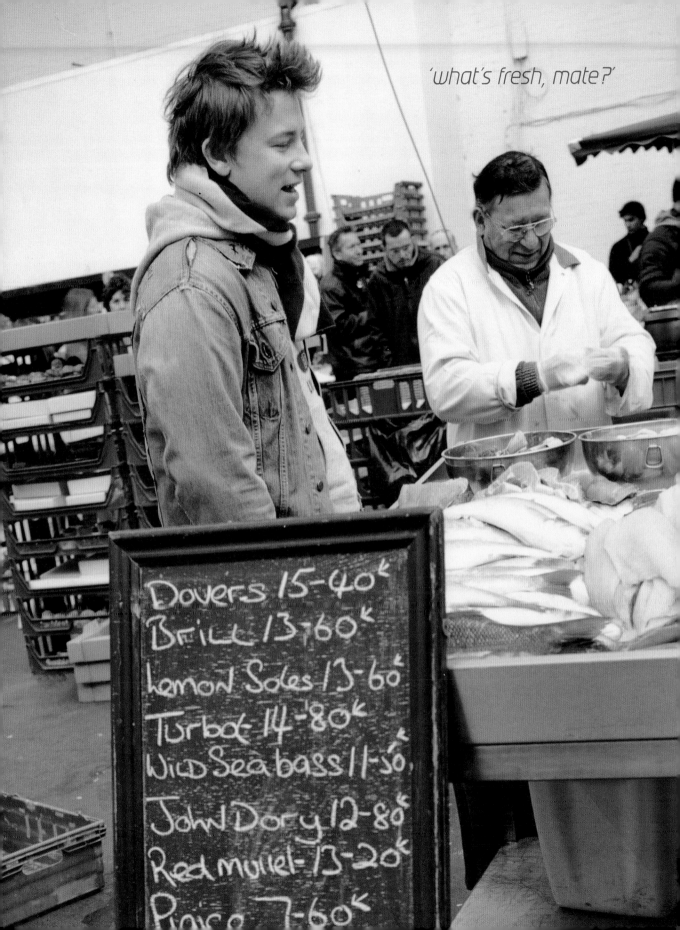

'what's fresh, mate?'

Dovers 15-40ᵏ
Brill 13-60ᵏ
Lemon Soles 13-60ᵏ
Turbot 14-80ᵏ
Wild Sea bass 11-50ᵏ
John Dory 12-80ᵏ
Red mullet 13-20ᵏ
Plaice 7-60ᵏ

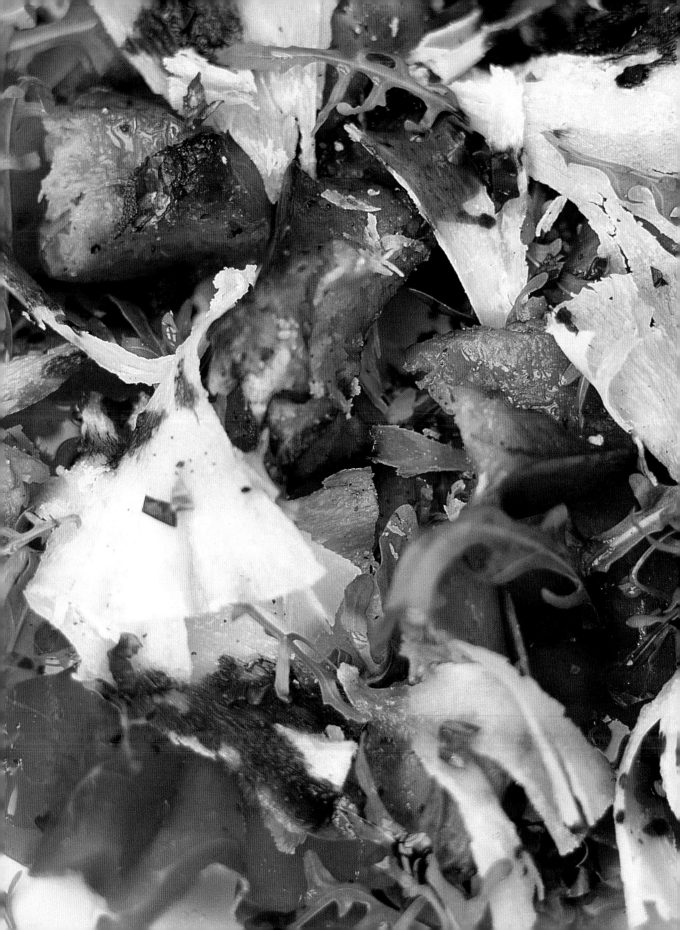

warm salad of roasted squash, prosciutto and pecorino

This is one of those easy salads with a twist. You may have tried a Parma ham, rocket and Parmesan salad with a little balsamic, but by adding warm roasted squash and trying it with Pecorino, which is slightly smoother than Parmesan, it's a real pleasure and even feels a bit posh.

Preheat your oven to 190°C/375°F/gas 5. Carefully cut your butternut squash in half, keeping the seeds intact. Remove the two ends and discard them. Cut each half into quarters and lay in a roasting tray. Rub with a little olive oil. In a pestle and mortar pound up a flat teaspoon each of salt, pepper and your chilli and coriander seeds. Scatter this over the squash. Roast the squash for half an hour or until soft and golden. Allow to cool a little.

Lay your prosciutto on 4 plates – let it hang over the rim of the plates and encourage it to twist and turn so it doesn't look neat and flat. Tear up your warm squash and put it in and around the ham. Sprinkle over the seeds and the rocket. Drizzle over the olive oil and balsamic, add a tiny pinch of salt and pepper, and use a vegetable peeler to shave over the Pecorino (see page 31). Easily done.

SERVES 4

1 butternut squash

olive oil

sea salt and freshly ground black pepper

1 small dried red chilli

1 heaped teaspoon coriander seeds

20 slices prosciutto or Parma ham

4 handfuls of rocket

6 tablespoons extra virgin olive oil

4 tablespoons balsamic vinegar

1 small block of Pecorino or Parmesan cheese

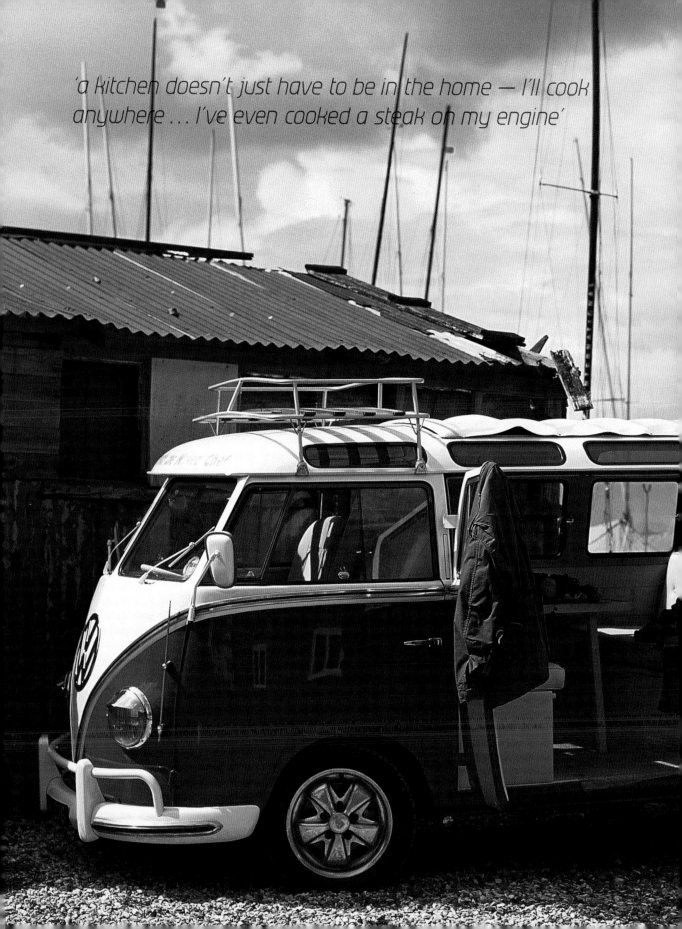

'a kitchen doesn't just have to be in the home — I'll cook anywhere ... I've even cooked a steak on my engine'

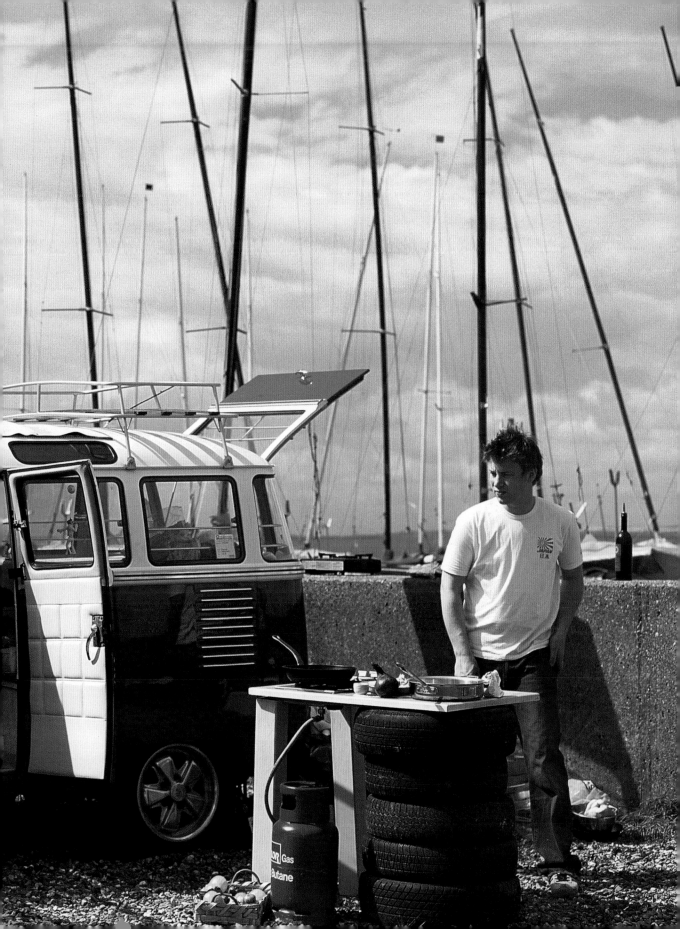

the proper french side salad

You know what I'm like – I'm the world's biggest lover of salads! When I worked in France we used to have brilliant cheap French salads, but on my last trip to Paris all I kept getting in restaurants were some miserable leaves served with bits of overcooked hard-boiled egg and big clumsy chunks of plain old tomato. I'm sure this was just bad luck, but it made me think about the good salads I'd had over there, with a cracking French dressing that didn't have any added sugar. I even saw a chef add some raw egg whites to a French dressing once to help it emulsify – a sackable offence.

Finely slice the shallots and put them into a small dish. Cover them with vinegar and let them sit for about 10-15 minutes. Pull off all the dark green frisée leaves and throw them away, as they are bitter. Then cut off all the yellow-white leaves down to the stalk. Wash these in ice-cold water with the chives and chervil, then dry them in a salad spinner and place them in a large salad bowl. Cook your green beans in salted boiling water until tender, then drain and allow to cool. I'm not a great fan of fridge-cold beans, but beans at room temperature or warm are fantastic in this salad, so add them to the bowl. Remove any sad-looking outer leaves from the gem lettuces and then cut them into 8 pieces (wash them if necessary, but they probably won't need it as the inner leaves will have been protected). Add to the salad bowl.

To make the dressing, first remove the shallots from the vinegar and sprinkle them over the salad leaves. Put 4 tablespoons of the leftover vinegar in a separate bowl, add the mustard and garlic with a small pinch of salt, then whisk in the oil until the dressing emulsifies. Taste and correct the seasoning. Dress the salad, give it a good toss and divide between 4 bowls. Serve immediately.

SERVES 4

*2 banana shallots or
6 normal-sized ones, peeled*

white wine vinegar

1 large frisée lettuce

1 bunch of fresh chives

*1 handful of fresh chervil,
leaves picked*

2 handfuls of fine green beans

2 gem lettuces

for the ultimate French dressing

1 tablespoon Dijon mustard

*1–2 cloves of garlic, peeled
and finely chopped*

*9 tablespoons extra virgin
olive oil*

*sea salt and freshly ground
black pepper*

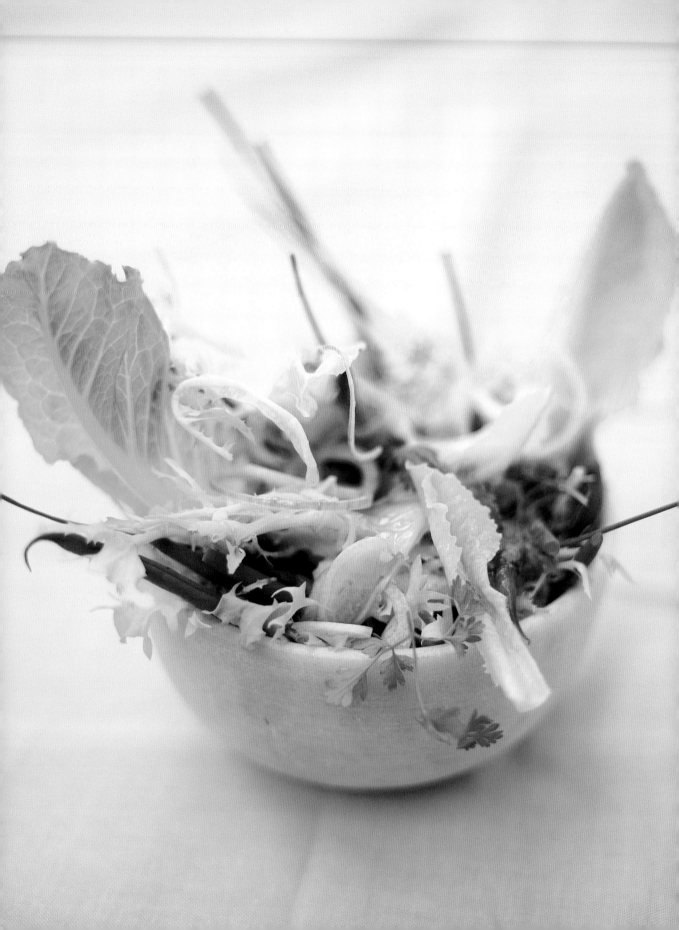

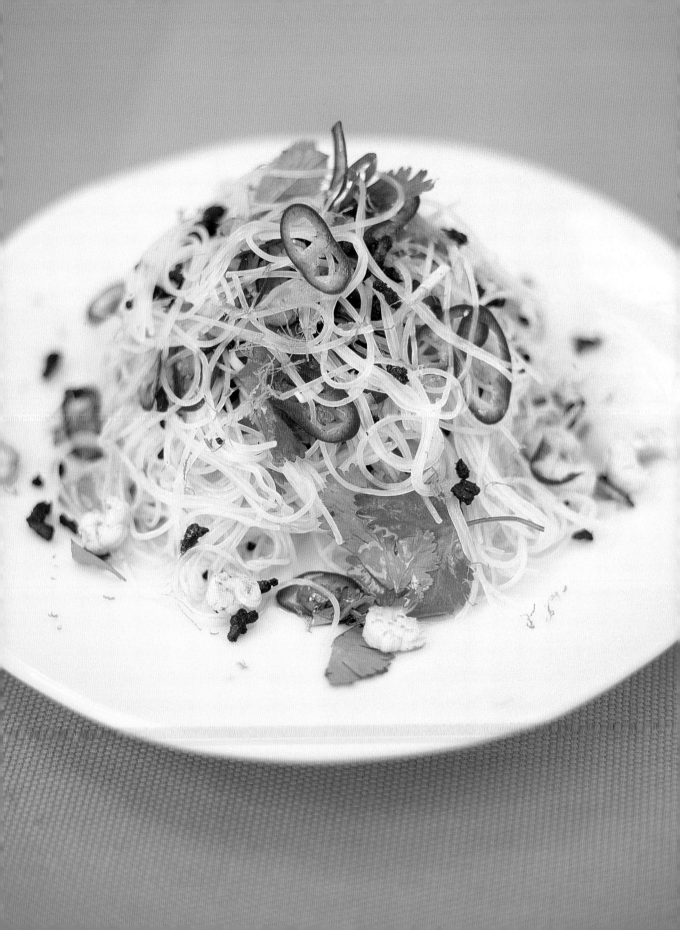

fresh asian noodle salad

This is one of those salads which tastes so amazing that you have to keep making it! It's spicy, zingy and really gets your tastebuds going.

Soak the noodles in a bowl of warm water until soft, then drain and put back in the bowl. In a hot wok fry the beef and five-spice in the olive oil until brown and crisp, then add the garlic, ginger, prawns and sugar and stir-fry for another 4 minutes. Remove from the heat and stir the wok mixture into the noodles. Add the spring onions, lime juice, fish sauce, chillies, coriander, mint and peanuts to the bowl. Toss well and correct the seasoning – it wants to be quite zingy with the lime juice. Sprinkle with some extra herb leaves if you like and serve cold.

Try this: You can modify the recipe by using a little wok-fried squid, shellfish or different minced meats.

SERVES 4

300g/10½oz cellophane noodles or beanthread noodles

200g/7oz minced beef

2 teaspoons five-spice

5 tablespoons olive oil

2 cloves of garlic, peeled and grated

2 heaped teaspoons of grated fresh ginger

150g/5½oz cooked peeled prawns

3 teaspoons sugar

1 bunch of spring onions, finely sliced

3 tablespoons fresh lime juice

1 tablespoon fish sauce

2 fresh red chillies, deseeded and finely sliced

1 handful of fresh coriander, chopped

1 handful of fresh mint, chopped

2 handfuls of roasted peanuts

sea salt and freshly ground black pepper

COOKING WITHOUT HEAT

In Mexico and Japan they have always used acidic marinades to cut through the richness of fish. On my last trip to America I saw some stunning ceviches – there are various interpretations of this but it basically means to use the acidic properties of citrus fruit or vinegar to partly cook meat or fish. This can be done at the last minute, which gives you a very light cure like when you put lemon juice on smoked salmon, making it go slightly opaque. I've even seen long-cured duck done for a few days in citrus juice, which had the effect of slow-roasting it. Amazing stuff. But what I find really exciting is the way that Thai people use essence of ginger and lime and fantastic things like that to cure any fish. Your inspiration should come from getting hold of really good fresh fish. Don't use any old rubbish – ask your fishmonger to tell you when the fish was caught and when it came into the shop. See page 14 for some tips on buying fresh fish.

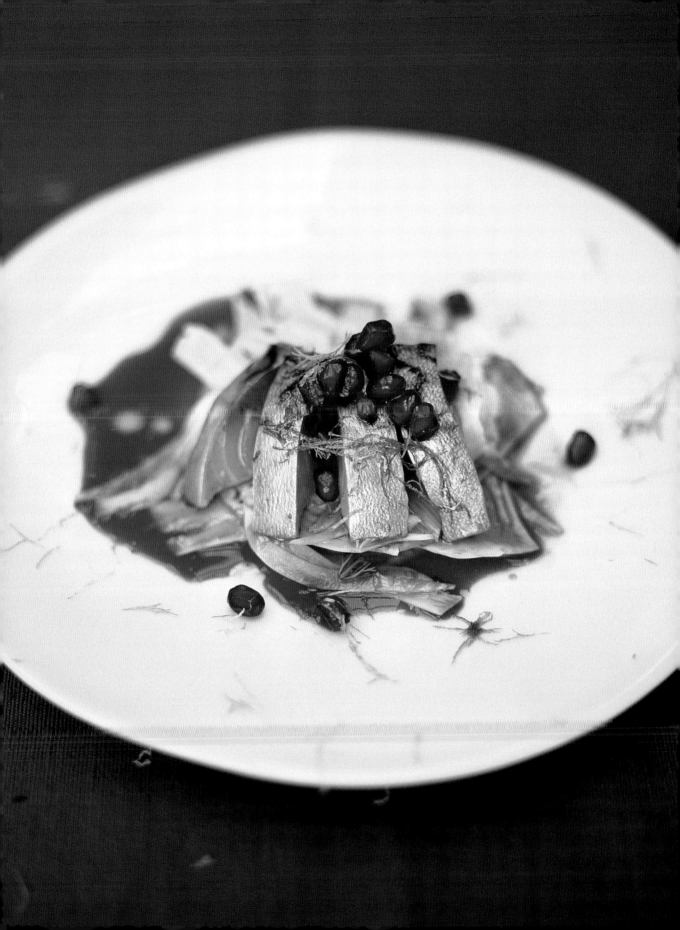

fresh mackerel cooked in pomegranate, lime juice and tequila with a crunchy fennel salad

This is a really unusual way to cook and serve fish. It's so tasty. If you're interested in cooking then you should challenge your tastebuds – and this is just the recipe to do it with! Obviously the finished dish is as good as the fish that you start off with, so get yourself some nice fresh mackerel and wow all your friends at your next dinner party.

You can make this on the morning of your dinner party. Heat the vinegar with a heaped teaspoon of salt in a saucepan until lukewarm. Remove from the heat. Place the 2 mackerel fillets in a tight-fitting dish and cover with the vinegar. Allow to sit all day (for around 7 hours), then drain and put to one side while you make your dressing. Juice 2 of the pomegranates by squeezing them over a sieve into a bowl, or use a lemon juicer, but be careful not to wear anything white when you juice them – when I do it I always cover myself in juice and I always get a rollicking from Jools. Add the lime juice, tequila, sesame oil and ginger to the pomegranate juice.

Place the fillets in half of your pomegranate juice mixture and allow them to sit for around half an hour, making sure both sides of the fish are covered. This will slowly 'cold cook' the mackerel and will give it a really fantastic flavour.

While the fish is 'cooking', finely slice the fennel and pick out the pomegranate seeds from the remaining pomegranate. You may think that this is a bit of a palaver but in fact all you have to do is break the pomegranate up and dislodge all the little capsules – it's quite easy and good fun. Divide the fennel on to 4 plates. Drain your mackerel and pat dry, then slice it up across the fillets as thin as you like. Place on top of your fennel, then sprinkle with the pomegranate seeds, fennel tops and lime zest. Carefully drizzle over some of the remaining pomegranate juice mixture and a little extra virgin olive oil to finish.

SERVES 4

285ml/½ pint white wine vinegar

sea salt

1 large mackerel (600g/1lb 6oz), cleaned, filleted and pinboned (see page 198)

3 ripe pomegranates

zest and juice of 2 limes

2 shots of tequila

1 teaspoon sesame oil

1 teaspoon grated fresh ginger

2 small bulbs of fennel, finely sliced and tops reserved

extra virgin olive oil

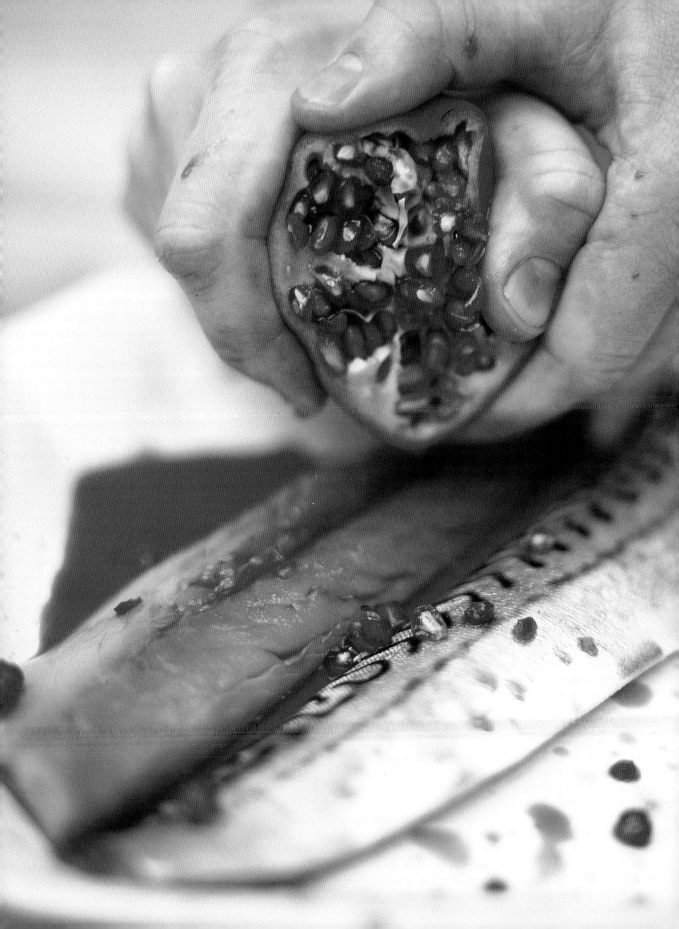

SEGMENTING CITRUS FRUIT

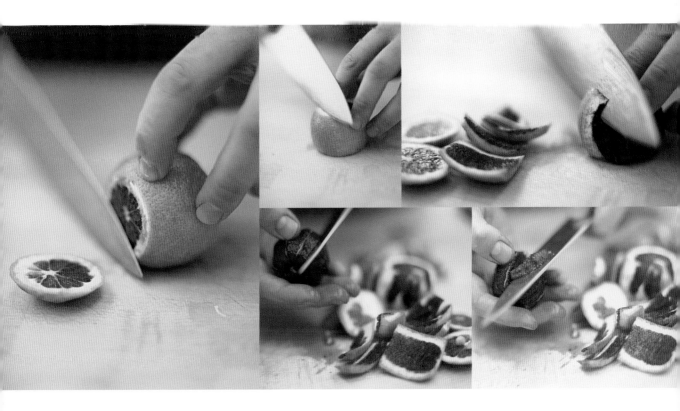

1. Remove both ends from the orange (or whichever citrus fruit you are using).

2. Turn the orange on to a flat edge and remove the first sliver of skin.

3. Twist the orange around to remove all the skin in slivers.

4. Insert your knife as close as possible to the connective white pith around each segment.

5. Then just twist your knife and ease the segment apart from the rest of the orange.

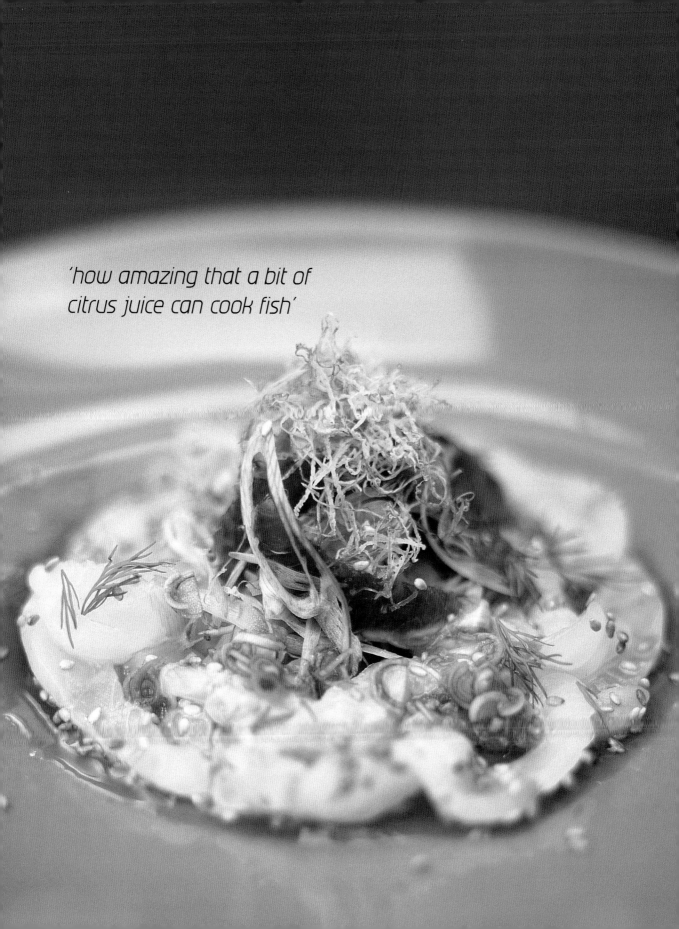

'how amazing that a bit of
citrus juice can cook fish'

quick-cooked white fish with blood orange, lemongrass and sesame seeds

This recipe is really flexible for all kinds of finely sliced white fish, such as brill, halibut, bass or turbot. Even red mullet is great. To get thin slices, use a really sharp carving knife. And it's such a simple fresh starter for any meal. This requires the freshest fish you can get your hands on. See page 14 for advice on shopping for fresh fish

Place your fillet of fish in front of you and, slicing away from you, cut it into the thinnest slices you can. A little trick we use in the restaurant to get the slices even thinner is to place them between 2 bits of clingfilm and bat them out very lightly with something flat until they are nice and thin. Divide the fish slices between 4 plates, in the centre of each. To make it look a bit more rustic try not to lay the fish flat on the plate – you can let some curl up and you can leave gaps in the middle to trap little pools of dressing.

To make the dressing, remove the tough outer part of the lemongrass, discard it and very finely slice across the pale tender ends. Put in a bowl with the juice of the 2 halved blood oranges. Add your ginger, a little pinch of salt, your olive oil and the lime juice. At this point you will need to taste. You want it to be nice and acidic, but if the limes are very sour you can mellow it slightly with a little extra olive oil, which won't hurt at all.

Finely slice your spring onions at an angle and mix with the orange segments and the sliced fennel. Lay this over the middle of the fish. Divide the tangy dressing between the 4 plates, making sure you drizzle it over the fish. Sprinkle with the lime zest and fennel tops and scatter over your sesame seeds. Serve straight away.

SERVES 4

600g/1lb 6oz trimmed white fish fillet, pinboned and skinned

2 sticks of lemongrass, trimmed

4 blood oranges, 2 halved and 2 segmented (see page 53)

1 tablespoon grated fresh ginger

sea salt

4 tablespoons extra virgin olive oil

zest and juice of 2 limes

4 spring onions

1 bulb of fennel, halved and finely sliced lengthways (herby tops put to one side)

4 tablespoons sesame seeds, toasted in the oven until golden

'it's great that world cuisine can be found in one city'

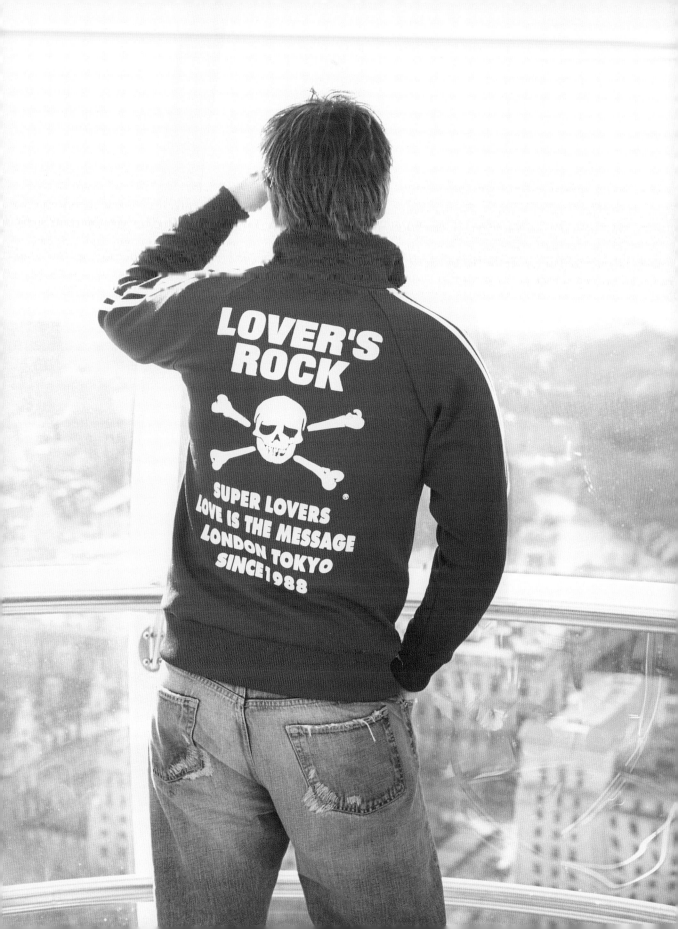

citrus seared tuna with crispy noodles, herbs and chilli

Tuna is a wonderfully rich, slightly fatty fish. Using grapefruit to sear it gives a really nice contrast of flavours. It's quick to prepare and it will definitely be a talking point when you have guests round for dinner. The noodles are a great part of this dish, but can be an optional extra.

Squeeze the grapefruit juice and pour into a sandwich bag with the fish sauce. Add the piece of tuna. Tie up the bag, squeezing out most of the air so the tuna is completely covered in the juice. Leave for 40 minutes, after which time the outside of the tuna will be pale and 'cooked'. Now carefully pour the grapefruit juice from the bag into a bowl, dry off the tuna and put to one side

For the dressing, mix the sesame oil, olive oil and chillies into the grapefruit juice. Use as much chilli as you like, and season to taste. Tear off a good handful of coriander and mint from the bunches and put to one side to use for garnish later. Finely chop the remaining herbs and really pat these around the tuna to encrust it. Wrap in clingfilm and place in the fridge until needed.

Boil the noodles for 1 minute until they are slightly flexible, drain and allow to steam dry and cool. Add a little olive oil to a hot non-stick pan, add your noodles and leave them until they are nice and crisp on one side. Now flip them over and do the same on the other side – it doesn't matter if some stick to the pan, just scrape them up and turn them over. Divide the crispy noodles between 4 plates. Slice your tuna up about 0.5cm/¼ inch thick – in Japan it's a sign of generosity to have nice thick slices of tuna, but I like them a little thinner as they are more delicate in the mouth.

Place the tuna on the noodles, sprinkle over the torn-up herbs that you put to one side earlier, sprinkle with the spring onions and then drizzle a couple of spoonfuls of the dressing over the tuna. Before your eyes you will see the cut sides of the slices of fish begin to change colour and 'cook'. Serve straight away.

SERVES 4

2 pink grapefruits

1 tablespoon fish sauce

500g/1lb 2oz piece of blue bigeye or very good yellowfin tuna

1 tablespoon sesame oil

6 tablespoons olive oil, plus extra for frying

2 or 3 fresh red chillies, very finely sliced

sea salt and freshly ground black pepper

1 large bunch of fresh coriander

1 small bunch of fresh mint

a couple of good handfuls of glass or cellophane noodles

4 spring onions, finely sliced at an angle

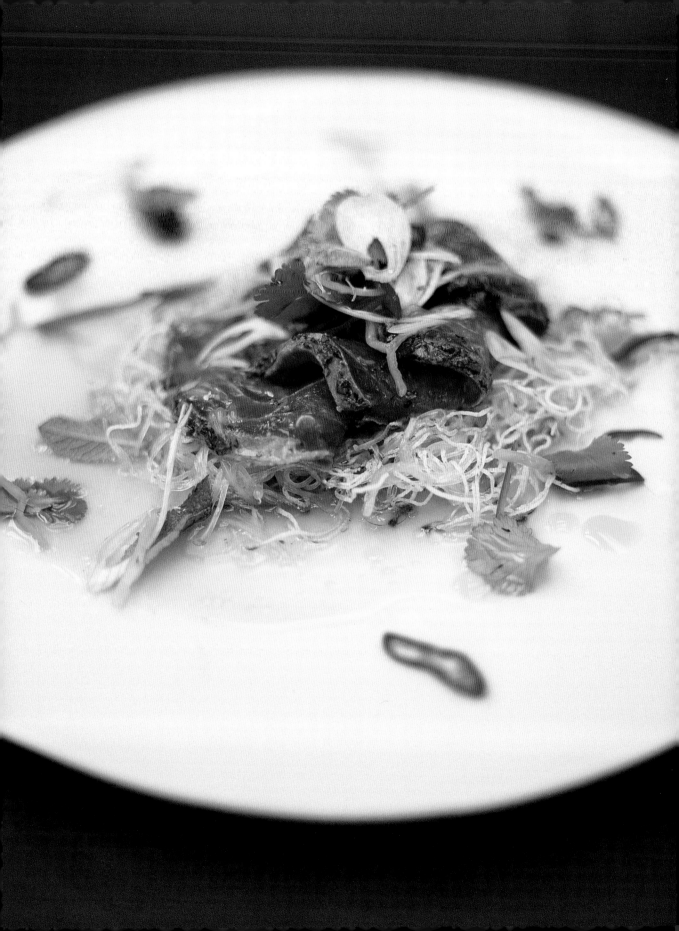

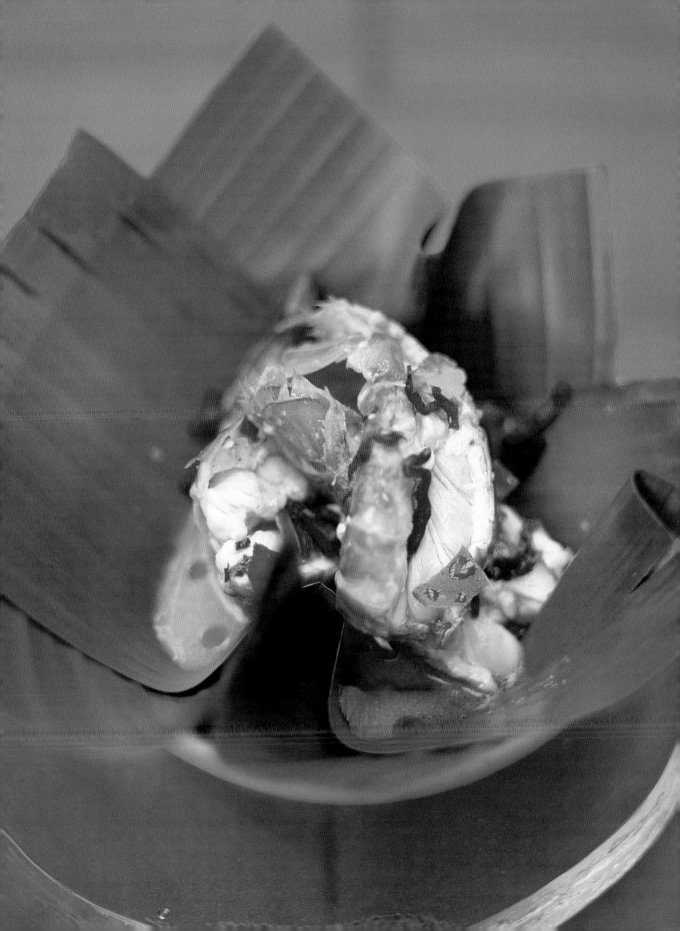

ceviche of raw crayfish with kaffir lime leaves, chilli and ginger

This is a great one and quite unexpected. I had something similar in a Spanish/Latino/Peruvian-style restaurant in New York where they specialize in ceviches. This is a good recipe to do as a canapé or pre-starter – you can whack some in the middle of the table and everyone can help themselves. It will really get the tastebuds going for dinner. You can buy fresh lime leaves and banana leaves in Asian grocery shops and some supermarkets.

Bash the lime leaves in a pestle and mortar with a pinch of salt (or use a metal bowl and the end of a rolling pin). Really bruise and break them up. Put them in a sandwich bag with the chillies, ginger, lime juice, sesame oil and extra virgin olive oil. Taste for seasoning – you may need a little salt.

Cut the crayfish or prawns down the back of each shell and open them up, removing the little vein in each as well as the head. This will help to make the fish look nicer but, more importantly, it makes the surface area bigger so that the acid can cook them quicker. Add the crayfish to the dressing in the sandwich bag, squeezing out all the air before tying it up and leaving it for half an hour.

Divide the crayfish between 4 bowls and drizzle the dressing over each bowl. Or you can use 4 small banana leaves if you want to. Hold them over a gas flame if you like so they become a deep green colour, and they'll smell fantastic. I normally slice the leaves up and squash them into a bowl with 3 crayfish on top so that all the lovely juices will be caught in the leaves and you can slurp them up.

SERVES 4

10 kaffir lime leaves

sea salt and freshly ground black pepper

2 fresh red chillies, finely sliced

2 teaspoons grated fresh ginger

juice of 3 limes

1 teaspoon sesame oil

4 tablespoons extra virgin olive oil

12 fresh large crayfish, langoustines or prawns

optional: 4 banana leaves

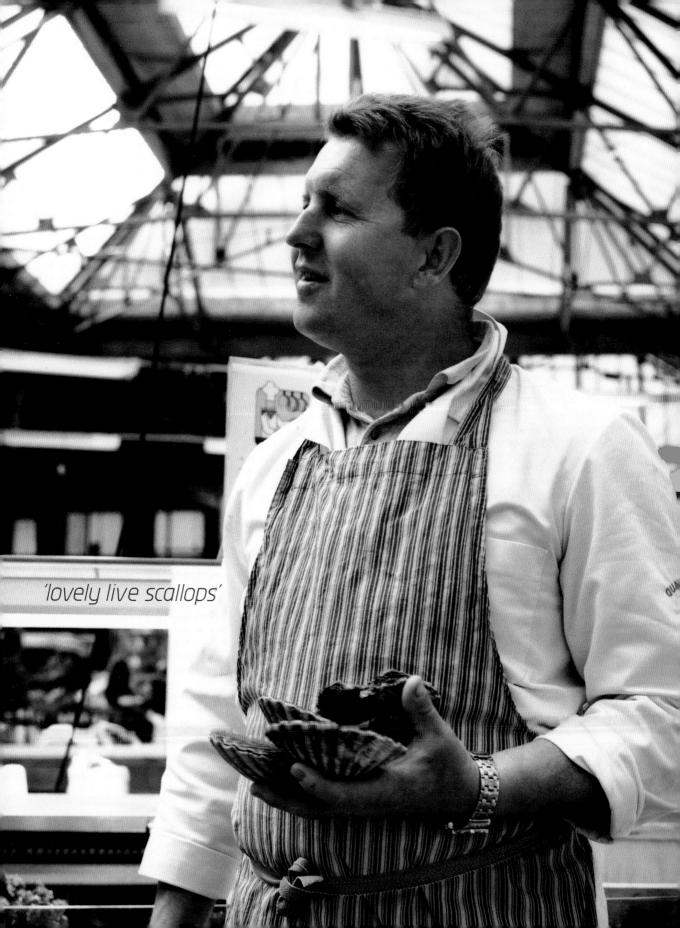

'lovely live scallops'

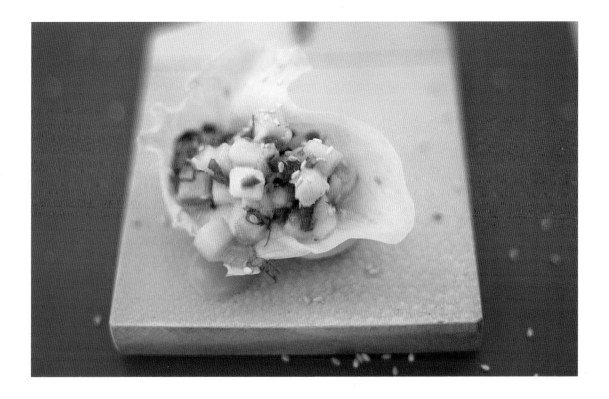

scallop spoons

This is a great little way to turn heads at a dinner party. Something as silky and delicate as a scallop is fantastic flavoured like this and served in a crunchy leaf.

By all means, get all your ingredients ready and prepared but don't mix together until the last minute or it won't taste as fresh. Finely dice and mix the scallops with the mango in a bowl. Add your spring onion and basil leaves and stir in, followed by the lime juice, olive oil, chilli and ginger. Check for seasoning. To serve, I love to divide little bite-sized portions of the mixture into small, crunchy iceberg lettuce leaves. Try and use the leaves from the centre of the lettuce as they are cup-shaped and will hold the filling really well.

Try this: Use gem lettuce or radicchio leaves or serve on dessert-spoons on a plate of cracked ice.

SERVES 4

6 large fresh scallops

½ mango, finely diced

1 spring onion, finely sliced

1 small handful of fresh basil, finely sliced (see page 114)

juice of 2 limes

3 tablespoons olive oil

½ fresh chilli, finely chopped

2 teaspoons grated fresh ginger

sea salt and freshly ground black pepper

1 iceberg lettuce

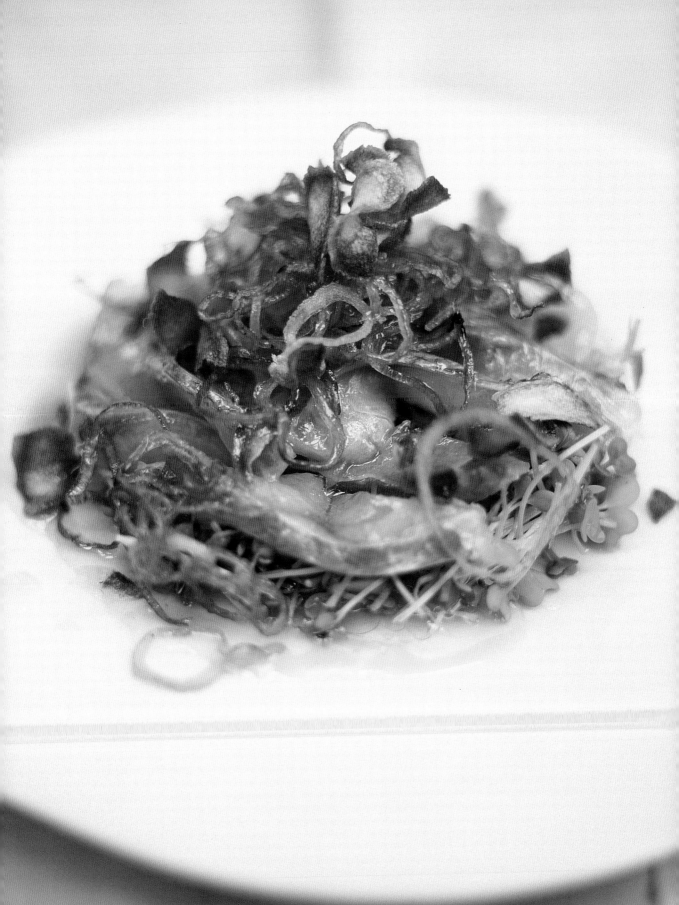

quick marinated red mullet with crispy ginger, shallots and a citrus dressing

Red mullet is a great fish to cook in this way. For me, the reason this dish works is that you've got the silky softness of the fish contrasting with the almost biscuity crispness of the ginger and the sweetness of the shallots. Really nice light tasty cooking.

Lightly season the fish on both sides and place in the fridge for half an hour to draw out any excess moisture. Put 3cm/1 inch of sunflower oil into a small, deep saucepan and place on a high heat. Place one slice of ginger in the oil. When it floats to the top and is sizzling nicely, the oil will be at the right temperature – about 170ºC. When ready, add all the ginger to the pan and fry on a medium high heat until crisp and nicely golden. Remove with a slotted spoon on to a kitchen towel and place to one side. Do the same with the shallots and remove when golden. Feel free to do them in a few batches so you get used to it. Allow the oil to cool down before you discard it. Divide the cress between 4 plates. Remove the fish from the fridge and pat dry. Using a sharp knife, thinly slice it across the fillet and divide it between the plates, draping it over the cress. Make sure it's not all flat and boring-looking. Mix your soy sauce with the lime zest and juice, coriander leaves and olive oil. Drizzle this over the fish, sprinkle over your ginger and shallots and tuck in.

Try this: If you want to make this look a little more delicate and cheffy, use a 15cm/6 inch pastry cutter as a frame or guide when placing your watercress and fish on the plates. It makes it all look a bit more professional.

Or this: You can actually use most fresh fish for this, so if you can't get red mullet try red snapper or whatever you fancy.

SERVES 4

400g/14oz red mullet fillets, pinboned and cleaned (see page 198)

sea salt and freshly ground black pepper

sunflower oil

2 thumb-sized pieces of fresh ginger, peeled and finely sliced

5 shallots, peeled and finely sliced

2 punnets of cress, trimmed and washed

2 tablespoons soy sauce

zest and juice of 2 limes

1 small handful of fresh coriander, leaves picked

6 tablespoons extra virgin olive oil

pomegranate and gin cocktail

This cocktail is great served at the end of a meal. The first time I had it was in a bar called MG Garage in Sydney, where they brought out frozen glasses, frozen gin and a tray full of pomegranates at the end of our meal. Since then I've used it as a good trick after a meal to clean the palate and relaunch the conversation. Buy a good-quality bottle of gin – you normally get what you pay for. Pop it in the freezer for an hour, along with a shot glass for each of your guests.

Peel some pomegranates and remove the beautiful deep purple-red capsules from inside. At the end of the meal, simply fill your shot glass with pomegranate seeds, pour in your iced gin and shoot the cocktail back. Don't swallow until you've crunched the pomegranate seeds and got a real burst of fragrance and flavour in your mouth. Then swallow the lot and continue the conversation . . . or have another one.

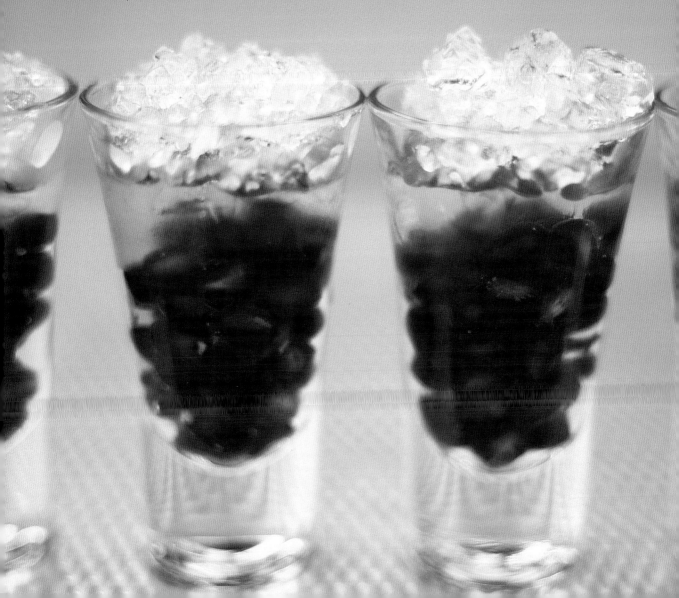

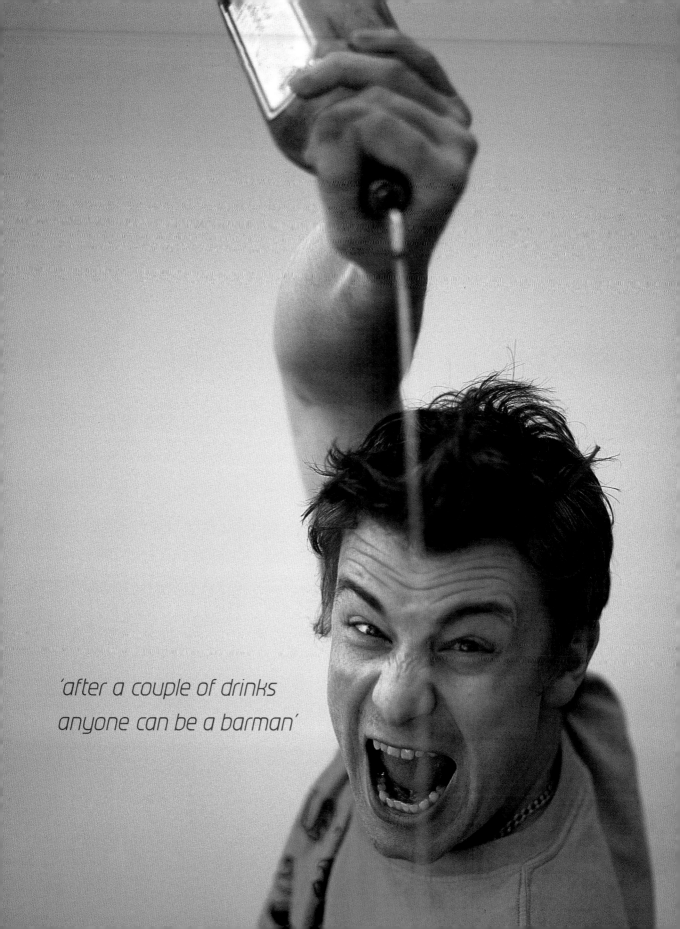

'after a couple of drinks
anyone can be a barman'

POACHING
AND
BOILING

POACHING

Poaching is a delicate and subtle way of cooking. You poach things below boiling point in just enough liquid to cover them, and that can be water, court bouillon (a flavoured stock made with wine, peppercorns and a wrap of herbs), stock or milk. Generally you use first-class cuts of meat and fish which need gentle cooking – you'll be surprised at the results of poaching a fillet steak, for example. It will taste really tender and clean.

BOILING

Boiling is a great method of cooking. It involves cooking stuff in a liquid at its boiling point. You can use water, court bouillon, milk or plain stock. Boiling liquid is a direct source of heat, so vegetables can be very quickly cooked, but be careful not to over-boil like my nan does or you'll end up with green water and grey greens! When boiling meat you're generally using tougher cuts, which will need to have their tough sinews melted away. In return you will get tender meat and a tasty stock.

barolo poached fillet steak with celeriac purée

I didn't try poached meat until a couple of years ago and to be honest the idea didn't appeal to me. A lot of chefs implied that cooking meat in good red wine was a waste, but how wrong they were. As well as Barolo, this dish works with many other red wines – especially nice spicy ones like Rioja or Shiraz. What I'm trying to say is that if you use rubbish wine in cooking it will come back to haunt you in the tasting.

First peel the celeriac down to the white, smooth flesh. Cut into rough 2cm/1 inch dice. Half fill a large saucepan with salted water and bring to the boil. Take another pan which will snugly fit your 4 steaks later, and add your chicken stock, wine, garlic, bunch of thyme, peppercorns and a pinch of salt. Bring this to the boil, then lower the heat to a gentle simmer. By this time your pan of boiling water should be ready, so add your celeriac, cover with a lid and boil fast for around 15–20 minutes until it's tender.

Place your 4 steaks side by side into the simmering wine and stock, making sure they are covered well by the liquid. Add a little water if needed, but if the pan is nice and snug the steaks should be well covered. As soon as they are in the pan, it generally takes about 6 minutes to cook rare, 8 minutes for medium and 10 for medium to well done. Depending on the thickness of the steaks and how cold they were when you put them in, there's always a bit of leeway on the timing, so the best thing to do is give them a little pinch to check how soft they are in the middle. Cover the pan with a cartouche (see page 174).

When cooked to your liking, remove them to a warm plate, cover and leave them to rest for a couple of minutes while you drain your cooked celeriac in a colander. Place it back in the pan, adding half the butter. Mash to a smooth purée and season well to taste.

To make a light sauce, all you need is 2 wineglasses full of the poaching liquor – you can freeze the rest. Bring this to the boil, then remove the thyme and peppercorns and mash up the garlic, which will be soft and sweet. Allow to boil for a couple of minutes. Remove from the heat, season to taste and add the rest of the butter. Shake the pan lightly so the melted butter dissolves into the wine – this will make a shiny lightly thickened sauce. Do not reboil as it will split. Serve each steak with a bit of mash and a little sauce.

SERVES 4

2 celeriacs

sea salt and freshly ground black pepper

4 x 200–225g/7–8oz fillet steaks, preferably organic and well marbled

570ml/1 pint chicken stock

½ bottle of Barolo or any other full-bodied red wine

6 cloves of garlic, peeled and kept whole

1 small bunch of fresh thyme

6 whole peppercorns

100g/3½oz butter

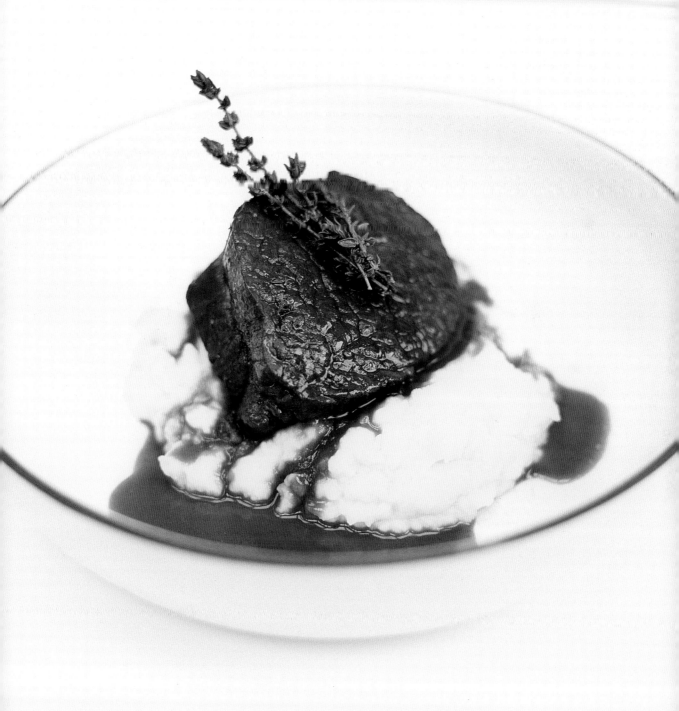

Try this: Any leftover cooking liquor can be sieved and kept in the freezer to use again or to make gravy from the goodness left in a roasting tray.

Or this: I prefer to serve this with celeriac mash because I think it's more interesting, but you can make any mash you like – Jerusalem artichoke, purple potato, or any other flavour.

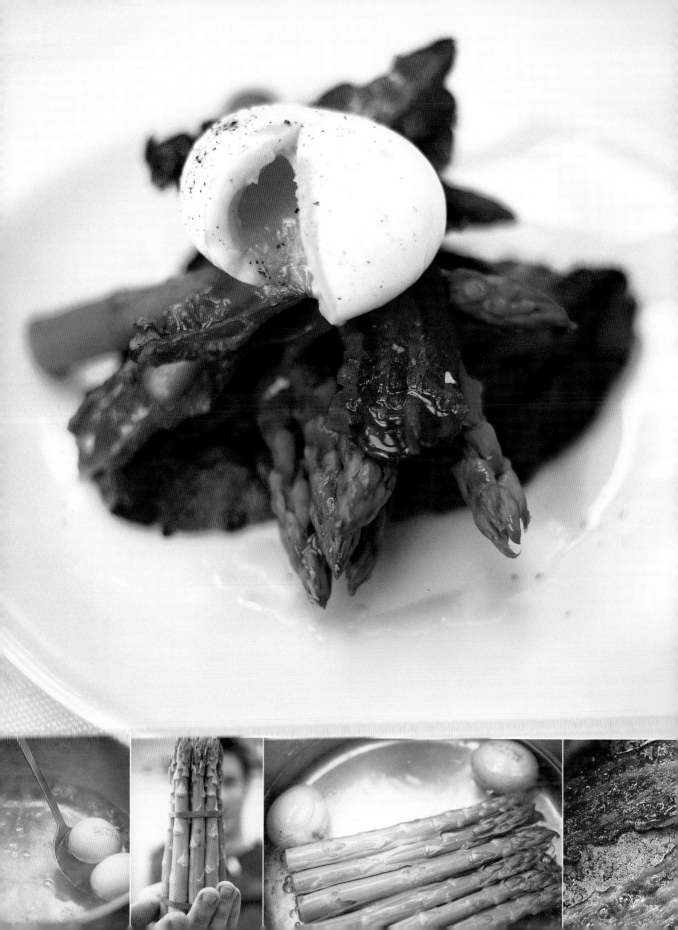

soft boiled egg with asparagus on toast

This is a great little brunchie snack. Apart from being quite healthy – or that's certainly how it makes you feel – you've got the great combination of silky soft asparagus with the soft egg and crunchy bruschetta and bacon. Anyone can make this. PS. Bruschetta basically means 'toast' in Italian.

Get some water boiling and your griddle pan on. Halve your tomatoes and place on a roasting tray, cut side facing up. Season, drizzle with a little oil and grill. When they start to colour, lay your slices of pancetta next to them, continue grilling until the pancetta is crisp and remove.

Carefully place your eggs and asparagus in the water and boil for just under 4 minutes. Depending on the thickness of the asparagus, you may want to fish it out a little earlier. Toast each piece of bread and put a slice on each of the 4 plates. Remove your eggs and asparagus from the water once cooked. In a bowl, toss the asparagus in the butter to coat. Peel your soft-boiled eggs. To make it really scrumptious get one half of tomato and rub and squash it into your bread, then divide your asparagus on top. Lay the pancetta over that and then top each carefully with an egg. Once secure, cut open the egg and allow all the lovely yolk to dribble down through the asparagus and on to the bread. Drizzle with olive oil and tuck in.

Try this: Use different eggs, such as goose and duck eggs, which are widely available in the supermarkets now. They will need slightly different cooking times depending on their size.

SERVES 4

2 ripe plum tomatoes

sea salt and freshly ground black pepper

extra virgin olive oil

8 slices pancetta or dry-cured smoky bacon

4 large free-range eggs

400g/14oz asparagus

4 good slices of rustic cottage-style bread

a knob of butter

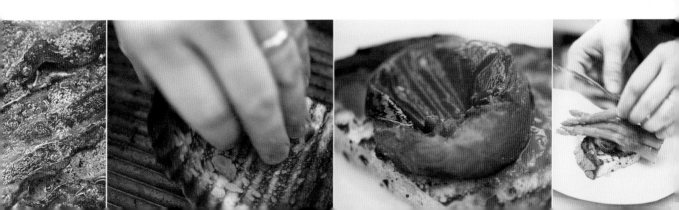

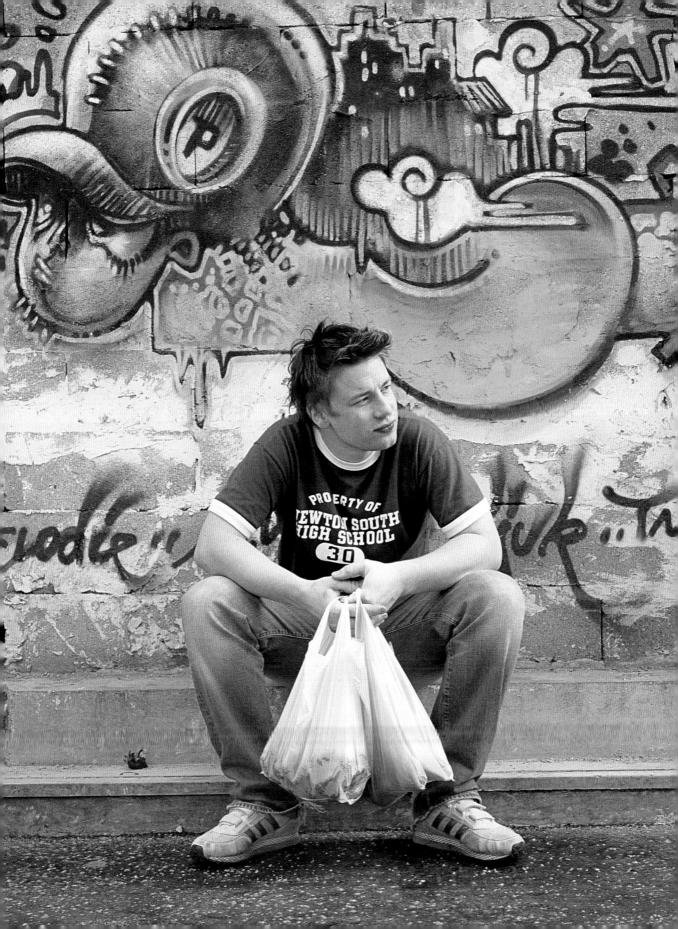

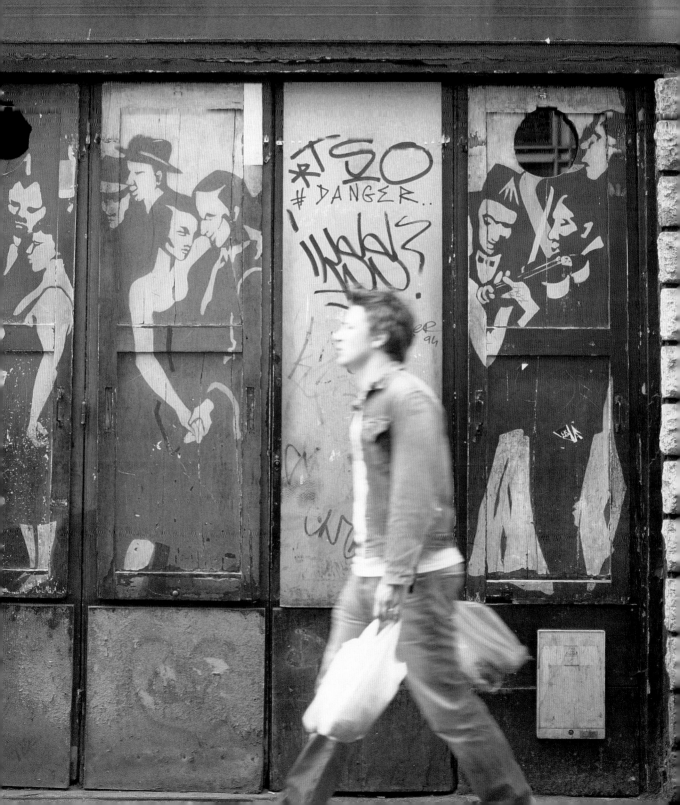

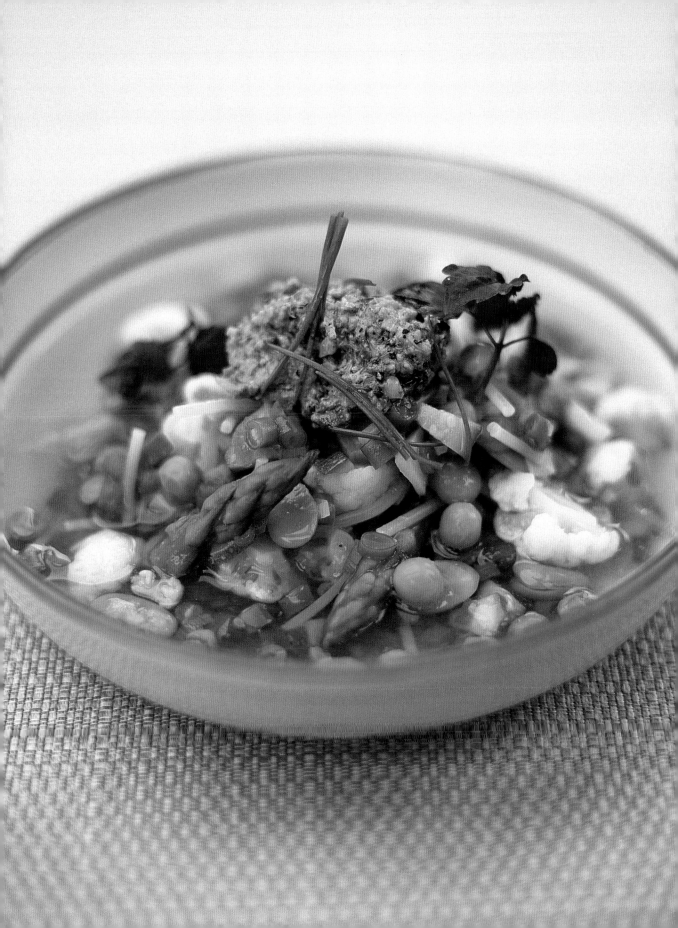

spring minestrone

There's a whole world of minestrones out there – most of which follow very strict, authentic recipes. Personally, I feel that a minestrone should always reflect the seasons: more cabbagy, frumpy ones in the winter and lighter, more colourful ones in the spring and summer. A minestrone can also be a whole meal if you want it to be, with pasta, stale bread or rice to bulk it out. To complement the spring vegetables, I've put a bit of a Genoese twist on it, with a spoon of fresh pesto added at the last minute, so the flavours explode in your mouth. Give it a bash.

First, if you're going to make pesto do it now. Bring a pot of stock to the boil. Then you need to get all the vegetables prepared and put to one side. The fennel has to be halved, sliced and finely chopped, the asparagus needs to have the woody ends removed, the stalks finely sliced and the tips left whole, the cauliflowers need to be divided into small florets, the courgettes need to be quartered lengthways and finely chopped and finally the tomatoes need to be blanched (see page 110). Cut them in half, remove the pips and finely slice. Now you're ready to rock and roll.

In a casserole-type pan (quite wide but not very deep) put 5 tablespoons of olive oil and heat the pan on a medium heat. Add the garlic, spring onions and fennel and gently fry without colouring at all for about 15 minutes. Then add the rest of your prepared vegetables, the pasta and your boiling stock. Bring to the boil, simmer for about 10 minutes, season, and serve in big bowls with a dollop of fresh pesto in the middle, a sprinkling of chopped basil and chives, and a drizzle of extra virgin olive oil.

Try this. As you can see, the idea of this soup is to celebrate all the vegetables that are available at the time, so feel free to modify the soup and make it your own.

And this: A good way to break up your spaghetti is to wrap it in a tea towel and then run it over the edge of your work surface.

Did you know? The fact that everything is finely chopped means that the cooking time is very quick and the soup remains light and fresh.

SERVES 6

6 heaped tablespoons fresh pesto (see page 106)

1.5 litres/2 3/4 pints good chicken, ham or vegetable stock

1 bulb of fennel

100g/3 1/2oz fine asparagus

2 Romanesco cauliflowers or 1 large cauliflower

6 baby courgettes

6 plum tomatoes

extra virgin olive oil

2 cloves of garlic, finely sliced

1 bunch of spring onions, finely chopped

100g/3 1/2oz green beans, finely sliced

100g/3 1/2oz yellow beans, finely sliced

100g/3 1/2oz peas, podded

100g/3 1/2oz broad beans, podded

100g/3 1/2oz spaghetti, broken-up

sea salt and freshly ground black pepper

1 small handful of green or purple basil

1 small handful of chives

roasted sweet garlic, bread and almond soup

I'm not quite sure where I got the inspiration for this recipe – I think it was actually when I was making bread one day and I incorporated some really sweet caramelized garlic and almonds into a focaccia. There's a slightly Spanish feel to the main ingredients – think of it as putting a bunch of old friends together and having a good party! My mother's initial reaction was, 'My God, that's a lot of garlic, you'll stink!' but don't let the amount put you off, as when garlic is roasted in its skin the pungent flavour is replaced by a jammy sweetness which is divine.

Roast the garlic cloves in a preheated oven at 180°C/350°F/gas 4 for around half an hour until soft to the touch. Meanwhile, take a large pot and slowly fry the white onion in 4 tablespoons of olive oil for about 10 minutes until really soft and translucent. Add the cream and the stock, bring back to the boil and simmer for 10 minutes, awaiting your garlic. Remove the garlic from the oven and allow to cool slightly before squeezing out all the sweet, golden paste. Whisk this into the soup. Discard the garlic skins.

Remove the crusts from your ciabatta, rip up the bread into small pieces and throw into the soup. Add the sherry vinegar, then allow the soup to simmer for 5 more minutes. Whizz it until smooth in your food processor with your toasted almonds. Season nicely to taste and serve in big bowls sprinkled with some orange segments, torn up coriander and mint, and drizzled with a good lug of extra virgin olive oil.

Try this: You can eat this cold in the summer – it's obviously going to be thick, which I think is a nice thing, but you can thin it with a little milk or stock if you want to.

And this: You may want to big up the sherry vinegar to give it that twang you get with a Spanish gazpacho soup.

Or this: There's a similar recipe from Spain where sliced white grapes are added to the soup – this contrasts really well with the garlic, so give it a go. A handful will do. Nice when eaten both hot and cold.

SERVES 6

3 large bulbs of fresh garlic, broken up and skins left on

1 medium white onion, peeled and finely chopped

extra virgin olive oil

285ml/½ pint double cream

1 litre/1¾ pints chicken or vegetable stock

1 large loaf of ciabatta bread

2 tablespoons sherry or white wine vinegar

200g/7oz whole blanched almonds, lightly toasted in the oven

sea salt and freshly ground black pepper

3 oranges, peeled and segmented (see page 53)

1 handful of fresh coriander, leaves picked

1 handful of fresh mint, leaves picked

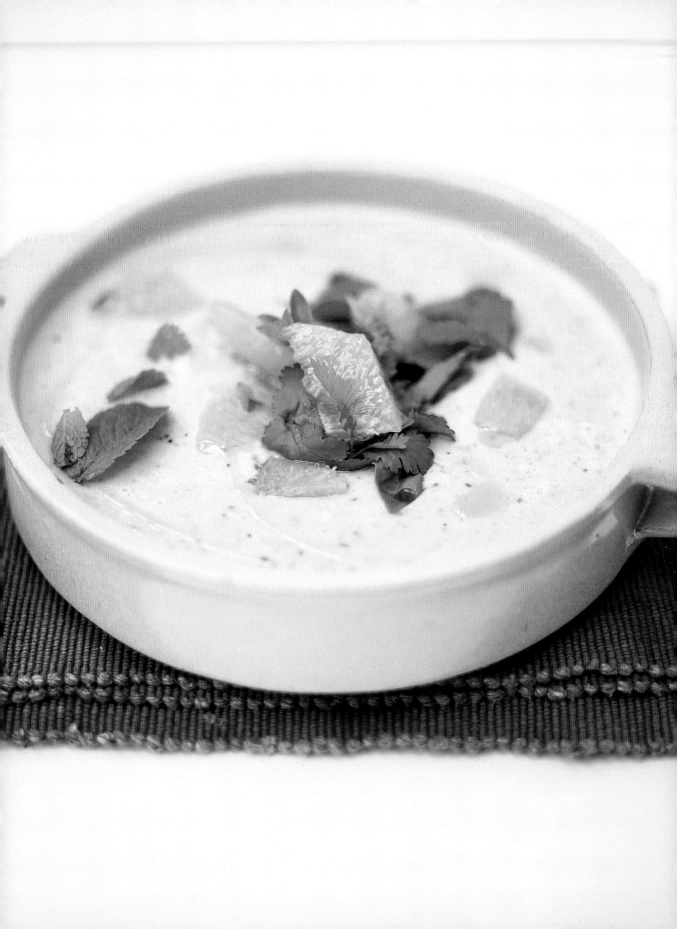

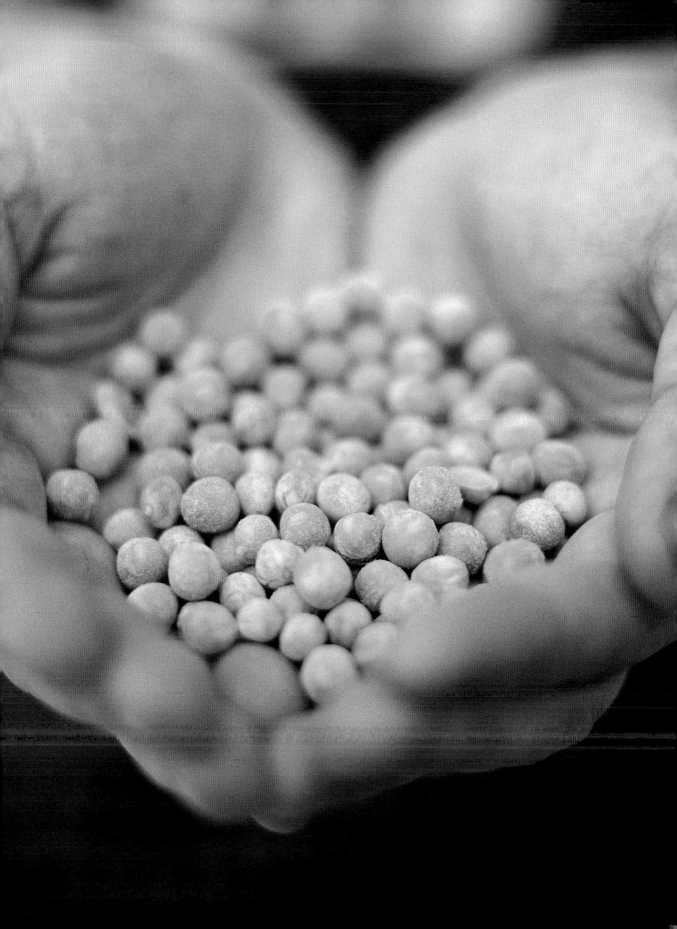

minted pea soup with crispy pancetta, bread and sour cream

This is a really addictive, thick soup that takes no time to make. I made it just at the start of summer, when the peas were really small, sweet and burst in your mouth. If you can do that then great, but in a way I think making a soup out of fresh peas is a bit of a waste really because spring peas are best just cooked for a couple of minutes in boiling water and served quite simply. I've got to be honest, when I made this with a packet of frozen peas (Bird's Eye seem to be the best) it was brilliant. With the nice hit of mint, you can serve this soup all year round and it will always work a treat.

Preheat your oven to 180°C/350°F/gas 4. Take the crusts off the bread and pinch off irregular dice-size pieces. Put these into a roasting tray and drizzle with a little olive oil, scatter over some of the mint leaves and season. Drape your pancetta over the top and cook until the bread and pancetta are crunchy and golden – around 15–20 minutes. Meanwhile, in a medium to large saucepan, slowly fry the spring onions and remaining mint in the butter for about 3 minutes until soft. Turn the heat up, add your frozen peas and the chicken stock and bring to the boil. Now lower the heat, add the double cream and simmer gently for 15 minutes.

The next thing is to liquidize the soup until it's very smooth (you may want to do this in batches). Correct the seasoning very carefully to taste – really think about this bit and get it just right. Remember: add, taste, add, taste. By this time your bread and pancetta should be nice and crisp, so ladle the soup into your bowls and sprinkle over your bread, mint leaves and pancetta. Add a little sour cream and drizzle with some peppery extra virgin olive oil. Lovely.

Try this: In the past I've used broad beans, spinach and asparagus as partners in crime – always nice.

Or this: You could try serving some simple ricotta-filled tortellini or ravioli, drizzled with a little of this soup. Toss the pasta in a bit of butter, crumble up the bread and bacon and sprinkle over the top.

SERVES 4–6

½ stale white loaf

extra virgin olive oil

1 large handful of fresh mint, leaves picked

sea salt and freshly ground black pepper

12 slices of thin pancetta or dry-cured smoky bacon

1 bunch of spring onions, ends trimmed and roughly chopped

2 knobs of butter

500g/1lb 2oz frozen peas

1.1 litres/2 pints chicken stock

100ml/3½fl oz double cream

4 teaspoons sour cream

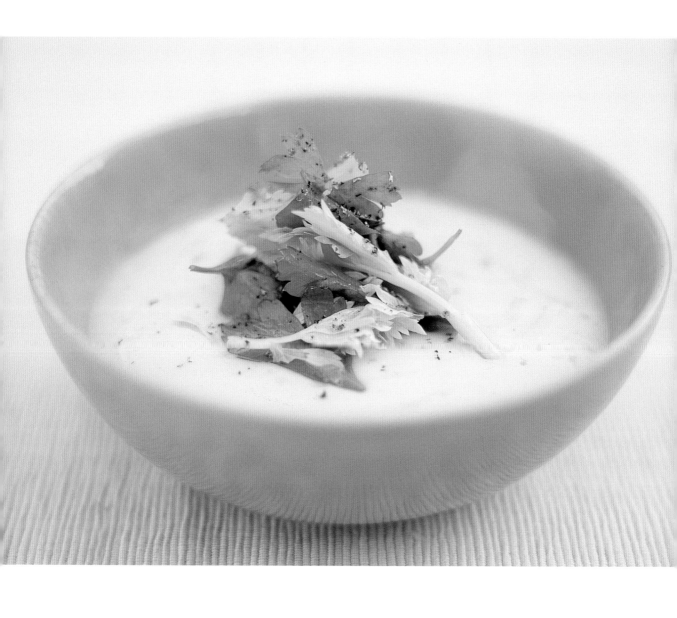

potato, celeriac and truffle oil soup

The fact is, I know using truffles at home is a little pretentious and very decadent, but even my local supermarket now stocks truffle oil. Admittedly it's more than likely not the real McCoy, but it does have a flavour you can't put your finger on – a kind of fragrant, garlicky, encapsulating smell which when used with subtlety is great. Truffle oil can be used for so many things – with a simple risotto or tagliatelle it's amazing. Then, when you've got the bug, treat yourself to the real thing, be it black or the exceptional white truffle.

In an appropriately sized pot, slowly fry the onion in the butter and olive oil for about 5 minutes until translucent and soft but not coloured at all. Get your bunch of thyme, tie it up with a little string and add to the pot with the celeriac, potatoes and stock. Bring to the boil and simmer for 40 minutes until the vegetables are tender. Add the cream, bring back to the boil, then remove the thyme and purée the mixture in a liquidizer or food processor. Season carefully to taste, adding the truffle oil tablespoon by tablespoon – the oil can vary in strength depending on the brand. Divide between your serving bowls. Feel free to improvise by adding croûtons, a little extra cream or, if you're really lucky, some real black or white truffles shaved over the top.

Try this: If you want to give an edge to this comforting soup, try dressing some chopped parsley and celery leaves with a little olive oil and lemon juice. Sprinkle over the soup at the last minute before serving.

SERVES 4–6

1 white onion, peeled and roughly chopped

1 good knob of butter

4 tablespoons extra virgin olive oil

1 bunch of fresh thyme

500g/1lb 2oz celeriac, peeled and roughly diced

500g/1lb 2oz floury potatoes, peeled and roughly diced

1.1 litres/2 pints chicken stock

100ml/3½fl oz double cream

sea salt and freshly ground black pepper

3–4 tablespoons truffle oil

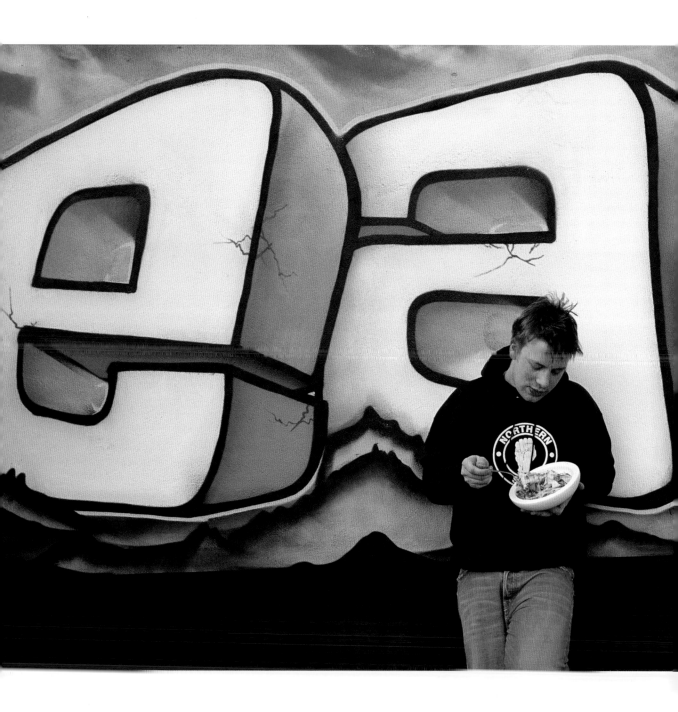

'as soon as the pasta's ready, eat it quick!!'

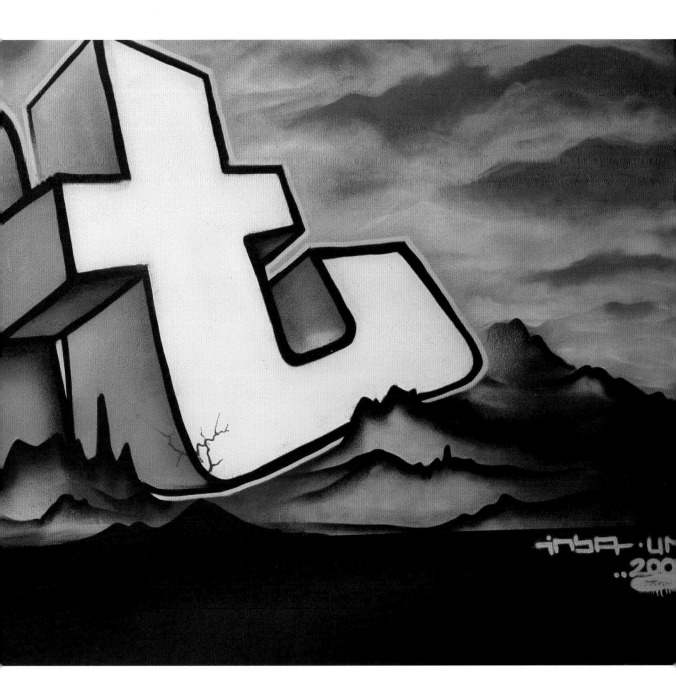

handy pasta recipe

I have done pasta before in my books, but I thought I'd give you a few more genius combinations.

Here is my basic pasta recipe. It's good for making so many different pastas, such as ravioli, tortellini, lasagne, pappardelle or tagliatelle. Please please don't read this and think, 'Oh, I can't do it.' I honestly have watched ten-year-old kids have a go and make half-decent ravioli. I've come home and within five minutes I've made my own pasta.

To make the pasta recipe less frightening, I'm going to be less strict on exact measurements, as all flours and eggs have different absorption rates and moisture levels.

You will need strong flour, preferably Tipo '00', which is an Italian phrase for milling the flour extra fine. I normally make at least enough for about 6 people at any one time – i.e. 600g/1lb 6oz flour and 6 eggs. If you want to make the pasta slightly yellower and richer, add 2 egg yolks per 100g/3½oz instead of 1 egg. And if you want to give the pasta a little more texture, use half strong flour and half semolina flour.

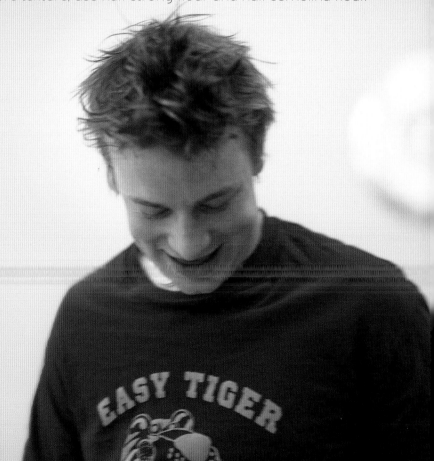

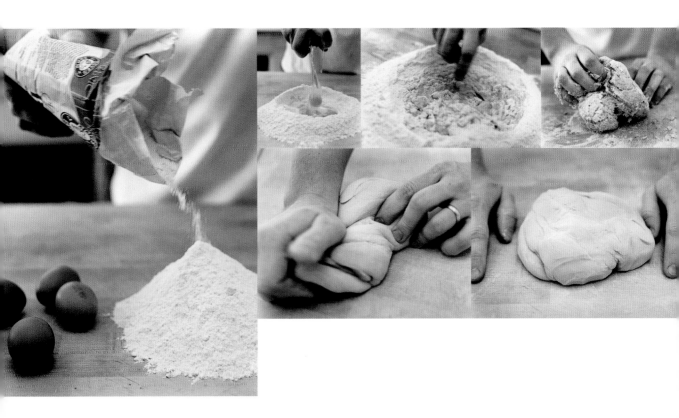

1. Place the flour on a board. You could always do this in a bowl.

2. Make a well in the centre of the flour and crack the eggs into it. Using a fork, beat the eggs until smooth.

3. Mix together with the flour as much as possible so it's not too sticky.

4. Then flour each hand and begin to knead.

5. This is the bit where you can let all your emotions out so go for it!

6. What you want to end up with is a nice piece of silky elastic dough. Cover it with clingfilm and leave it to rest for about half an hour while you make your fillings.

TURNING PASTA DOUGH INTO A SHEET

It's amazing the number of different things you can do with a sheet of pasta, so get stuck in and have a go at making one!

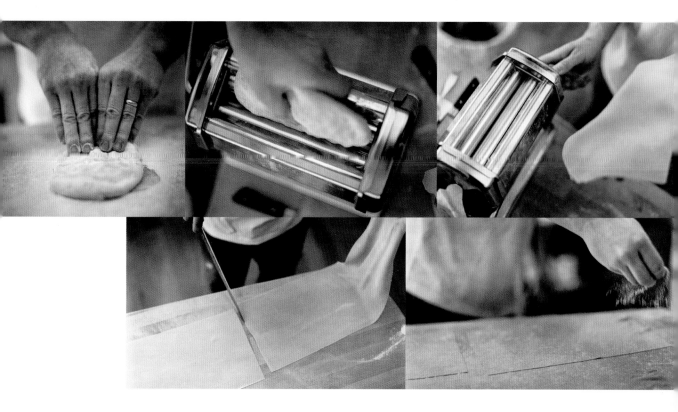

1. Divide your dough in half. Cover one half with clingfilm and place in the fridge until ready to use it. Push the other piece of dough out with your hand.

2. Run it through your pasta machine on the thickest setting for a few times, folding it in half each time until you have a nice, elastic, silky dough.

3. Keep rolling the pasta through the settings, reducing the thickness each time until it's as thick as a beer mat.

4. If the pasta gets too long to work with, cut it in half.

5. You now have your pasta sheet and can start to shape it.

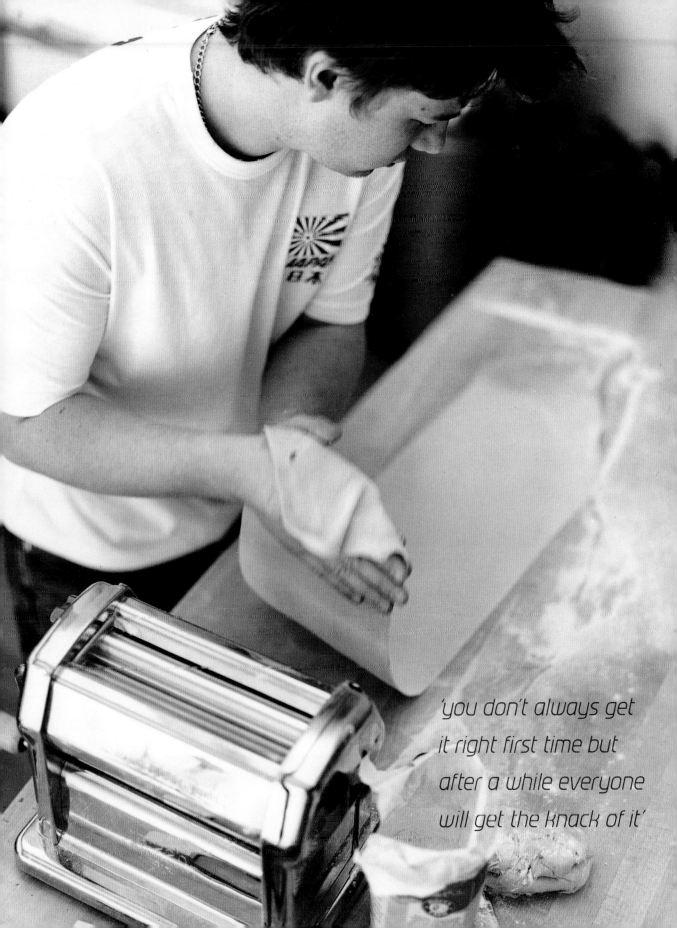

'you don't always get
it right first time but
after a while everyone
will get the knack of it'

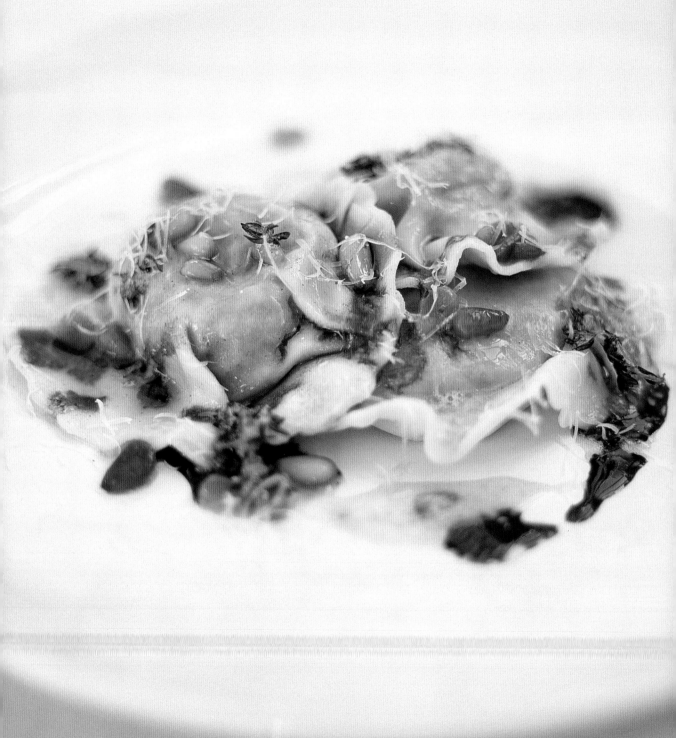

ravioli of roasted red onions, thyme, pinenuts and maris piper potato

This was a pasta I tried in a restaurant in Tuscany in late November, when I was over there buying olive oil for the restaurant. It's quite a robust ravioli but one of the best I've had in a long time. Although it's a winter ravioli I eat this any time of the year.

Make your pasta into a sheet (see page 88).

Preheat the oven to 200°C/400°F/gas 6. Put the onions in a small roasting tray and add the thyme, 12 tablespoons of balsamic vinegar and a few good lugs of olive oil, then cover well with a piece of wet greaseproof paper. Prick your potatoes and place on another tray. Place both trays in the oven for around 40 minutes, until the onions are really soft and sweet and the potatoes are cooked through. The spuds may need a bit longer, depending on their size. If so, just remove the onions while you wait for the potatoes. When cooked, allow the onions and potatoes to cool slightly, then scoop the fluffy potato out of the skins into a bowl.

Finely chop the onions, then spoon them into the bowl with the potato, including all the juices from the tray. Add 3 knobs of butter and Parmesan, then mix up and season very well to taste. Allow to cool. Roll the filling up into marble-sized balls – use your hand or a teaspoon to do this – and fill your ravioli. See page 92 for a good demonstration of how to do this.

To serve, cook the ravioli in salted boiling water for 3–4 minutes. At the same time, in a hot non-stick pan, lightly toast the pinenuts in little lug of oil and the last knob of butter. Fry until the nuts are lightly golden, then remove from the heat and add a couple of swigs of balsamic vinegar. Add the ravioli to the pan, toss and serve with a little more grated cheese over the top.

Try this: You should really cook your ravioli as near to making them as possible. So if you want to serve them at a dinner party, I would suggest that after making them you place them in boiling water for 1 minute, drain and cool them carefully in cold water, then drain again and toss in a little olive oil. These can then be kept for up to a day – cook them for 3 minutes before serving.

SERVES 4

1 x basic pasta recipe (see page 86)

2 red onions, peeled and quartered

1 small handful of fresh thyme, leaves picked

balsamic vinegar

extra virgin olive oil

around 400g/14oz large Maris Piper potatoes, washed and unpeeled

4 good knobs of butter

1 handful of grated Parmesan cheese, plus a little extra

sea salt and freshly ground black pepper

1 handful of pinenuts

SHAPING INTO RAVIOLI

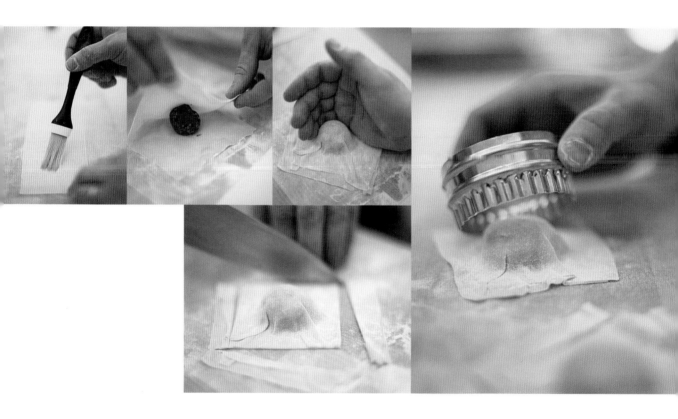

1. Cut the pasta into 18 x 9cm/7 x 3½ inch strips, then brush or spray each strip with a little water.

2. Add a teaspoon of filling to the centre of one side of each pasta strip, then fold over in half.

3. Mould the pasta carefully around the filling, pushing out any air bubbles.

4. You can cut the ravioli into squares with a knife . . .

5. . . . or into circles with a pastry cutter.

SHAPING INTO CARAMELLA

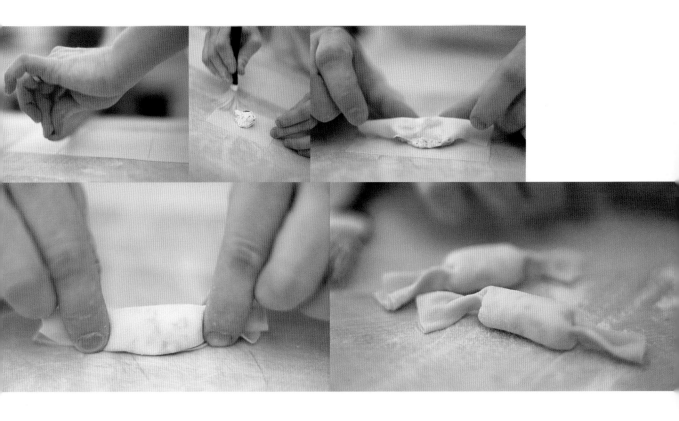

1. For caramella cut the pasta into 10 x 6cm/4 x 2½ inch rectangles.

2. Fill the middle with a teaspoon of the filling and brush lightly with water.

3. Roll up.

4. Pinch hard to secure at each end.

5. Keep on a flour-dusted tray in the fridge until you need them, and try to cook them as fresh as possible.

caramella of mint and ricotta

This is a really lovely summer pasta which is easy to make. Caramella means 'sweetie' in Italian, and the finished pasta looks like a sweetie in its wrapper.

Make your pasta dough (see page 87). While the dough is resting, make your filling by mixing together the ricotta, lemon zest, nutmeg, mint and Parmesan – you may want to reserve a little Parmesan and mint for serving – and then carefully season to balance the flavours. Squeeze a little lemon juice into the mix to loosen it a bit. If you're partial to a little bit more Parmesan, mint or lemon, then do personalize the dish to your liking. Roll good teaspoons of the mix into little balls ready to fill your caramella. For good pictures of how to shape and fill the pasta, see page 93. Make as many as you can, but I like to serve about 4 per person.

If you're not going to cook the caramella straight away, put them on to a flour-dusted tray and place in the fridge until you're ready. To serve, place in boiling salted water for 3–4 minutes, then drain, reserving some of the cooking water. Melt 3 good knobs of butter in a non-stick pan with the juice of ½ a lemon and a couple of tablespoons of the reserved cooking water. Season a little, and toss the pasta in this flavoured butter. Serve straight away with a little extra Parmesan and mint scattered over the top.

SERVES 4

1 x basic pasta recipe (see page 86)

340g/12oz crumbly buffalo ricotta cheese

zest of 1 large lemon

juice of 1 lemon

¼ nutmeg, grated

1 handful of mint leaves, finely sliced (see page 114)

2 handfuls of grated Parmesan cheese

sea salt and freshly ground black pepper

3 knobs of butter

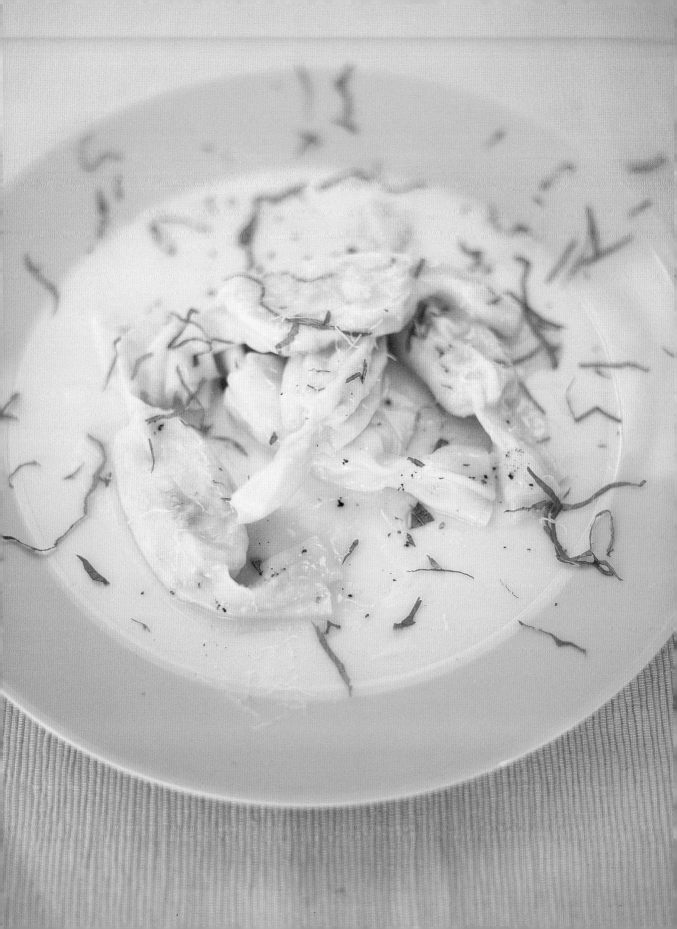

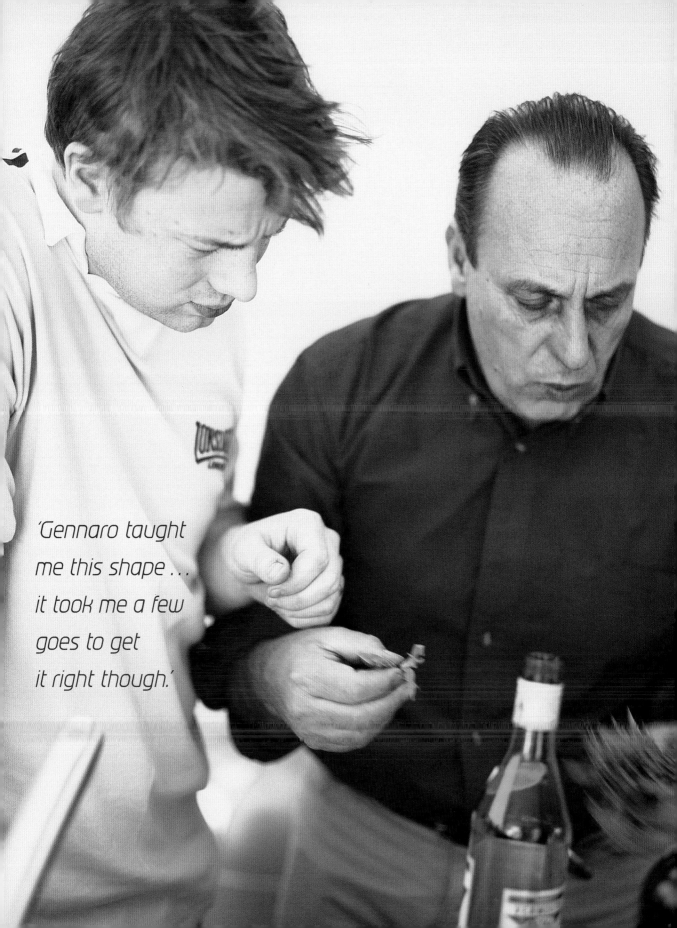

'Gennaro taught
me this shape ...
it took me a few
goes to get
it right though.'

SHAPING INTO CULURZONES

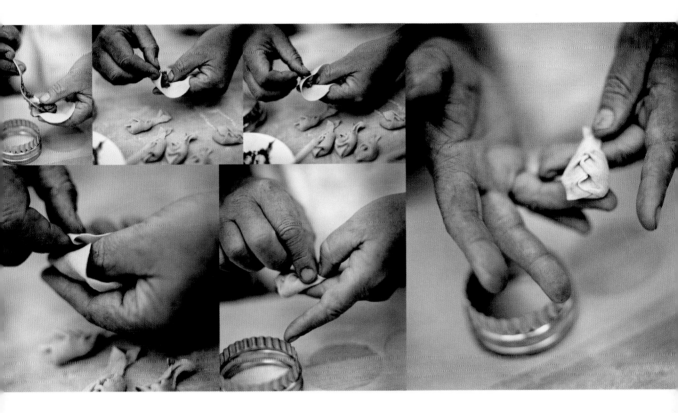

1. Cut a circle with a pastry cutter and place a teaspoon of filling at one end.

2. Bend the end over and keep the filling in place with your thumb.

3. Begin to fold over the sides and push against your nail to secure . . .

4. . . . all the way up . . .

5. . . . until the end and give it one last pinch.

6. So, so beautiful!

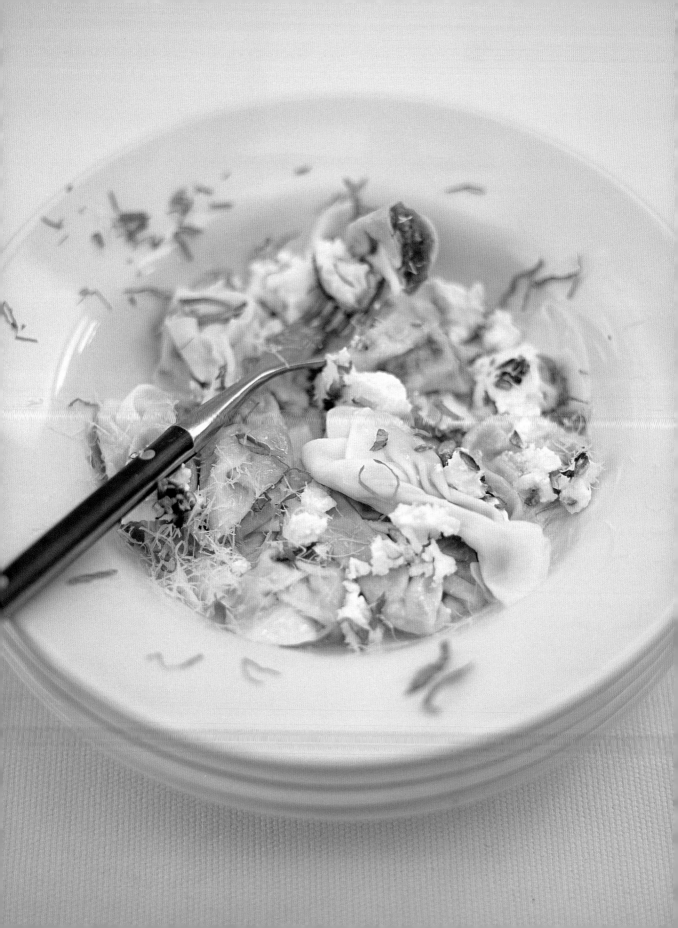

sardinian culurzones with butternut squash and baked goat's cheese

Here's a beautiful sexy little pasta that my mate Gennaro Contaldo makes. Culurzones are ravioli or folded pasta shapes classically served with three cheeses and mint. You can make this dish using caramella-shaped pasta or the more usual ravioli shapes (see pages 92–3) if you like, but this one is exciting – the way the pasta is almost plaited together means that it holds the cheesy, buttery sauce better.

Make your pasta dough (see page 87).

Preheat the oven to 190°C/375°F/gas 5. Remove the seeds from both halves of your butternut squash and put them to one side. Grate the squash using a cheese grater and pound up the coriander seeds and chilli in a pestle and mortar (or use the end of a rolling pin and a metal bowl). Mix the squash with the pounded spices, rosemary and 3 tablespoons of olive oil, then lay it out flat on a tray. Bake for around 30 minutes until it looks dried out but is really intense and sweet.

Roughly chop the squash seeds. Rub the goat's cheese with a little olive oil and pat and press the squash seeds and oregano around the cheese. Place in an ovenproof dish. Bake the goat's cheese for about 20 minutes or until lightly golden – it will taste fantastic and be really crumbly.

Allow the squash mixture to cool slightly, then season well to taste. This is now ready to be used as the filling. See page 97 for some good pictures of how to shape and fill the culurzones.

Cook the culurzones for 3–4 minutes in boiling salted water until they float to the surface. Put the butter in a non-stick pan and heat. When it foams toss in your culurzones and then divide them between your serving plates. Sprinkle with a little Parmesan and sliced basil and crumble over your baked goat's cheese.

Try this: Sometimes, Italians contrast the savoury sweetness of the squash with something called mostarda di Cremona, which is a mustard-spiced selection of preserved fruit, and quite hot! And bashed-up cantucci biscuits, which are usually served with coffee. These are just mixed in with the squash before the pasta is filled.

SERVES 4

1 x basic pasta recipe (see pages 86–7)

1 butternut squash, peeled and halved

1 tablespoon coriander seeds

1 dried red chilli

3 sprigs of fresh rosemary, leaves picked and roughly chopped

extra virgin olive oil

100g/3½oz goat's cheese

1 teaspoon dried oregano

sea salt and freshly ground black pepper

3 knobs of butter

1 handful of grated Parmesan cheese

1 small handful basil leaves, sliced (see page 114)

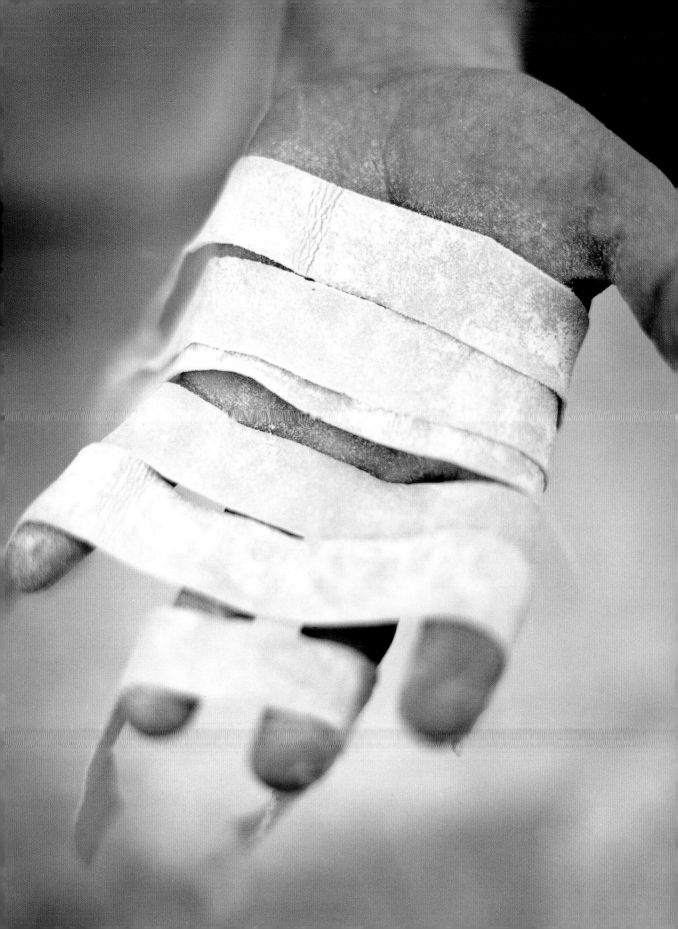

SHAPING LASAGNETTI, PAPPARDELLE, TAGLIATELLE AND TAGLIERINI

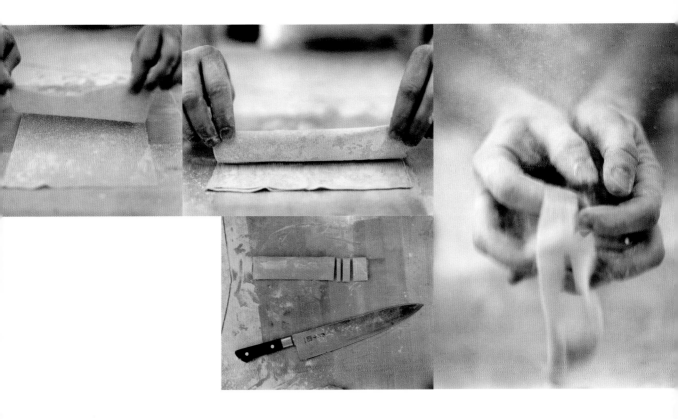

1. Cut your sheet of pasta into 20cm/8 inch lengths. Dust well with flour then fold in half.

2. Fold in half again and then once more, dusting with flour each time.

3. Cut into 5cm/2 inch pieces for lasagnetti, 2cm/³⁄₄ inch for pappardelle, 1cm/¹⁄₂ inch for tagliatelle and 0.5cm/¹⁄₄ inch for taglierini.

4. Make a cage with your fingers and shake until the pasta separates out.

pappardelle with amazing slow-cooked meat

For this recipe you can use beef, venison, wild boar and even pigeon or hare. In Italy, if a family had to feed 8 people out of this, then they would cook more pasta and add a little more water – as always, a little meat can go a long way.

In a hot casserole-type pan fry your meat in a little olive oil – it doesn't matter if it's cut into large 5cm/2 inch chunks if it's venison, beef or wild boar, or left whole if a pigeon, or jointed into 5 or 6 pieces if you're using a hare. Fry the meat until golden brown then add your herbs, onions, garlic, carrot and celery. Turn the heat down and continue to fry for 5 minutes until the vegetables have softened. Add your red wine and continue to simmer until the liquid has almost cooked away but left you with a fantastic colour and fragrance.

Add the plum tomatoes, the pearl barley and just enough water to cover the meat by 1cm/½ inch. Make yourself a cartouche of grease-proof paper (see page 174). Wet it under the tap, rub it with a little olive oil and place it over the pan. Put a lid on the pan as well, as this will retain as much moisture as possible while cooking. Cook on a really low heat for about 2–3 hours, depending on the tenderness and type of meat. It's ready when you can literally push the meat off the bone and it will flake away in tender oxtaily strands. At this point season carefully to taste and allow to cool slightly before removing the meat from the pan. Using 2 forks, pull apart all the lovely pieces of meat, throwing away any skin and bones. Put the meat back in the pan on a low heat.

It's now ready to serve, so cook your pappardelle in a pan of boiling, salted water for 3 minutes if using fresh pasta and according to the packet instructions if using dried. Once it's cooked, drain it in a colander, saving some of the cooking liquid in case the sauce needs a little loosening. Remove the stewed meat from the heat and stir in the butter and Parmesan with a little of the cooking water – this will make it juicy and shiny. Toss together with your pasta and serve immediately.

Try this: Serve sprinkled with a little finely chopped fresh rosemary and some grated Parmesan.

SERVES 4

800g/1lb 12oz braising meat (see above), seasoned

extra virgin olive oil

1 handful of fresh rosemary and fresh thyme, leaves picked and finely chopped

1 small red onion, peeled and finely chopped

4 cloves of garlic, peeled and finely chopped

1 carrot, peeled and finely chopped

1 celery stalk, finely chopped

2 wineglasses of Chianti

2 x 400g/14oz tins of plum tomatoes

2 tablespoons pearl barley

salt and freshly ground black pepper

400g/14oz fresh or dried pappardelle (for fresh, see page 101)

100g/3½oz butter

2 handfuls of grated Parmesan cheese

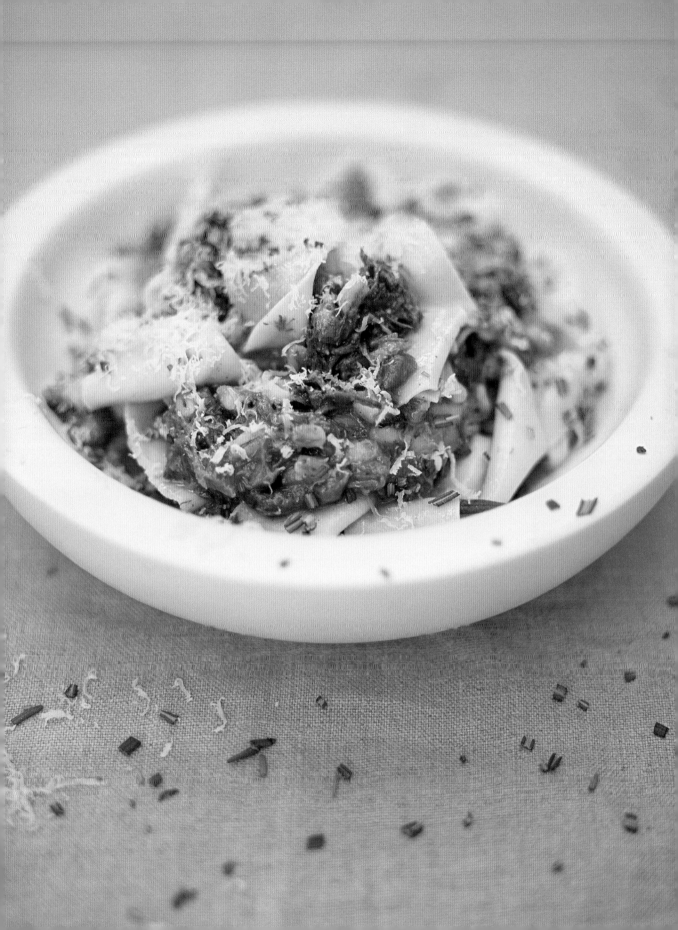

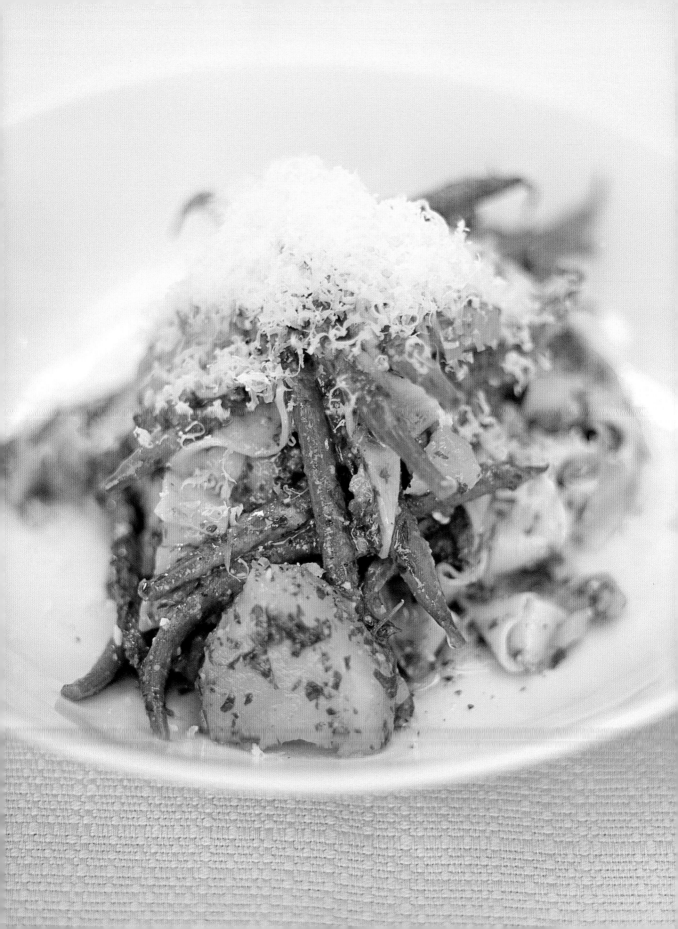

tagliatelle genovese

This is one of the all-time classics from Genoa in Italy, really beautiful fresh home made pesto with pasta, cooked broken potatoes and green beans. The reason I've included it in the book is that two years ago I taught one of my mates, Wally, how to make pesto from scratch. He's not a great cook, but he got the hang of it quickly and made it really well. Since then he's stretched from an inch to a mile and has done barbecued veg with pesto, grilled fish with pesto and roasted chicken with pesto, and I think that's the key really. To be a good cook you don't need to know everything – you just need to be able to do something well. Even though it might sound a bit odd to us to have potatoes and pasta in the same dish, in Italy they manage to pull it off with such amazing results that you really should try it.

First of all, make your pesto. Season to taste and put to one side. Slice the potatoes 1cm/½ inch thick and put them into a large pan of salted water – the idea is to cook the pasta in this pan as well, so make sure it's big enough. Bring to the boil, cook until the potatoes are tender but still holding their shape, then add the pasta to the same water. If you're using fresh pasta then add the beans at the same time, as they will both need about 3 minutes; if using dried, add the beans 3 minutes before the pasta is done. Don't worry too much about the potatoes breaking up, as very often when you are served this in Genoa, the beans are a little overcooked and sometimes the potatoes have broken up into small pieces but the flavour remains sublime. And it adds to the whole character of the dish.

Once the potatoes, pasta and beans are cooked, drain in a colander, saving some of the cooking water. Now place the potatoes, pasta and beans in a large bowl with your pesto. Toss together, coating the pasta, then add a bit of the cooking water to give you a loose light sauce – you don't want it to be too claggy. Season well to taste and serve straight away with extra grated Parmesan on the table and a nice bottle of white.

SERVES 4

1 x pesto recipe (see page 106)

salt and freshly ground black pepper

200g/7oz of Maris Piper or Desirée potatoes, peeled

400g/14oz fresh or dried tagliatelle (for fresh, see page 101)

1 handful of fine green or yellow French beans, tops removed (leave the wispy ends on)

1 handful of grated Parmesan cheese

pesto sauce

There are no real rules for pesto – as long as you make it fresh and use the best ingredients it'll always taste superb. The key to getting it right is to keep tasting and adding cheese or oil until you have the right semi-wet but firm mixture.

Pound the garlic with a little pinch of salt and the basil leaves in a pestle and mortar, or pulse in a food processor. Add a bit more garlic if you like, but I usually stick to ¼ of a clove. Add the pinenuts to the mixture and pound again. Turn out into a bowl and add half the Parmesan. Stir gently and add olive oil – you need just enough to bind the sauce to get it to an oozy consistency.

Season to taste, then add the rest of the cheese. Pour in some more oil and taste again. Keep adding a bit more cheese or oil until you are happy with the taste and consistency. It may need a squeeze of lemon juice at the end, but it's not essential.

SERVES 4

¼ of a clove of garlic, chopped

3 good handfuls of fresh basil, leaves picked and chopped

1 handful of pinenuts, very lightly toasted

1 good handful of grated Parmesan cheese

extra virgin olive oil

sea salt and freshly ground black pepper

optional: small squeeze of lemon juice

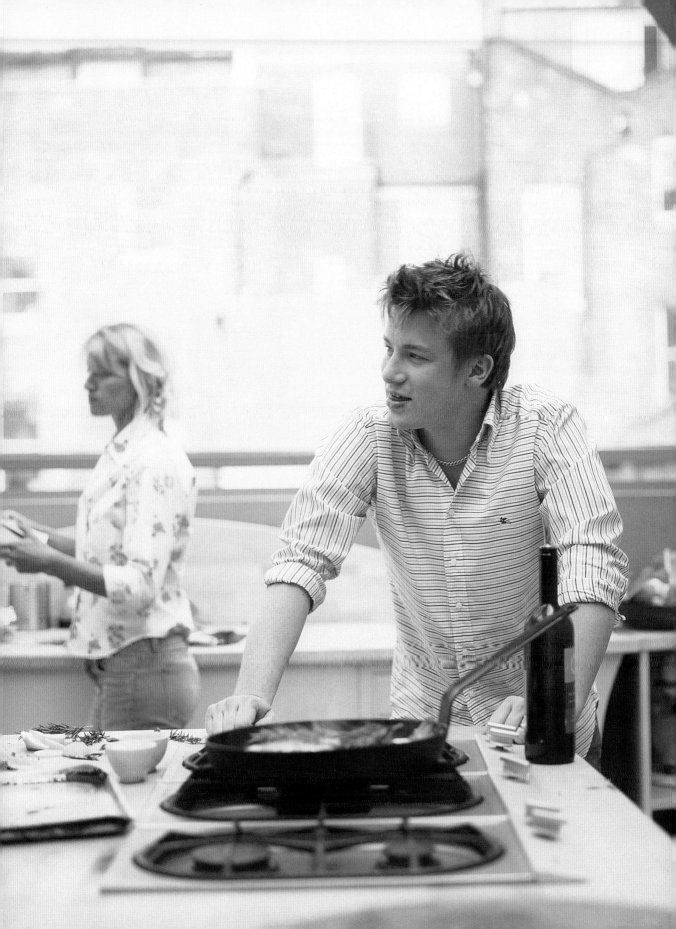

taglierini with a simple sweet tomato sauce and shrimps

Taglierini is a similar shape to fettuccine or egg noodles and lends itself well to creamy, buttery or light tomato-based sauces and especially little seafood numbers like this one. Feel free to use tagliatelle as well.

Blanch and skin the tomatoes (see pages 110–11), then halve them and chop into small pieces.

Put a pan of salted water on to heat for the pasta. Put the butter and a couple of lugs of olive oil in a second pan, and fry the prawns, garlic, lemon zest and tomatoes for a couple of minutes. Add the booze and allow to flame if you like. (The flame should go out after about 30 seconds, so don't worry!) Add the cream, allow to simmer gently for a couple more minutes and then remove the pan from the heat. Season the sauce carefully with salt, pepper and the lemon juice.

Put the pasta into the boiling water – fresh will need only 3 minutes and dried will need to be cooked according to the packet instructions. If your sauce has cooled down then reheat it now. When the pasta is cooked, drain it in a colander and then toss with the parsley in the pan in which it was cooked. Check the seasoning, then divide on to your serving plates with the sauce on top. Serve straight away, telling your guests to stir the pasta up in their bowls every so often to keep the pasta moist.

Try this: Crumble over a little ricotta or feta cheese – just a little bit – both of these cheeses have a nice texture, go really well with prawns and make it look great.

And this: A handful of spinach added at the end gives a nice vibe – the heat will wilt it into the sauce.

Or this: You can use tinned tomatoes for this dish but you won't get the freshness or lightness that you get from fresh tomatoes.

SERVES 4

8 plum tomatoes

sea salt and freshly ground black pepper

2 good knobs of butter

extra virgin olive oil

300g/10¹/₂oz small peeled prawns or shrimps

1 clove of garlic, peeled and finely chopped

zest and juice of 1 lemon

2 shots of Vecchia Romana or Cognac

150ml/5¹/₂fl oz double cream

400g/14oz fresh or dried taglierini (for fresh, see page 101)

1 large handful of fresh parsley, roughly chopped

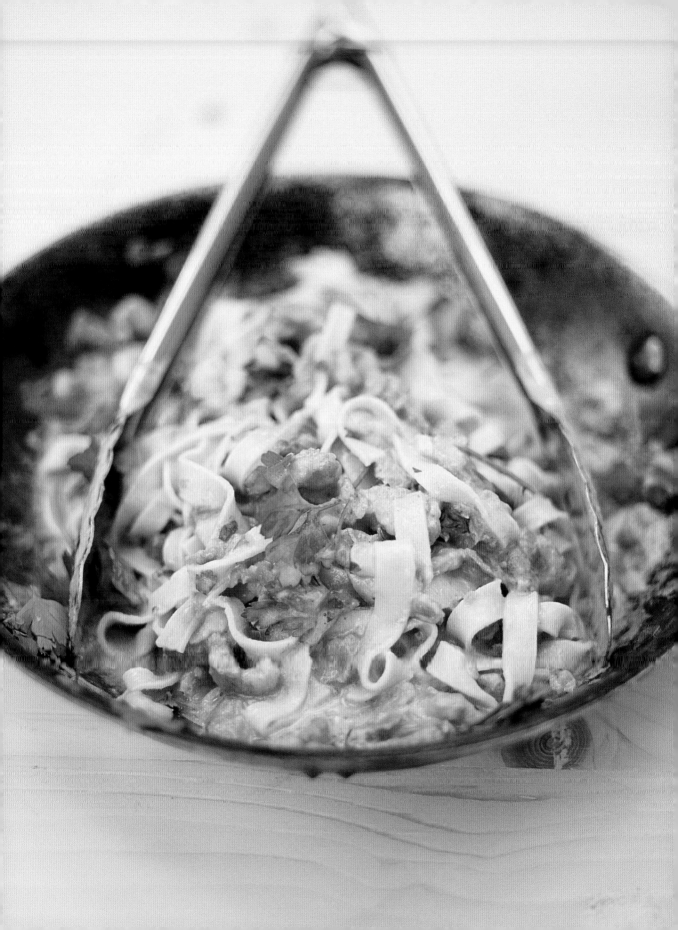

BLANCHING TOMATOES

This is one of the first things you learn at college, when you make tomato concassé, which is basically peeled, deseeded and finely chopped tomatoes. However, it's also handy for peeling cherry or plum tomatoes before roasting them as their skins aren't digestible. Also good for removing the skins of peaches and plums, etc.

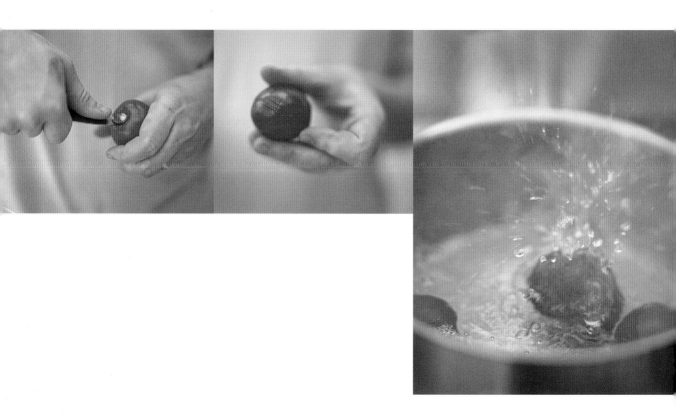

1. Using a small knife, remove the core from the tomato.

2. Lightly score the other end with a criss cross.

3. Carefully plunge the tomatoes into boiling water and boil for around 30 seconds until the skins begin to peel away.

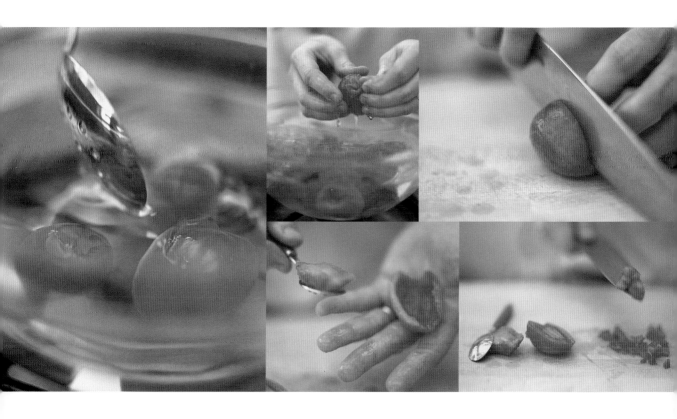

4. Remove the tomatoes with a slotted spoon and cool in cold water

5. Remove the skins.

7. Using a spoon, scoop out the seeds.

6. Cut the tomatoes in half.

8. Then you can slice or chop the tomatoes as you like.

'sourcing olive oil in Italy, November 2001. we had
lunch with the adorable Cassini family.'

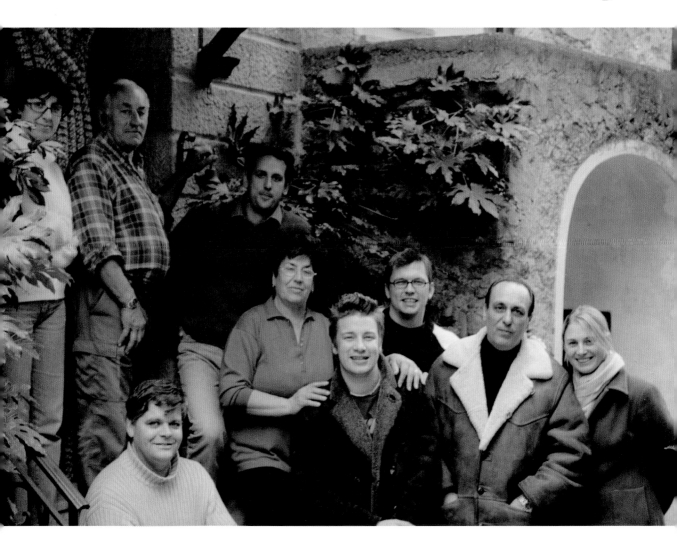

From left to right: Elisa Cassini, Rinaldo Cassini, David Gleave the wine don, Vittorio Cassini,
Elina Cassini, me, my best mate Jimmy Doherty, Gennaro Contaldo the Italian stallion, and my
editor the lovely Lindsey Jordan.

lasagnetti with chickpeas, parma ham, sage, cream and butter

I had a soup in Italy made by the Cassini family's lovely mother, Elina, whose son Enzo is the manager of Zafferano restaurant in London. Her other son, Vittorio, makes fantastic extra virgin olive oil under the Zafferano brand, which can be bought in Sainsbury's. Mrs Cassini made this amazing soup using massive dried chickpeas, and prosciutto hock with broth. Since the day I ate it, I've wanted to adapt it into a pasta recipe and so here it is. Lasagnetti is basically a smaller version of lasagne. If you're not going to make fresh lasagnetti, you can buy fresh lasagne sheets prepacked and cut them in half lengthways, or use some tagliatelle. If you've got time then dried chickpeas soaked overnight will give the best results but you can use tinned ones.

Soak your chickpeas overnight in water. Drain, then bring to the boil in fresh water and simmer for about 40 minutes until tender. Add the tomato and potato to the water as this will flavour and soften the chickpea skins. Once tender, put to one side. Put a couple of lugs of extra virgin olive oil in a casserole-type pan and fry the Parma ham and the bacon until lightly golden on both sides. Add the sage leaves and stir around until lightly crisp as well. Add your butter, leeks and garlic and slowly fry until the leeks are nicely softened. Drain the chickpeas, discarding the tomato and potato and reserving the cooking liquid, and add to the pan. At this point mush up about a quarter of them to give a pasty, smooth consistency to the sauce. Give them a good stir and pour over the chicken stock, or you could use the cooking liquor from the chickpeas. Add the cream, bring to the boil, then simmer slowly for 15 minutes to let all the flavours mix. Carefully correct the seasoning.

Cook your lasagnetti in some boiling, salted water. Drain, saving some of the cooking water, and throw the pasta into the chickpea pan – this can now be taken off the heat. Add most of the Parmesan and carefully stir the whole lot together. Add some of the reserved cooking liquor to loosen the pasta. Divide between your plates and serve immediately with the rest of the Parmesan sprinkled over the top and a good drizzle of peppery extra virgin olive oil.

Try this: If you have any dried porcini mushrooms, soak them in boiling water for a few minutes then drain and add with the leeks and garlic to give a lovely intense flavour.

SERVES 4

150g/5½oz dried chickpeas

1 tomato

1 small potato, peeled

extra virgin olive oil

8 slices of Parma ham

4 rashers of smoked streaky bacon or pancetta, sliced

1 handful of fresh sage, leaves picked

100g/3½oz butter

2 leeks, trimmed, washed and finely sliced

1 clove of garlic, finely chopped

285ml/½ pint chicken stock

100ml/3½fl oz double cream

sea salt and freshly ground black pepper

400g/14oz lasagnetti (see page 101) or dried lasagne

1 good handful of grated Parmesan cheese

SLICING HERBS AND LEAVES

Normally I rip up herbs as this tends to bruise more of the flavour out, but sometimes there is call for delicate, finely sliced herbs or salad leaves like spinach – the French call this 'chiffonade'.

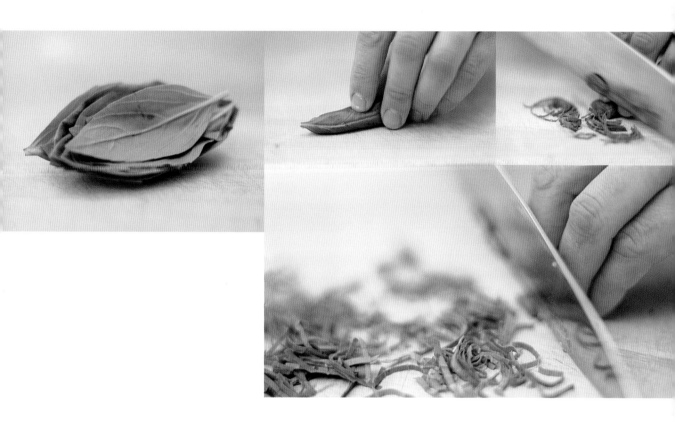

1. First pile your leaves on top of each other.

2. Roll them up like a cigar and hold them together.

3. Finely slice, making sure you tuck in your fingers.

4. Never do this in advance to any herb – always make sure it's done at the last minute or the herbs will wilt and turn black.

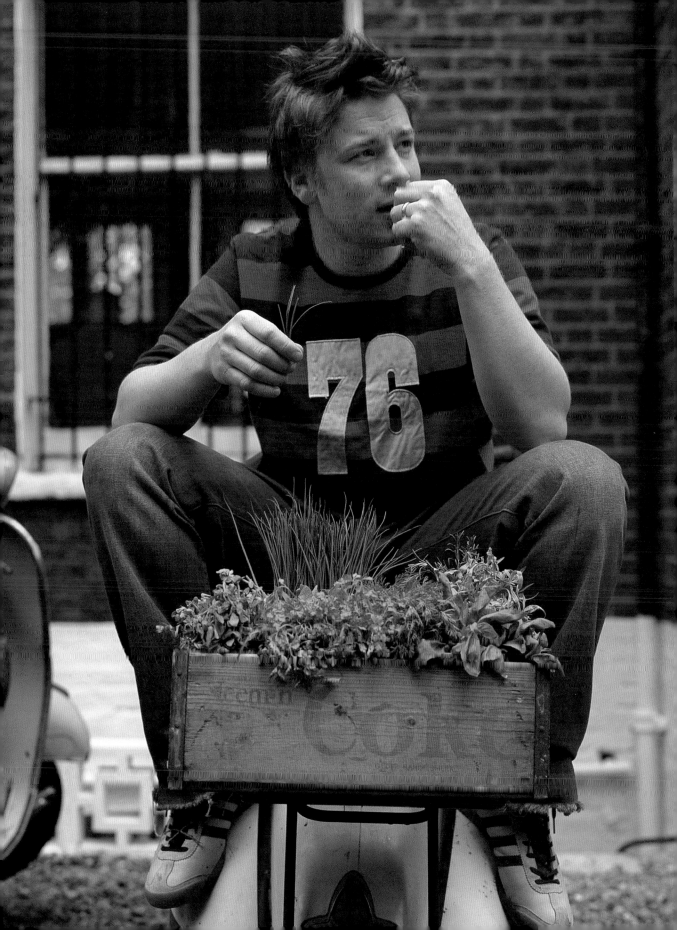

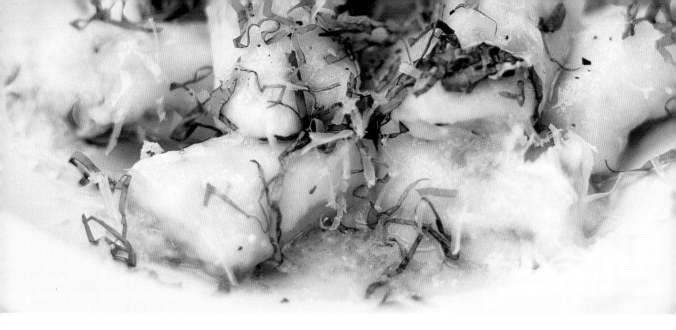

the easiest, lightest and most flexible gnocchi

I've made gnocchi with potatoes and with semolina – in fact, I've made just about every type of gnocchi possible! However, it's the lightness that you're after and this recipe is so easy.

Stir together the ricotta, Parmesan, basil and lemon zest and season to taste with salt, pepper and nutmeg. Empty most of the semolina into a little tray so it's about 1cm/½ inch deep. Take a dessertspoon of the ricotta mixture. To smarten up its shape you want to scrape it from one spoon to another. Do this a few times. It's called 'quenelling' in French and is a classic thing to do in cooking. (They don't have to be perfectly shaped, so don't worry too much about this!) When your gnocchi is shaped, place on to the semolina base in the tray. When they're all done, sprinkle the rest of the semolina on top and give the tray a gentle shake to ensure the gnocchi is covered. Leave for 2 hours before turning them over on to their other side. Leave them in the tray for at least 2 hours, but preferably overnight, in the fridge to set, making sure they don't touch. The semolina will stick to the ricotta forming a coating to protect it from the boiling water that you're going to put it in. To cook the gnocchi, add to a large pan of boiling salted water for 2 minutes or until they float to the surface.

To serve, you can simply toss the gnocchi in a little butter and then sprinkle with a little extra Parmesan and basil.

SERVES 4

500g/1lb 2oz ricotta cheese, preferably buffalo

2 handfuls of grated Parmesan cheese

1 handful of fresh basil, thinly sliced (see page 114)

zest of 1 lemon

sea salt and freshly ground black pepper

½ a nutmeg, grated

1.5 kg/3½lb fine semolina flour

gnocchi with fresh tomato and morel sauce

Dried morels have a slightly smoky flavour which is a really nice contrast to the fresh ricotta. Feel free to use fewer morels mixed with other cheaper mushrooms if you like.

Make your gnocchi. When they have firmed up in the semolina, just cover the morels with boiling water and let them soak for 15 minutes to soften up, then drain them. Get a pan hot, add the olive oil, and fry the garlic. When it has softened, add your morels and tomatoes. Simmer slowly for 5 minutes. Try and break up some of the morels if you can. Cook your gnocchi in boiling salted water for 2 minutes while you season the sauce to taste with salt, pepper, basil and Parmesan. Stir in the butter. With a slotted spoon, remove the gnocchi from the water and stir into the tomato and morel sauce. Divide between your serving plates and sprinkle with a little extra Parmesan.

SERVES 4

1 x basic gnocchi recipe (see opposite page)

1 handful of dried morels

4 tablespoons olive oil

1 clove of garlic, peeled and finely chopped

8 plum tomatoes, peeled, deseeded and finely chopped (see pages 110–11)

sea salt and black pepper

1 handful of fresh basil, rolled and sliced (see page 114)

2 handfuls of grated Parmesan

1 knob of butter

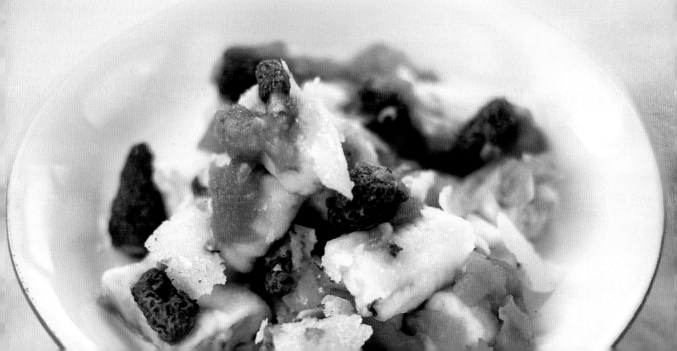

risotto

This is a great recipe for making risotto. You want it to be smooth, creamy and oozy, not thick and stodgy.

Stage 1: Heat the stock. In a separate pan heat the olive oil and butter, add the onions, garlic and celery, and fry very slowly for about 15 minutes without colouring. When the vegetables have softened, add the rice and turn up the heat.

Stage 2: The rice will now begin to lightly fry, so keep stirring it. After a minute it will look slightly translucent. Add the vermouth or wine and keep stirring – it will smell fantastic. Any harsh alcohol flavours will evaporate and leave the rice with a tasty essence.

Stage 3: Once the vermouth or wine has cooked into the rice, add your first ladle of hot stock and a good pinch of salt. Turn down the heat to a simmer so the rice doesn't cook too quickly on the outside. Keep adding ladlefuls of stock, stirring and almost massaging the creamy starch out of the rice, allowing each ladleful to be absorbed before adding the next. This will take around 15 minutes. Taste the rice – is it cooked? Carry on adding stock until the rice is soft but with a slight bite. Don't forget to check the seasoning carefully. If you run out of stock before the rice is cooked, add some boiling water.

Stage 4: Remove from the heat and add the butter and Parmesan. Stir well. Place a lid on the pan and allow to sit for 2 minutes. This is the most important part of making the perfect risotto, as this is when it becomes outrageously creamy and oozy like it should be. Eat it as soon as possible, while the risotto retains its beautiful texture.

SERVES 6

approx. 1.1 litres/2 pints stock (chicken, fish or vegetable as appropriate)

1 knob of butter

2 tablespoons olive oil

1 large onion, finely chopped

2 cloves of garlic, finely chopped

½ head of celery, finely chopped

400g/14oz risotto rice

2 wineglasses of dry white vermouth (dry Martini or Noilly Prat) or dry white wine

sea salt and freshly ground black pepper

70g/2½oz butter

115g/4oz freshly grated Parmesan cheese

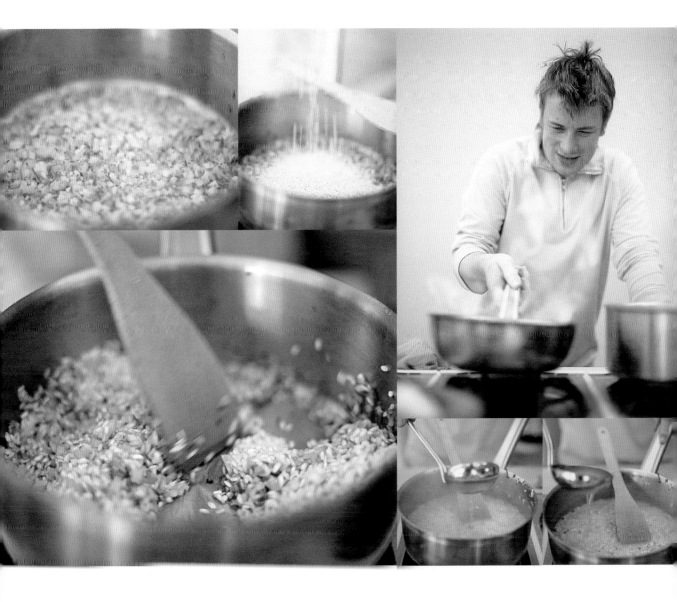

1. Slowly fry the vegetables.

2. Add the rice.

3. Keep stirring until the rice is translucent.

4. Add the white wine or vermouth and cook down. It might flame at this point, which is great!

5. Add the stock one ladle at a time.

6. Keep stirring until the rice is cooked.

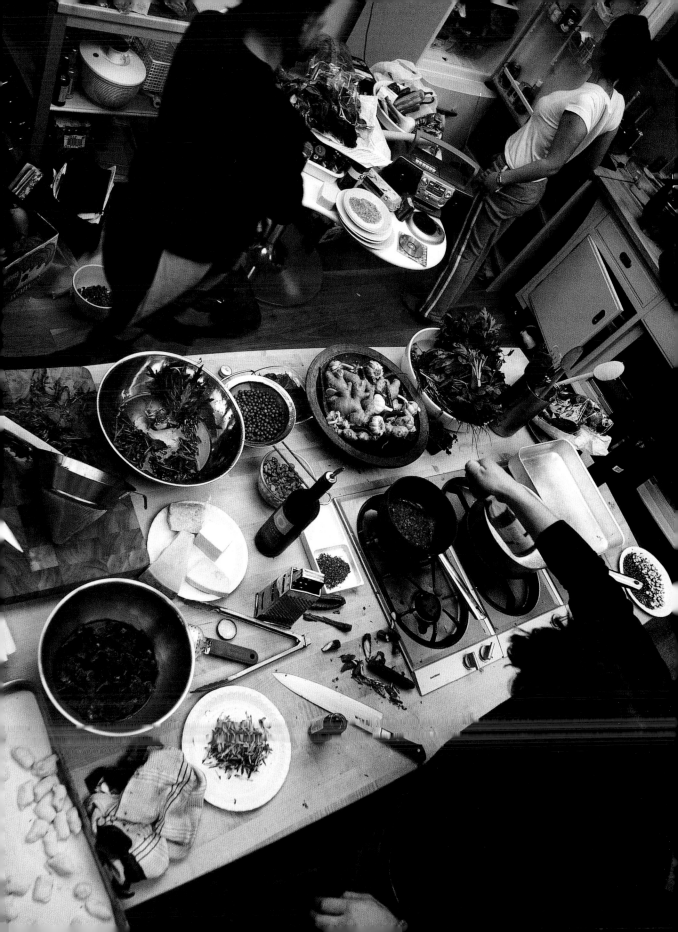

easy chicken stock

Stock is usually one of those things that even chefs don't have time for at home, but here is a really easy recipe for a good chicken stock. I find that I tend to make this after we've had our Sunday roast – I just throw the carcass in a pan with any root veg and herbs I happen to have. However, you'll probably get a cleaner-tasting stock if you use raw carcasses.

Place the chicken carcasses, garlic, vegetables, herbs and peppercorns in a large, deep-bottomed pan. Add the cold water and bring to the boil, skim, then turn the heat down to a simmer. Continue to simmer gently for 3–4 hours, skimming as necessary, then pass the stock through a fine sieve. Allow to cool for about half an hour, then refrigerate. Once the stock is cold it should look clear and slightly amber in colour. I usually divide it into small plastic containers at this point and freeze it. It will keep in the fridge for about 4 days and in the freezer for 2–3 months.

Try this: If you still think you can't be bothered to make stock, then use some good chicken bouillon, or simply buy it premade.

MAKES 4 LITRES/7 PINTS

2kg/4 ½lb raw chicken carcasses, legs or wings chopped

½ a head of garlic, unpeeled and bashed

5 sticks of celery, roughly chopped

2 medium leeks, roughly chopped

2 medium onions, roughly chopped

2 large carrots, roughly chopped

3 bay leaves

2 sprigs of fresh rosemary

5 sprigs of fresh parsley

5 sprigs of fresh thyme

5 whole black peppercorns

6 litres/10 ½ pints cold water

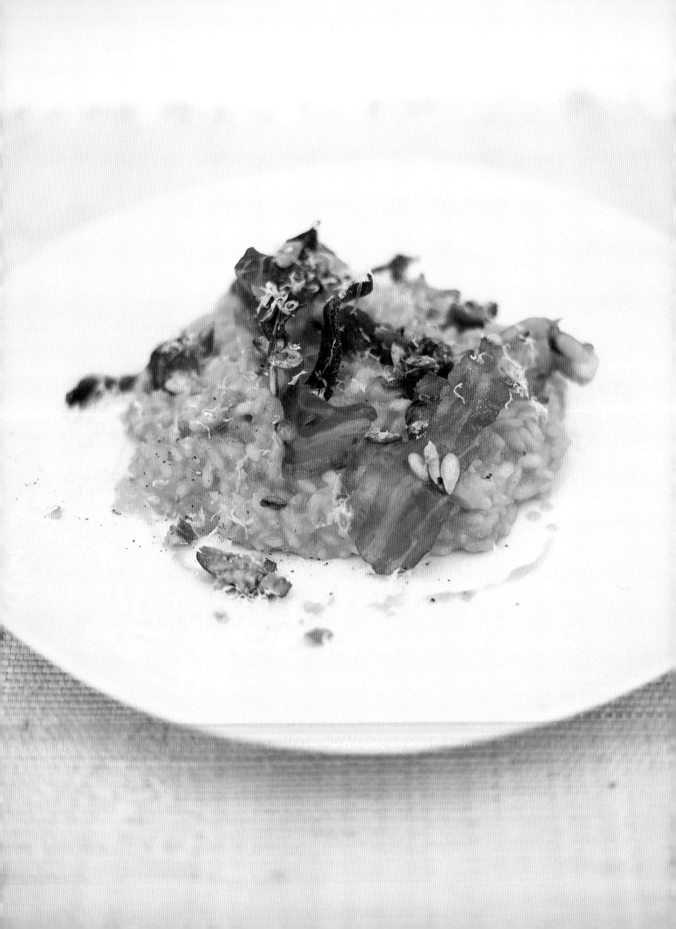

roast squash, sage, chestnut and pancetta risotto

If I could pick a load of ingredients that just shout out 'Bonfire Night! Christmas! Cosy!' it would have to be all the ones in this risotto. It's so damn good – cook it when all the ingredients are in season.

Preheat your oven to 190°C/375°F/gas 5. Carefully cut your butternut squash in half and scoop out the seeds. Put these to one side. Cut the squash lengthways into 0.5cm/¼ inch slices. Bash up your coriander and chillies with a pinch of salt and pepper in a pestle and mortar (or use a metal bowl and the end of a rolling pin). Dust this over your squash with a tablespoon of olive oil. Toss around until completely coated. Line up snugly in a roasting tray and bake for around 30 minutes until the flesh and skin are soft to the touch. Now get all your ingredients ready and start making your basic risotto.

Remove the squash from the oven and lay your pancetta over it. Mix the squash seeds, chestnuts and sage leaves with a little olive oil, salt and pepper. Sprinkle over the squash and pancetta and place back in the oven for about 5–10 minutes until the pancetta is crisp.

Once the squash has cooled down a little, shake off the pancetta and chestnuts and finely chop the squash – it will be quite mushy but that's fine. I go for half of it fine and half chunky. Add this to the risotto at the end of Stage 3. Carry on as normal through the basic recipe, season to taste and serve with the pancetta, chestnuts, sage leaves and squash seeds sprinkled over the top. Lovely served with a big dollop of mascarpone cheese on the side.

Try this: Place a grater and a block of Parmesan cheese in the middle of the table so that everyone can help themselves.

SERVES 6

1 x basic risotto recipe (see page 118)

1 butternut squash

1 level tablespoon coriander seeds

2 small dried chillies

sea salt and freshly ground black pepper

olive oil

12 slices of pancetta or dry-cured smoky bacon

100g/3½oz chestnuts (vac-packed are fine)

a bunch of fresh sage, leaves picked

optional: 6 heaped tablespoons mascarpone cheese

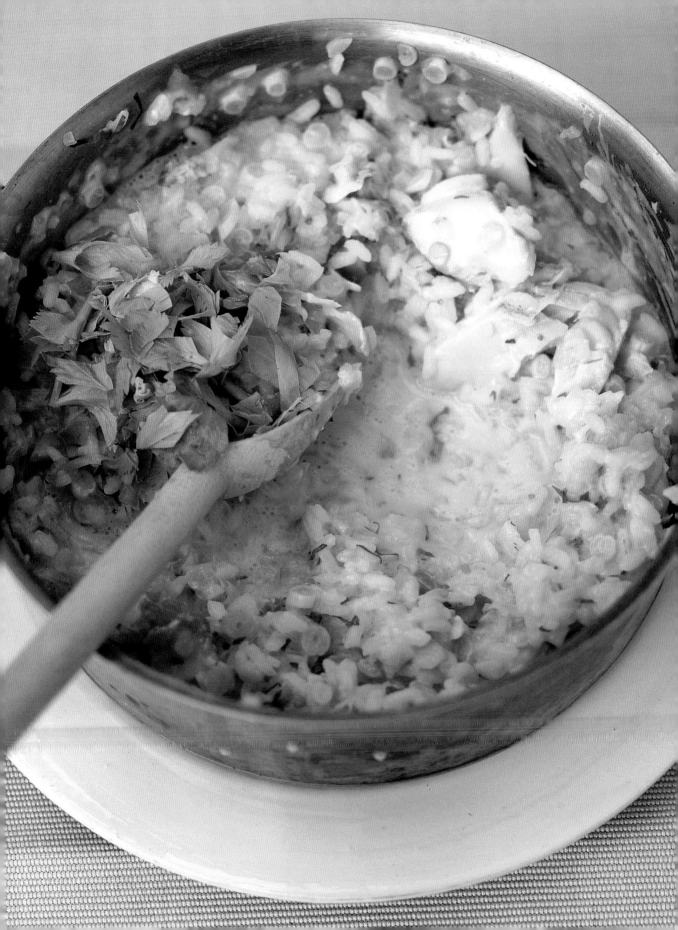

yellow bean, vodka and smoked haddock risotto

The thing about risottos is that you can never have enough combinations, and just when you think you've done them all you come up with a new one that hits the spot. The use of vodka instead of wine leaves you with a fragrant freshness when the risotto is cooked, which marries fantastically well with smoky flakes of haddock and the al dente crunch of fine yellow beans. As there is fish in this risotto you don't want to include any Parmesan, so bear this in mind. If you're a risotto fan you've got to give this a try.

Start your basic risotto, adding the vodka at Stage 2 instead of the wine. Then lightly poach your haddock in the milk and stock from the basic recipe with a couple of bay leaves, covered with a lid. Simmer for around 5 minutes and remove from the heat. At Stage 3 of the basic recipe, I like to add the poaching liquor to the rice and then I carry on as normal through the recipe. At the end of Stage 3 flake in your smoked haddock, add the beans and carry on as normal through to the end of the recipe. Don't serve with any Parmesan sprinkled over – serve sprinkled with the celery leaves. Add a dash of vodka and a squeeze of lemon to lift the flavours. Lovely.

SERVES 6

1 x basic risotto recipe (see page 118) minus the Parmesan

4 shots of vodka (in place of the wine in the basic recipe)

700g/1½lb smoked haddock, undyed

565ml/1 pint milk

2 bay leaves

255g/9oz yellow beans, stalks removed, finely sliced

1 handful of yellow celery leaves, from the heart

STEAMING AND COOKING IN THE BAG

STEAMING

Steaming's a cracker — it's great at transmitting subtle flavour even though it's through the slightly indirect method of hot steam. This can be done at varying pressures — for example, the Japanese will steam slowly in a bamboo basket, and my nan has a pressure cooker that heats, cooks and nukes anything at a very high temperature. This basically means that cooking times can be reduced by up to half while keeping the food moist and succulent.

COOKING IN THE BAG

This method was first recognized in France — known as cooking *en papillote*, or in greaseproof paper. Even though this still works well, these days tinfoil is much easier to use, more pliable and definitely a better conductor of heat. This is a fantastic way to cook, because you get a variation of cooking methods happening inside the bag, from boiling to steaming to even a bit of baking, and most importantly you don't make any mess because you chuck the bag away when you've finished.

steamed sea bass, green beans with a white wine, vanilla, cream and garlic sauce

Steaming is a great way to appreciate how delicate fish can be. You can try this recipe with all sorts of white fish, but for me sea bass is a bit more of an event and really gets me going. I suppose the real twist here is using the vanilla as a savoury flavouring, though in the history of cooking it's not a new thing. It's a very simple dish to make, and it sounds, looks and tastes like you've been grafting all afternoon.

Put half of the vanilla seeds into a bowl with the lemon zest and the olive oil. Mix up well and rub this marinade over your sea bass fillets and into the score marks. Bring a large pot of salted water to the boil and add the clove of garlic. Allow to boil for 3 minutes, then lay your 4 marinated fish fillets next to each other in a colander, bamboo steamer or normal steamer and throw your green beans into the water. Place your steamer on top, making sure the fish is not in direct contact with the water – it just wants to get the steam – and cover. When the water comes back to the boil, both the fish and the beans will need about 4–5 minutes to cook. If your fish fillets are thick they may need a bit longer, so put them on a bit before the beans. You can check to see if they're done by inserting a knife tip.

While everything's cooking, put a separate pan on a high heat and add the wine, the rest of the vanilla seeds and the vanilla pods. Boil until the liquid has reduced by half, then add the double cream. Remove the garlic from the beans, mash it up and stir it into the cream sauce. Carry on reducing the sauce until it coats the back of a spoon nicely. Season well to taste, then serve the fish and beans with the sauce, removing the vanilla pods. Sprinkle with the celery leaves.

Try this: If you remove the vanilla pods and whizz up the sauce in a liquidizer, you get a thick cappuccino effect to the sauce which visually and texturally is quite nice.

Or this: Sometimes I make this a bit more substantial by scrubbing some new potatoes, boiling them in the steaming water until cooked and then carrying on with the recipe as above, using the same water for the beans.

SERVES 4

seeds from 2 vanilla pods
(see page 304)

zest of 1 lemon

2 tablespoons extra virgin
olive oil

4 x 225g/8oz sea bass
fillets, scored

sea salt and freshly ground
black pepper

1 clove of garlic, peeled

4 handfuls of fine green beans,
tops removed

1 wineglass of white wine

150ml/5½fl oz double cream

yellow leaves from 1 celery
heart (or use chervil)

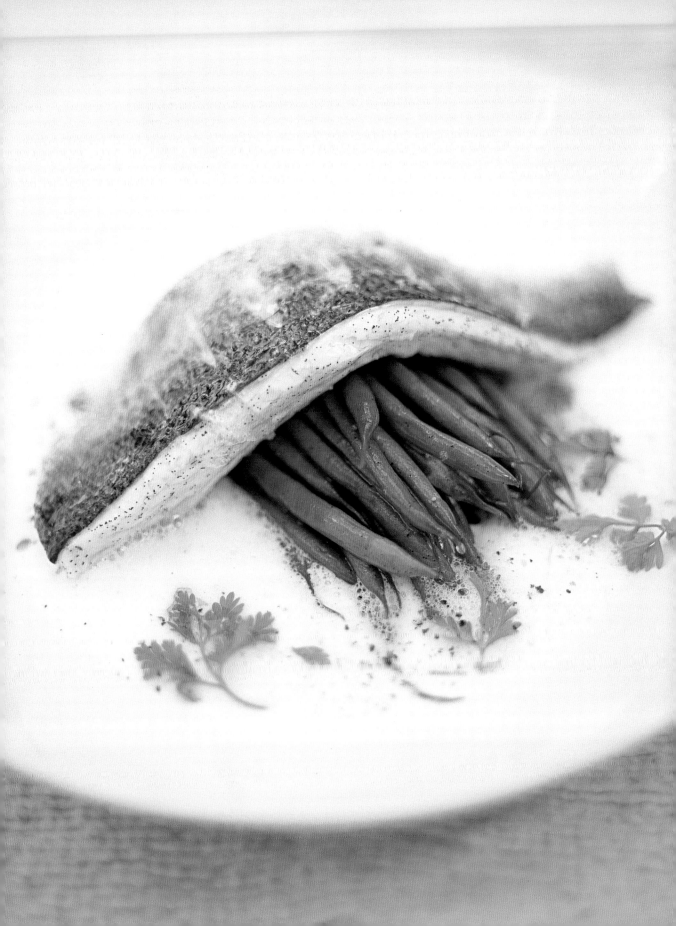

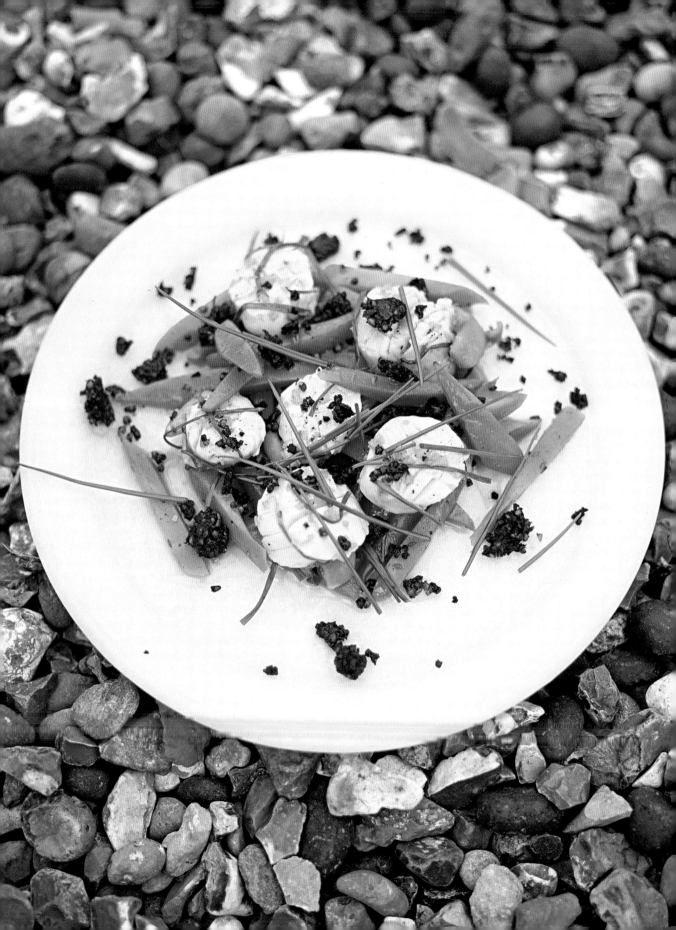

steamed scallops with spiced carrots, crumbled crispy black pudding and coriander

You may think this sounds like an odd combination of flavours, but we put a similar dish on the menu at Monte's last year and it was great. I wanted to steam some scallops as they were so big and sweet. My mate Ben had just come back from Morocco and he suggested these spicy carrots. We were both trying to think of something to pull the dish together – something that would give it a bit of texture and make it nice and moreish – and we came up with black pudding. If you can't get hold of good scallops, you can do exactly the same with medallions of monkfish. And black pudding is easy to find these days.

Preheat the oven to 220°C/425°F/gas 7. In a casserole-type pan, slowly fry all the spices with the garlic in about 6 tablespoons of olive oil for about 30 seconds, then add the carrots. Stir well and add a pinch of salt and sugar and a couple of large wineglasses of chicken stock or water. Put a lid on the pan then bring to the boil and simmer slowly for around 40 minutes or until the carrots are tender. (Make sure the pan doesn't boil dry.)

Meanwhile, split the black pudding lengthways and tear it open. Sounds a bit painful but this will help to make it go really crispy. After the carrots have been cooking for about 20 minutes, put the black pudding in the oven in a small dish or on a tray for about 15–20 minutes until crispy. Put about 2.5cm/1 inch of water in a pan, then, using a colander, bamboo steamer or other type of steamer, place over the heat and get it to a slow steam.

Score your scallops on one side in criss cross fashion, season with a little salt and pepper and sprinkle with the orange zest. Steam for about 5–6 minutes, depending on the size of the scallops. You don't want to overcook them or they'll go rubbery.

Remove the cinnamon stick, then divide the carrots between the plates, place the scallops on top, then crumble over a little black pudding. Scatter over the chives (or use basil or coriander). Make a dressing with the orange and lemon juice and the same amount of olive oil. Drizzle this over and serve straight away.

SERVES 4

½ a cinnamon stick

1–2 dried red chillies, crumbled

½ teaspoon ground cumin

1 teaspoon five-spice

½ a nutmeg, grated

2 cloves of garlic, peeled and finely sliced

extra virgin olive oil

1.2kg/2½lb carrots, peeled and roughly sliced into small batons (see page 266)

sea salt and freshly ground black pepper

a pinch of sugar

2 wineglasses of chicken stock or water

200g/7oz black pudding

12–16 large scallops, trimmed and ready to cook

zest and juice of 1 orange

1 bunch of fresh chives, basil or coriander

juice of ½ a lemon

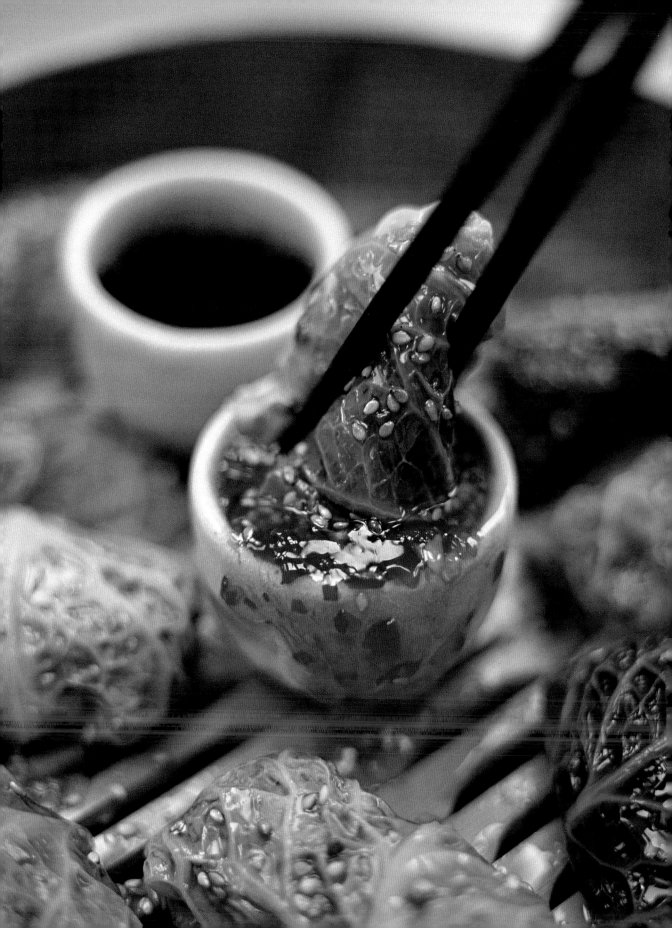

chinese chicken parcels

When Jools was pregnant this was one of her favourite things to eat, along with bananas dipped in Marmite!

Remove and discard the core and outer leaves from the cabbage, undo the remaining cabbage leaves and place them in a pan of salted boiling water for 2 minutes to soften. Cool them in a bowl of cold water, drain and put to one side.

In a food processor, whizz up your garlic, ginger, spring onions, coriander, chilli and fish sauce with a good pinch of salt. Then add the chicken, water chestnuts, lime zest and juice and sesame oil and pulse until you have a minced meat consistency.

Place a heaped dessertspoonful of the flavoured mince on to one end of each cabbage leaf. Fold it up and tuck in the sides, then roll up. Rub a bamboo steamer, colander or normal steamer with a little olive oil and place in the cabbage parcels. They may try to unfold themselves, but once you start putting them next to each other they will hold in place. When they're all in, sit the steamer over a pan of boiling water, making sure the water doesn't touch the parcels and that it's just the steam that's cooking them. Put a lid on top and steam for about 6 minutes until cooked. If you're worried about the cooking time, take one of the parcels out and cut it in half to make sure that the heat has penetrated and that they're cooked.

When they're done, I like to serve them in the bamboo steamer. I move a couple of the parcels out of the way and put in a dish of sweet chilli jam, jelly or sauce – you can get these in all supermarkets and delis. The parcels are also good dipped in soy sauce and sprinkled with the sesame seeds.

SERVES 4

1 Savoy or Chinese cabbage

sea salt

2 cloves of garlic, peeled

1 thumb-sized piece of fresh ginger, peeled

1 bunch of spring onions, trimmed

1 handful of fresh coriander

1–2 fresh red chillies

1 tablespoon fish sauce

4 trimmed boneless chicken thighs, skin removed, roughly chopped

1 handful of water chestnuts

zest and juice of 2 limes

1 teaspoon sesame oil

extra virgin olive oil

sweet chilli jam, jelly or sauce

soy sauce

1 tablespoon toasted sesame seeds

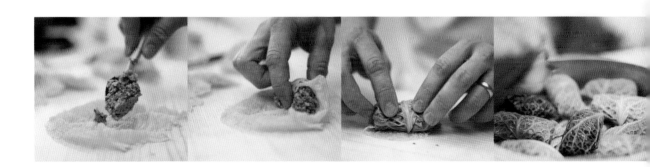

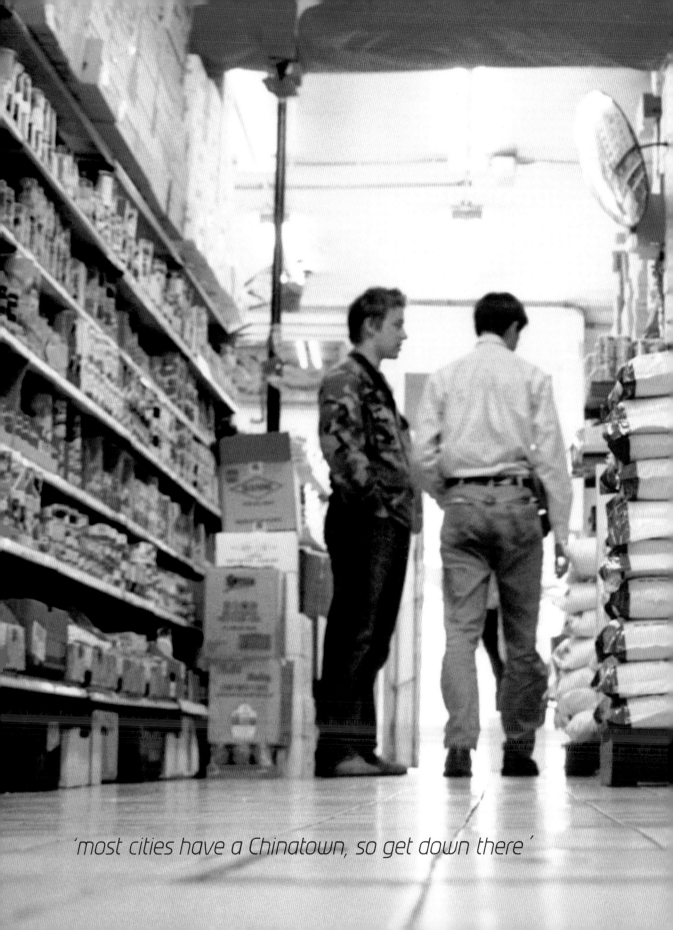

'most cities have a Chinatown, so get down there'

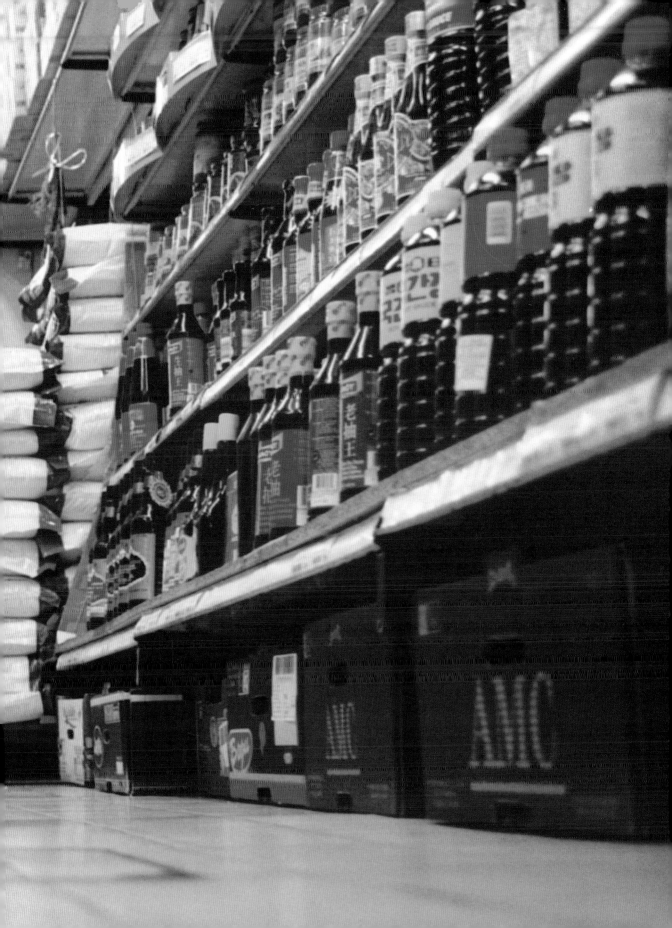

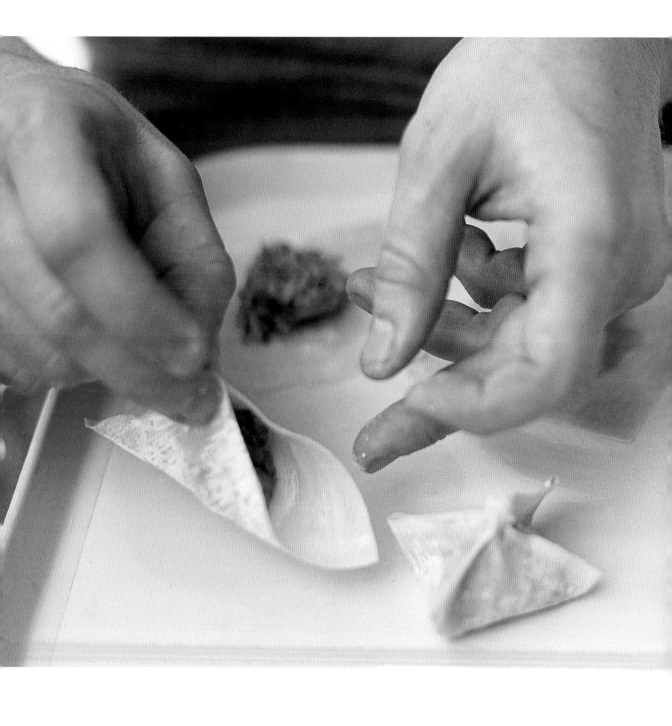

steamed prawn wontons with red chilli and spring onion

These are very simple and tasty little darlings to make. They're really open to variation using different herbs and flavourings. You might find them a little fiddly to make, but once you get the hang of it nothing will stop you!

Finely chop the ginger, garlic, coriander, chillies and spring onions and place with the prawns in a food processor. Pulse until everything is mixed together, then add the sesame oil and soy sauce. Pulse again, then tip into a mixing bowl and season with salt and pepper.

Lay the wonton wrappers out on a dry surface and put a small teaspoon of filling in the middle of each one. Brush the exposed wonton pastry with a little water and bring the edges up over the filling, squeezing them at the top so they stick together and encase the filling completely. The truth is, there are lots of different ways to shape the parcels – as long as the filling is completely sealed you can make any shape you fancy.

Put the wontons in a bamboo steamer, colander or normal steamer in one layer and steam gently over a pan of boiling water for about 7 minutes, or until the prawn filling is cooked and slightly pink (open one up to check if you want to). These are lovely served with little bowls of soy sauce, sweet chilli sauce and sesame oil for dipping.

MAKES AROUND
16 WONTONS

2cm/³/₄ inch piece of fresh ginger, peeled

2 cloves of garlic, peeled

1 small handful of fresh coriander

2 fresh red chillies, deseeded

5 spring onions

300g/11oz raw tiger prawns, shelled

1 tablespoon sesame oil

2 tablespoons soy sauce

sea salt and freshly ground black pepper

1 packet of pre-rolled wonton wrappers

STEAMING AND COOK ↓G IN THE BAG

137

steamed pork buns chinese style

I really love these steamed buns. Try getting the lime leaves to steam them on – you can usually buy them either fresh or frozen from good supermarkets and Asian stores.

Heat a large frying pan and add a splash of olive oil. Season the chops with salt, pepper and the five-spice and fry on both sides until browned and cooked through. Add the garlic, ginger and chillies and continue to fry for a minute. Add the orange juice, reduce by half, then pour the contents of the pan into a bowl and leave to cool.

Empty the yeast into a second bowl and add half the tepid water. In another bowl, sieve the flours and the salt together and rub in the butter. When the yeast has bubbled up, pour in the rest of the water and then add that to the flour and butter. Mix to form a soft dough. Leave to prove in a warm place, covered with clingfilm, until it has doubled in size, then break it into pieces about the size of a walnut and shape into little round balls.

Put one of the chops into a food processor, together with all the juice remaining in the mixing bowl, and pulse until fine. Cut up the other chop coarsely by hand to give you good texture, and add all the pork back to the bowl with the hoi-sin, the sesame oil and the chilli sauce. Mix well.

What I like to do for extra fragrance is line the bottom of a bamboo steamer, colander or your normal steamer with lime leaves. Take one of the risen dough balls and flatten it out on the palm of your hand until it measures about 6cm/2½ inches in diameter. Press it down in the middle so it's slightly cup-shaped, and put a teaspoon of the pork mix in the middle. Gently wrap the sides of the dough up around the filling, pinch and seal it up, and place sealed-side down on the lime leaves in the steamer. Repeat with the other dough balls. Leave a gap of about 2cm/¾ inch between the buns to give them room to puff up (you could steam them in 2 or 3 layers at once, or in batches, depending on your steamer). Allow the buns to sit and prove for 5 minutes before you steam them. Put the lid on and steam over a pan of boiling water for about 10 minutes, until the buns are cooked and the filling is hot (cut one open to check). Serve with little bowls of soy sauce and sweet chilli sauce to dip the buns in.

MAKES 8 BUNS

for the filling

olive oil

2 x 200g/7oz pork chops, deboned

sea salt and freshly ground black pepper

1 tablespoon five-spice

3 cloves of garlic, peeled and sliced

2.5cm/1 inch piece of fresh ginger, peeled and sliced

2 dried chillies, crumbled

1 wineglass of fresh orange juice

6 tablespoons hoi-sin sauce

1 tablespoon sesame oil

1 tablespoon sweet chilli sauce

optional: 1 handful of fresh lime leaves

for the buns

1 x 7g sachet of dried yeast

200ml/7fl oz tepid water

250g/9oz plain flour

100g/3½oz cornflour

1 teaspoon salt

50g/1¾oz butter

to serve

soy sauce

sweet chilli sauce

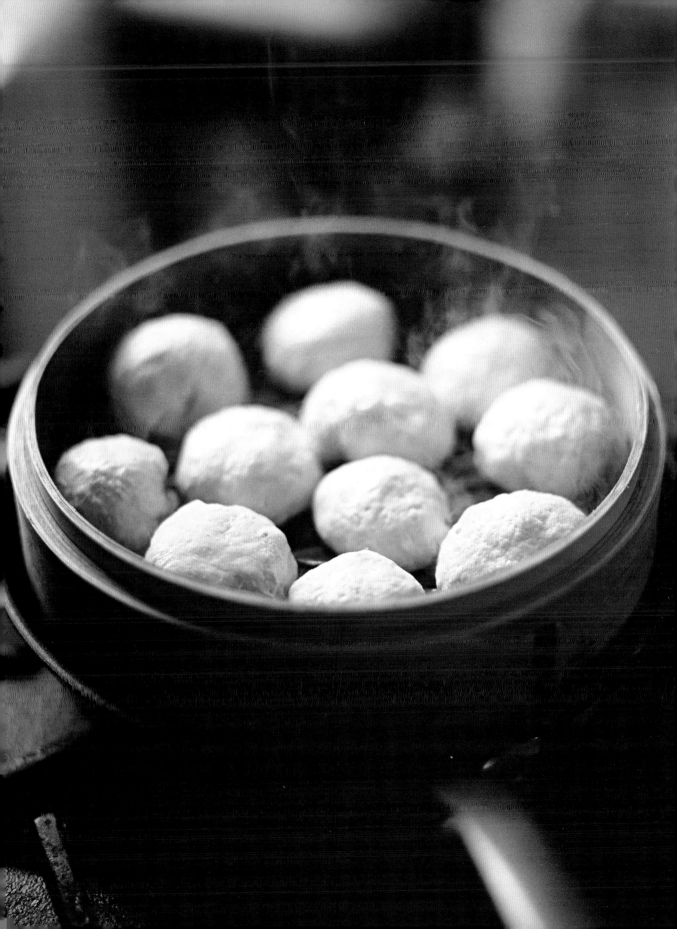

haddock baked in the bag with mussels, saffron, white wine and butter

This is a really good way to bake haddock or any white fish – cod, hake, even monkfish. Get your fishmonger to cut you a nice fillet. This method doesn't make the skin go crispy, but it's still quite good to cook it with the skin on as it flavours and protects the fish from losing moisture. There's no real spice that can give such flavour, colour and smell to a dish as quickly as saffron. It's an amazing ingredient to work with – not cheap, but a little goes a long way. The mussels work so well cooked like this, but make sure that you completely de-beard them before you cook them.

Preheat the oven and a roasting tray to 250°C/475°F/gas 9. First of all, you need to make your 4 tinfoil or greaseproof paper bags. Do this by taking 4 x A5-sized pieces of foil or greaseproof paper, fold each one in half, then fold up the 2 ends tightly, giving you an 'envelope'.

Put the wine in a bowl, then add your saffron and let it soak for 5 minutes. This will start to bring out the flavour and colour. Divide the parsley between the bags and place the fish on top. Cut the butter into 4 pieces and place one on top of each fish. Divide the mussels between the bags then carefully pour some of the infused white wine into each bag. Make sure you don't spill any and be careful not to let it ooze out of the bag. Sprinkle in the spring onions, then seal up. Remove the hot roasting tray from the oven and carefully lay the bags side by side on it – ensure the corners of the bags are bent upwards so that no liquid can escape. Place the roasting tray on the hob to get the bags going – they should start sizzling a little bit and steam will begin to build up inside. Place the tray in the oven for 12 minutes – the bags will puff up.

Take the tray to the table and let each guest open up their own bag. Serve simply with some boiled potatoes and nice greens. And put a little dish on the table for people to put their tinfoil and mussel shells in.

SERVES 4

2 wineglasses of white wine, preferably Chardonnay

1 large pinch of saffron

1 handful of fresh parsley, roughly chopped

4 x 225g/8oz haddock fillets, bones removed

100g/3½ oz butter

1 bunch of spring onions, trimmed and finely sliced

2 large handfuls of mussels, cleaned and beards removed

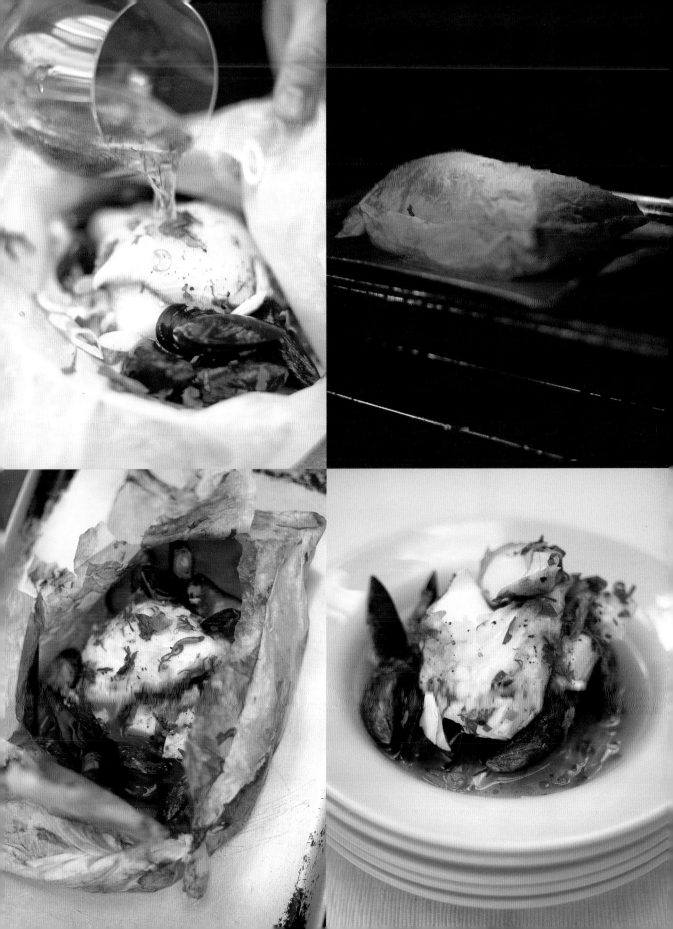

steamed squid

The great thing about this dish is that everything cooks at the same time. Once it's all in the steamer it only takes about 7 or 8 minutes, so it's damn quick too! Dried salted black beans are fantastically tasty and you should be able to get hold of them at Asian food shops, or use a jar of black beans instead.

Finely chop the spring onions, chilli, lemon, coriander and mint, mix together and season with a little salt and pepper. Using a teaspoon, stuff the mixture loosely into the squid – they're now ready to cook.

Put some water into a pan and bring to the boil to get ready to steam – you can use one of the 25cm/10 inch bamboo steamers which are really cheap to buy, or a covered colander over some boiling water. Line the bottom of the steamer evenly with the pak choi leaves. Sprinkle the sugar-snap peas over the top. Gather the yellow beans together in a big bunch, cut the ends off them and then slice them up finely. Scatter these over the peas. Sprinkle the black beans over, followed by the ginger. Place the squid on top, put the lid on and steam for 7–8 minutes.

Meanwhile mash the 2 tablespoons of black beans in a pestle and mortar then add all the other dressing ingredients and stir well. Place your steamer on a plate, then pour the dressing over your squid and eat it straight out of the steamer.

Try this: Feel free to flavour and scent the steaming water with things like star anise and other spices or herbs. This makes a really subtle difference.

Or this: Mix a little wok-fried minced chicken in with the vegetables before stuffing the squid and steam for a little longer. This makes it a little more substantial – check that the filling is cooked before tucking in.

SERVES 2

3 spring onions

1 fresh red chilli

¼ of a lemon

1 handful of fresh coriander

1 small handful of fresh mint

sea salt and freshly ground black pepper

4 medium squid with their tentacles, cleaned

2 heads of pak choi, washed and leaves separated

1 handful of sugar-snap peas

1 handful of yellow or green beans

1 handful of dried salted black beans, washed

1 thumb-sized piece of fresh ginger, grated

for the dressing

2 tablespoons dried salted black beans, washed

2 teaspoons sugar

2 tablespoons rice wine vinegar

2 tablespoons sweet chilli sauce

2 teaspoons sesame oil

2 tablespoons vegetable oil

a pinch of black pepper

a little fresh coriander, chopped

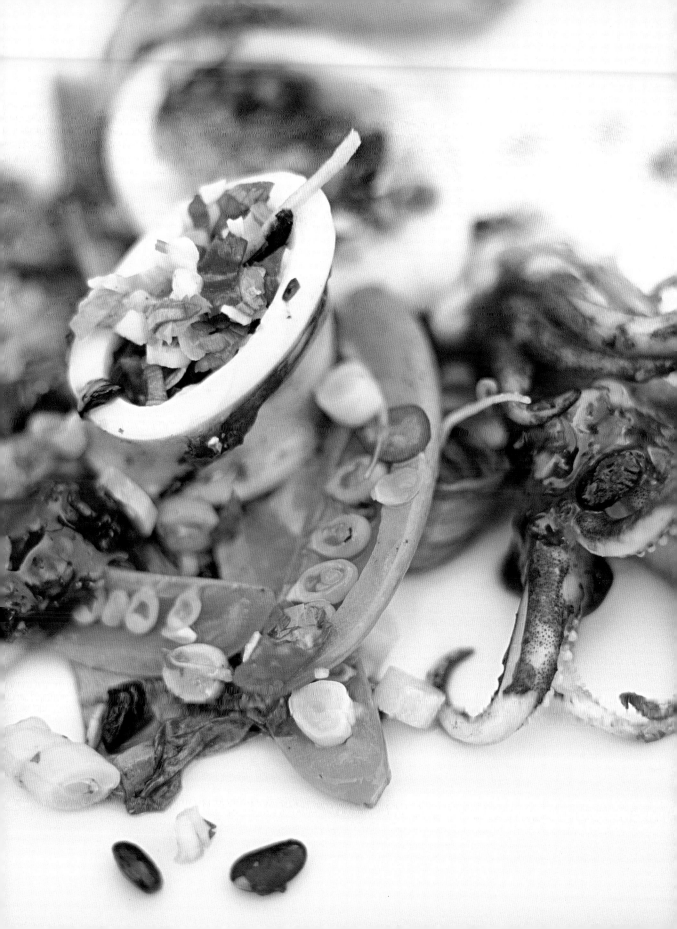

CHOPPING AND SLICING

The most important thing about using a knife is not to take off all your fingers! So here are a few key rules to get you used to your chopper, which can only be a good thing as it makes life easier in the kitchen. Do get yourself a few good knives and make sure you keep them sharp, or you will end up putting too much body weight on to them and you'll have an accident.

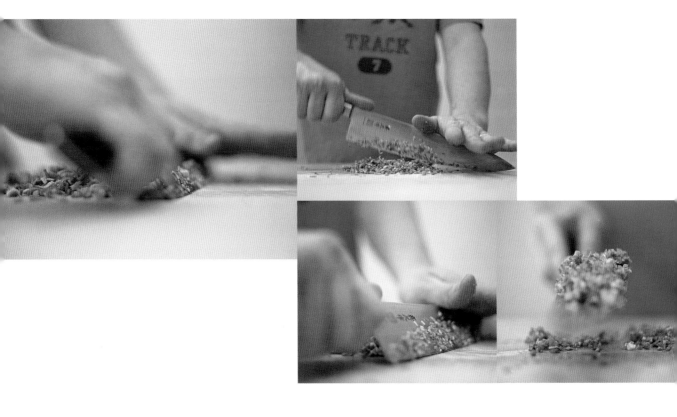

1. There are many techniques for how to chop things – whether you're preparing herbs, meat or vegetables – but for me the one I'm showing you here is the safest and quickest.

2. Firmly hold the handle. Lay your other hand completely flat along the pivot point (where the knife curves).

3. As you chop, stuff will tend to fly all over the board, so every now and again use the knife as a scraper to bring it all back into the centre.

4. You can use the knife to pick up whatever you're chopping, to save your hands getting dirty.

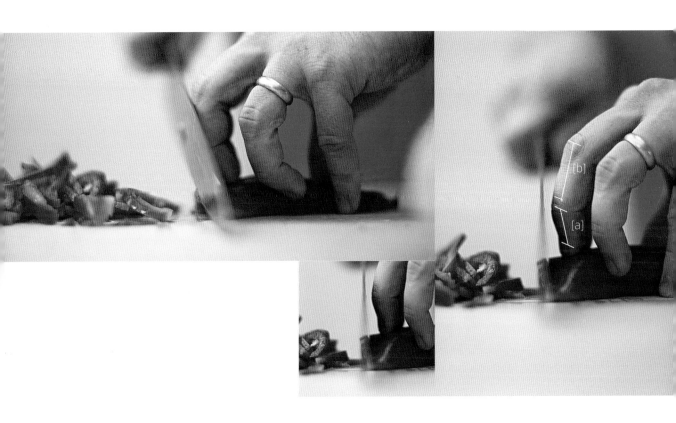

1. It's tempting to want to slice really quickly but the thing to do is start off slowly and get to know your knife. Practice makes perfect!

2. Get your vegetable on to a flat edge, or slice a piece off it to make a flat edge. This is important so it doesn't move about.

3. The theory is that if you tuck your fingertips in they won't get cut (see [a] above). Then use the upper part of your finger as a flat surface and guide your knife up and down (see [b] above). P.S. Don't forget to keep pulling your thumb back as you move along the vegetable.

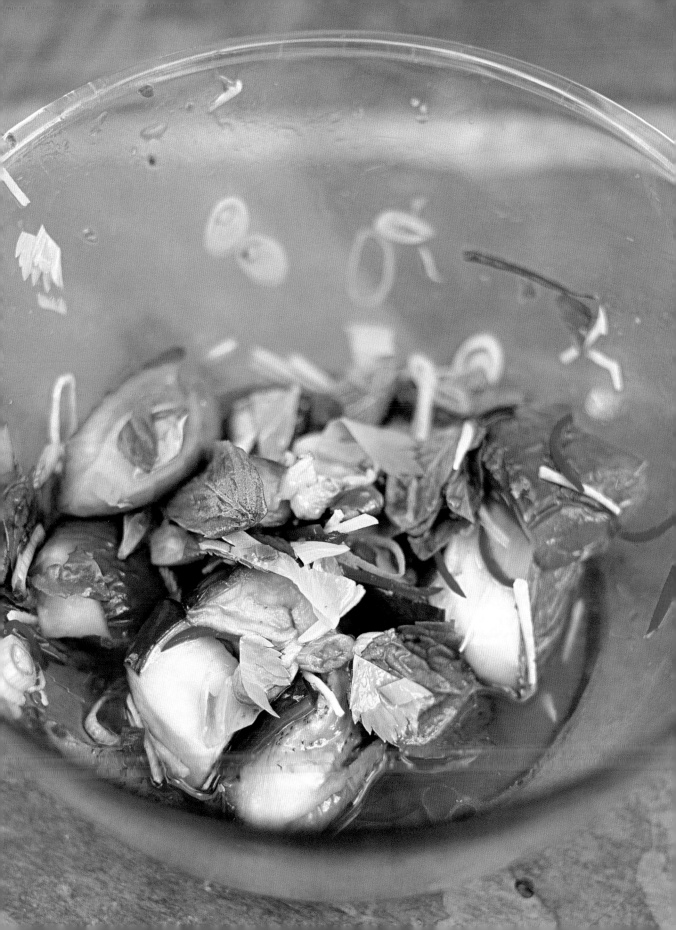

steamed aubergine

This is a great way to cook aubergines, and probably one that not a lot of people would think of doing. To me, steamed aubergine sounds horrible but, believe me, this recipe is fantastic. Aubergines are usually fried or roasted, which makes them soak up loads of oil, but steaming means they go really soft and tender so that they're lighter to eat – which means you can eat a lot more! All round the world there are so many different varieties of aubergines – long, round, purple, green – so keep your eyes peeled and try cooking them all.

Put some water in a pan and bring it to the boil. Slice the aubergines in half lengthways and place them in your steamer with the cut side facing up. Steam them for about 10 minutes – to check whether they're ready, simply squeeze the sides gently and if they're silky soft then they're done. Remove them from the steamer, place them in a colander and leave to cool.

Now make your dressing by mixing all the ingredients together. When the aubergines are warm this is the perfect time to flavour them. Cut them up into rough 2.5cm/1 inch dice, then dress them and toss. Serve immediately as a salad, tapas dish or as a vegetable next to any simple cooked fish. Just really tasty!

SERVES 4

2 medium purple aubergines

for the dressing

2 teaspoons sugar

4 tablespoons soy sauce

3 tablespoons sweet chilli dipping sauce

2 teaspoons sesame oil

zest and juice of 1 lemon

4 spring onions, sliced

2 fresh red chillies, finely chopped

1 large handful of fresh coriander, roughly sliced

1 large handful of fresh basil, roughly sliced

1 large handful of fresh mint, roughly sliced

1 large handful of yellow celery leaves

sea salt and freshly ground black pepper

skate baked in the bag with artichokes, purple potatoes, capers and crème fraîche

Potatoes and artichokes are always such a winning combination with fish, so I've put them in this dish, using fantastic purple potatoes which I've seen in the supermarket – if you can't find them, ask your local store to get some in. They are a great colour and, served in this way, might help in getting your kids to eat fish if they're not keen. They're not floury and they're not waxy, just somewhere in the middle, so they're great for baking and boiling. Buy the skate as fresh as you can – it doesn't matter if the pieces are large or small, as you'll want to cut them up anyway. Steaming skate makes it really soft, so it will just fall off the bone when done. This dish is just as good when eaten cold as a salad.

First make your 4 tinfoil or greaseproof paper bags. Do this by taking 4 x A5-sized pieces of foil or greaseproof paper, fold each one in half then fold up the 2 ends tightly, giving you an 'envelope'. Preheat the oven to 250°C/475°F/gas 9. Boil your spuds until cooked, then drain and put to one side to cool. Slice them up roughly. Peel back the artichoke leaves, remove the chokes with a teaspoon, then rub the artichokes with lemon juice to stop them discolouring and slice very finely. Put the artichokes and potatoes in a bowl with the melted butter, thyme, parsley and capers and season well. Toss together and divide between the bags. There'll be a little butter left over in the bottom of the bowl, so you can add a little olive oil to it and use this to rub on to the skate pieces.

Season the fish then place on top of the potatoes and artichokes. Add a glass of wine to each bag with a sprig of rosemary, tightly sealing the final side and pulling up the corners so that the liquid is contained. Bake on a roasting tray in the preheated oven for 15 minutes. By this time the bags will be beautifully puffed up. Serve at the table so that your guests can open their bags themselves, leaving a plate of really flavoursome vegetables, fish and juice. Serve with a dollop of crème fraîche seasoned with a little salt and pepper, and a nice green salad.

SERVES 4

1kg/2lb 3oz purple potatoes, scrubbed

5 medium to large globe artichokes

1 lemon

4 heaped tablespoons butter, melted

1 handful of fresh thyme, leaves picked

1 large handful of fresh parsley, chopped

4 heaped tablespoons capers in oil or brine, drained

sea salt and freshly ground black pepper

extra virgin olive oil

4 x 225g/8oz skate pieces, trimmed and halved

4 small wineglasses of white wine

4 small sprigs of fresh rosemary

4 tablespoons crème fraîche

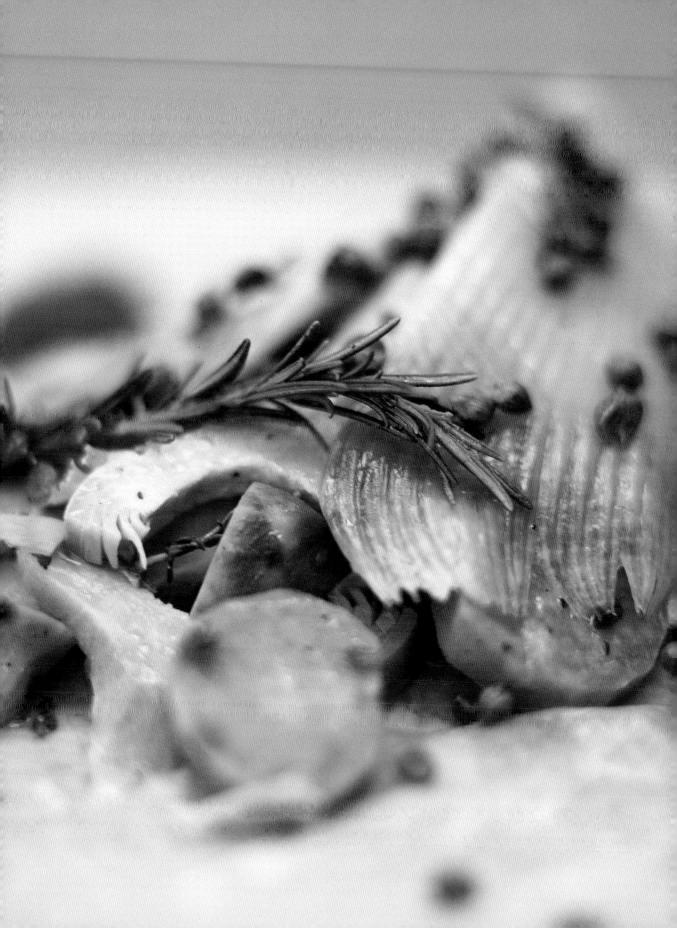

STEWING AND BRAISING

Stewing and braising for me are great cooking methods. I love stuff I can make in a big pot to serve at large dinner parties. I like to mush up the leftovers and put them in a cannelloni or lasagne, like the Italians do – they never have any waste! Whenever I eat a good stew it always makes me feel homely, hearty and comforted. Apart from that, it's great for turning cheap cuts of meat into a delectable feast and all the nutrients and vitamins are kept within the pot.

Whether you're stewing or braising, start off by browning your seasoned and floured meat in a hot pan or tray in the oven – this seals the meat, which gives you good flavour and colour. You can make a classic combination or you can make up your own. By using wine, stock, different vegetables and beans, you can assemble your own stew to reflect what's available in your cupboard or in season. And if you're not a great cook, you'll find it quite hard to overcook braised or stewed dishes. Both can be thrown together in minutes and can be cooking all day so that when you get home there is a beautiful welcoming smell to greet you, as well as a great meal.

Braising is generally about cooking portions or large pieces of meat, whereas stewing normally involves smaller pieces of tougher meat. Classically, stews are cooked on the hob most of the time, whereas braising is done in the oven, both covered with lids.

special chicken stew

This recipe is based on the classic French fricassee of chicken that I spent so many years as a student preparing. I've been lucky enough to see authentic ones cooked in France, and the Italian version of the same. A fricassee means floured meat fried and turned into a stew, using the flour as a thickening agent. In this recipe I've bastardized an old original, using individual spring chickens, but you can use a jointed whole chicken (see page 162).

Preheat the oven to 180°C/350°F/gas 4. Season your baby chickens inside and out and stuff each of them with the parsley and tarragon stalks. Using your forefinger, carefully part the skin from the breast meat and smear a teaspoon of wholegrain mustard into each bird. Rub the flour all over the chickens so they are covered in a thin layer. Keep any flour that falls off.

In a snug-fitting casserole-type pan, fry your chickens in 3 good lugs of olive oil on all sides for 10 minutes until golden. Remove them to a plate and then fry off the onion, garlic and celery in the pan. Add the butter and spare flour and continue to fry for about 4 minutes, scraping off any goodness that is on the bottom of the pan. Add your 2 glasses of white wine and allow the liquid to reduce by half, then put the chickens back into the pan. Now pour in your stock – it should come to about half-way up the chickens. Make yourself a cartouche (see page 174). Wet it so it's flexible then tuck this in and around the pan.

Place in the oven and cook for around 50 minutes to an hour until the chickens have crisp skin and the thigh meat falls off the bone. Remove the chicken to some nice serving bowls – ones that can hold a bit of sauce – and place your pan back on the hob. Add the lettuces, grapes, parsley leaves and tarragon leaves and simmer for a couple more minutes. Correct the seasoning carefully and spoon this sauce next to the chicken.

Try this: A fricassee can also be made successfully using white fish

Or this: Sometimes I tie the birds up (see page 228) to stop the legs sticking out all over the place when they cook.

SERVES 4

salt and freshly ground black pepper

4 spring chickens or poussins

1 small handful of fresh parsley, leaves picked, stalks kept

1 bunch of fresh tarragon, leaves picked, stalks kept

4 teaspoons wholegrain mustard

2 heaped tablespoons plain white flour

extra virgin olive oil

1 white onion, peeled and finely chopped

2 cloves of garlic, peeled and finely sliced

1/2 celery heart, trimmed back and finely sliced

2 good knobs of butter

2 wineglasses of crisp white wine

565ml/1 pint stock

4 gem lettuces, quartered

1 small bunch of seedless grapes, washed and halved

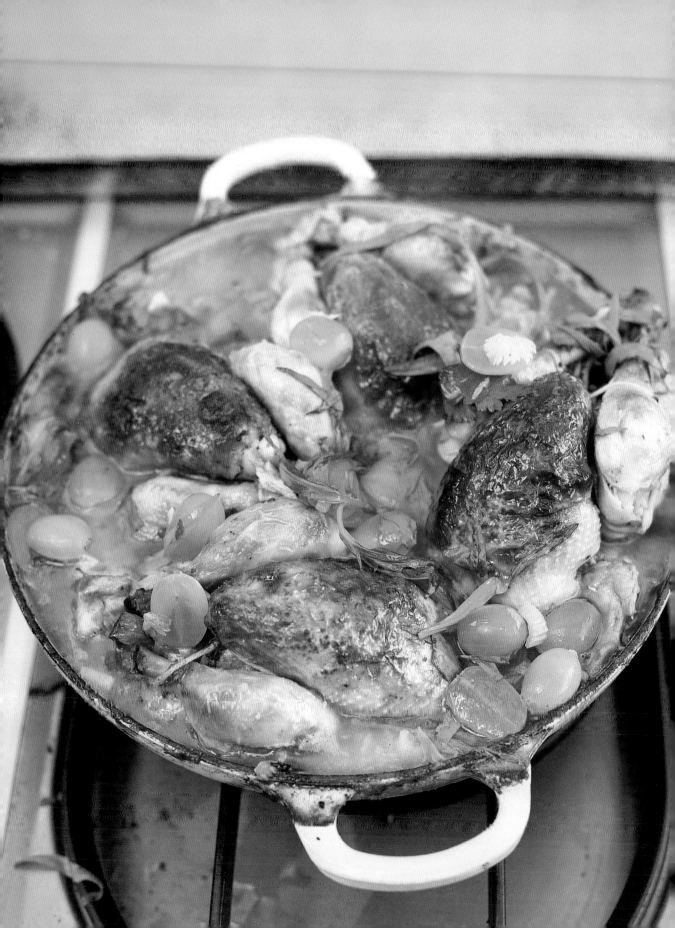

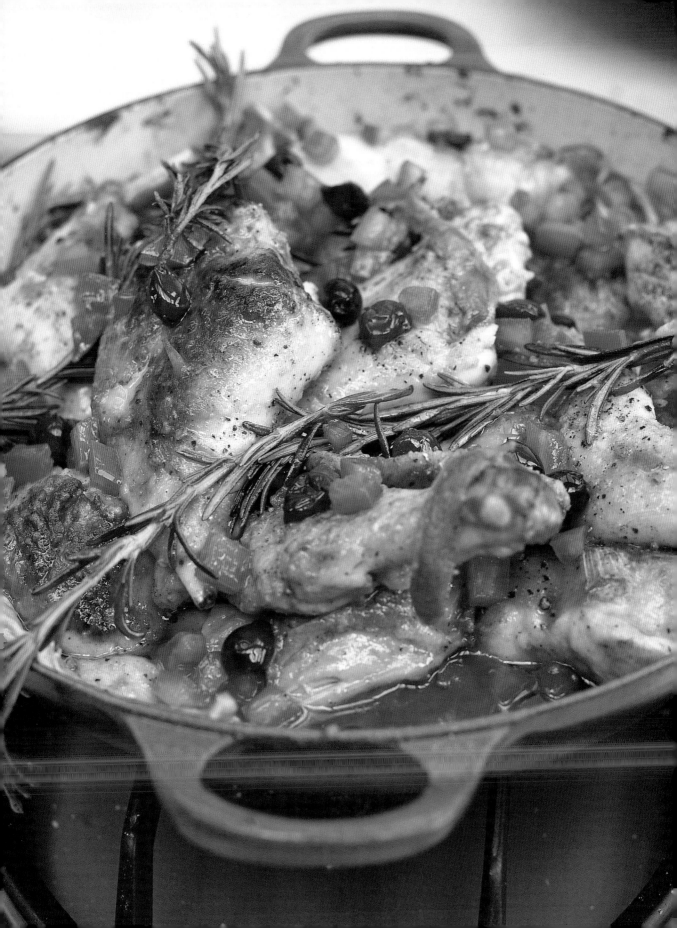

ligurian braised rabbit and rosemary with olives and tomatoes

The main reason that a lot of people don't eat rabbit is because they had one as a pet or think of them as sweet little things. Which is right, they are sweet – but they taste sweet as well! I know for a fact that Jools won't even try rabbit on principle and I'm not going to argue with her – I gave up many years ago!

This dish cooks quite quickly, especially if you find yourself a nice young 1kg/2¼lb rabbit (preferably no bigger). It will feed 2 people and will be so tender. With this dish, less is definitely more – for instance, fewer olives are better than overdoing it with loads, as you'll get a really subtle flavour. Ask your butcher to joint your rabbit for you.

In Liguria this is always made and served with the stones still in the olives, which is great because they taste so much better that way. If you don't like the idea of having stones in them then feel free to remove them yourself, but please don't buy those horrible stoned olives as they have absolutely no taste at all.

Preheat your oven to 190°C/375°F/gas 5. Toss your rabbit joints in the flour with plenty of salt and pepper. Place the rabbit in a hot, appropriately sized casserole-type pan with the olive oil and fry until the meat is nice and golden on one side. Then turn the joints over, add your rosemary and garlic and continue to fry until the garlic has softened but not coloured. Add the white wine and wait for it to come to the boil before adding the rest of the ingredients. Put a lid on or make a cartouche (see page 174) and tuck this over the pan. Place in the oven for 25 minutes. All the lovely flavoured liquor will cook into the rabbit, making it extremely tender and very tasty, leaving you with a little intensely-flavoured sauce. If you find that the sauce is a bit too watery, then keep the pan on the heat and reduce it a bit more.

Try this: Serve the rabbit with some dried cannellini beans which have been soaked overnight then boiled until tender with a little chunk of potato, a piece of tomato and some herbs to tenderize and flavour them. Then drain, discard the potato and tomato, season the beans to taste and dress with some good peppery extra virgin olive oil.

Or this: Also nice with some steamed greens.

SERVES 4

2 x 1kg/2¼lb rabbits, jointed

2 heaped tablespoons flour

sea salt and freshly ground black pepper

4 tablespoons extra virgin olive oil

1 bunch of fresh rosemary sprigs

6 cloves of garlic, skin on and squashed

½ bottle of white wine

4 anchovy fillets

1 handful of small black olives, stones left in

3 ripe plum tomatoes, halved, deseeded and finely chopped

moroccan lamb stew

I made this dish up the other day on a kind of Moroccan vibe, when I was mucking about with ways of marinating and tenderizing a neck fillet of lamb, which is a really tasty and cheap cut of meat. I trimmed the meat of all sinews, bashed it flat using a rolling pin, and made 2 incisions down the length of each fillet, but not quite to the end, so it looked almost like a tripod. I then marinated it with lots of spices and herbs and plaited it, to give a contrast between crispy and soft meat which I thought would be interesting. You don't have to plait the meat but it does increase the surface area, meaning the marinade can get right in there. Needless to say, Jools thought I was mucking around with it too much and being very camp – you decide!

Preheat the oven to 190°C/375°F/gas 5. Pound up your cumin, coriander and fennel seeds with the dried chillies, rosemary, ginger and a pinch of salt and pepper, stirring in a couple of tablespoons of olive oil. Smear half of this marinade over your lamb before you plait it. Rub and massage it in, then put the meat to one side while you mix the rest of the marinade in a bowl with the sweet potatoes, onions and garlic.

Brown your 4 marinaded pieces of meat on both sides in a pan with a little olive oil. Add the sweet potato mixture to the pan and remove the lamb to the empty bowl while you fry your veg for about 4 minutes until the onions are slightly soft. Add your tomatoes, give the pan a shake and place the meat on top. Add 3 wineglasses of water, the cinnamon stick, bay leaves and dried apricots, and braise in the preheated oven (I suggest you do this with the lid off to give it a little colour) for 1 hour 15 minutes. Now pour the boiling water over the couscous and allow it to be absorbed. Then fork the couscous through, season with salt, pepper, a lug of olive oil and a swig of wine vinegar, cover with tinfoil and place in the oven for 5 minutes to steam.

Roughly chop the fresh coriander and stir it through the stew just before serving. Divide between 4 plates with the couscous and spoon over a good dollop of natural yoghurt.

SERVES 4

½ teaspoon cumin seeds

1 tablespoon coriander seeds

1 teaspoon fennel seeds

3–4 small dried chillies

1 small bunch of fresh rosemary, leaves picked and finely chopped

2 thumb-sized pieces of fresh ginger, peeled

sea salt and freshly ground black pepper

extra virgin olive oil

4 smallish neck fillets of lamb, prepared as above

4 sweet potatoes, peeled, cut into 2.5 cm/1 inch dice

2 red onions, peeled and roughly chopped

4 cloves of garlic, peeled and sliced

12 ripe plum tomatoes, each cut into 8 pieces

1 stick of cinnamon

2 bay leaves

1 handful of dried apricots

285ml/½ pint boiling water

350g/12oz couscous

a little wine vinegar

1 large bunch of fresh coriander

4 tablespoons natural yoghurt

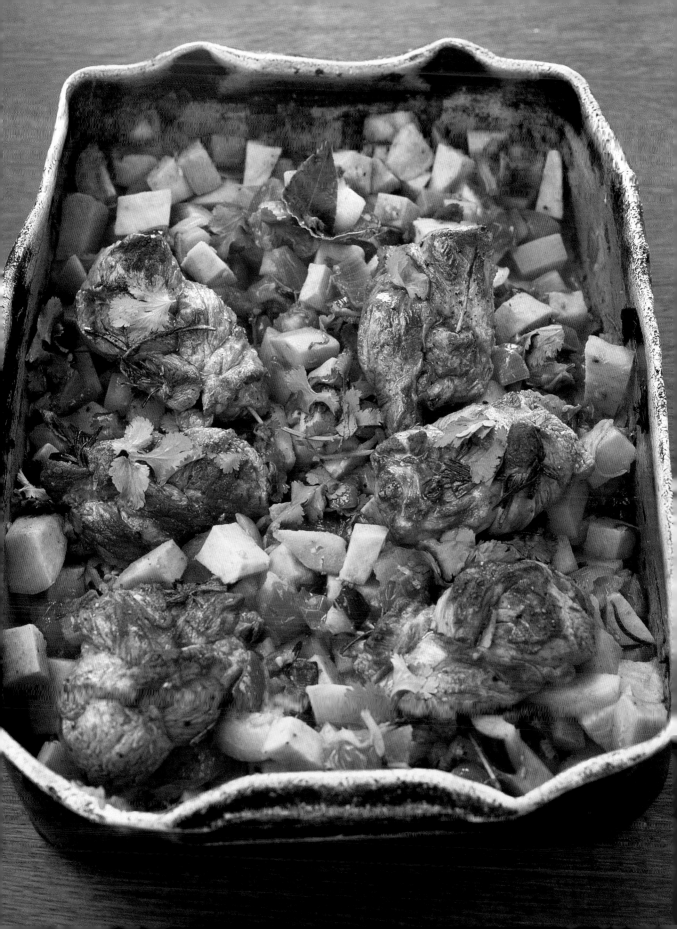

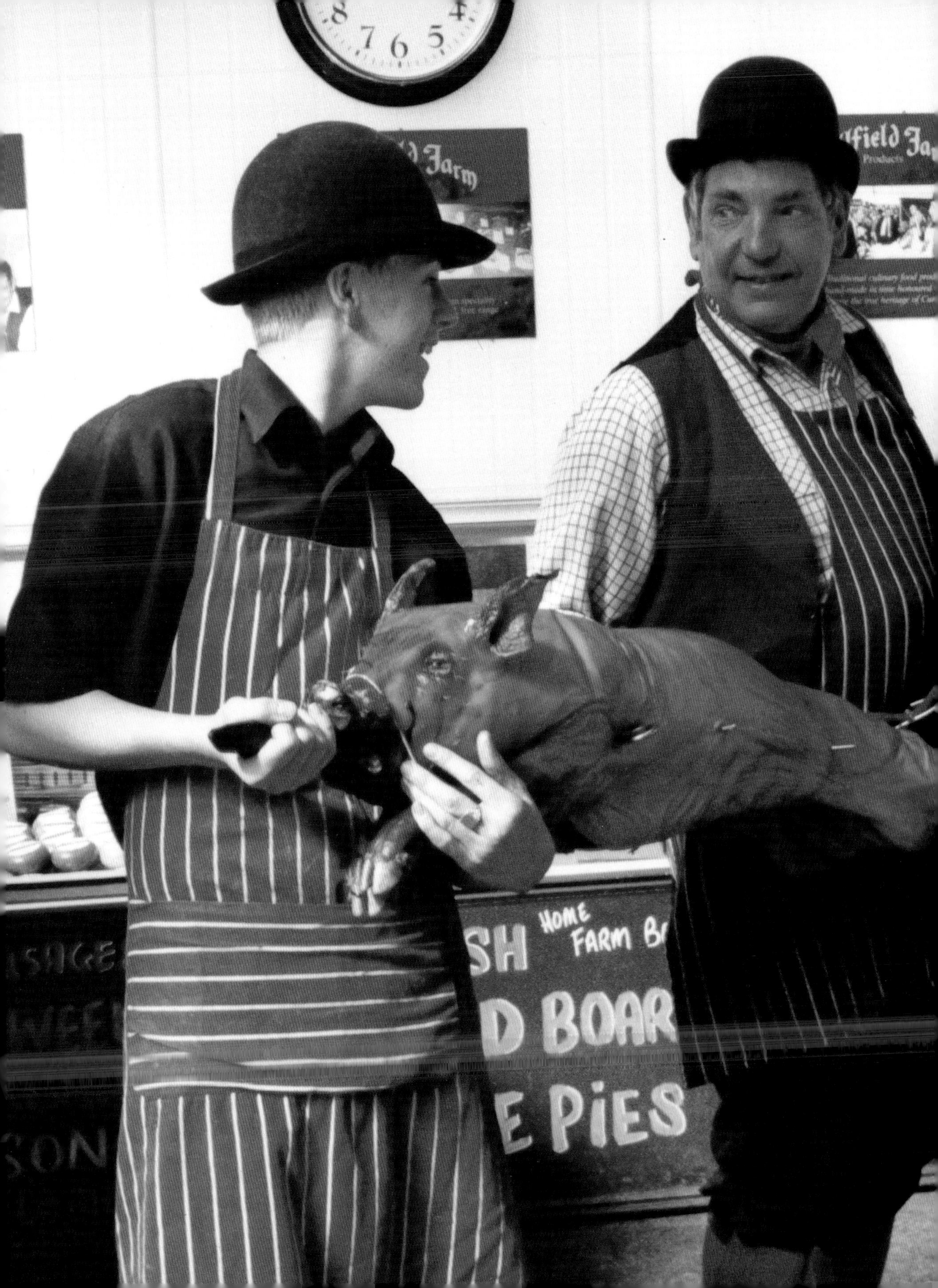
HOME
FARM
PIES

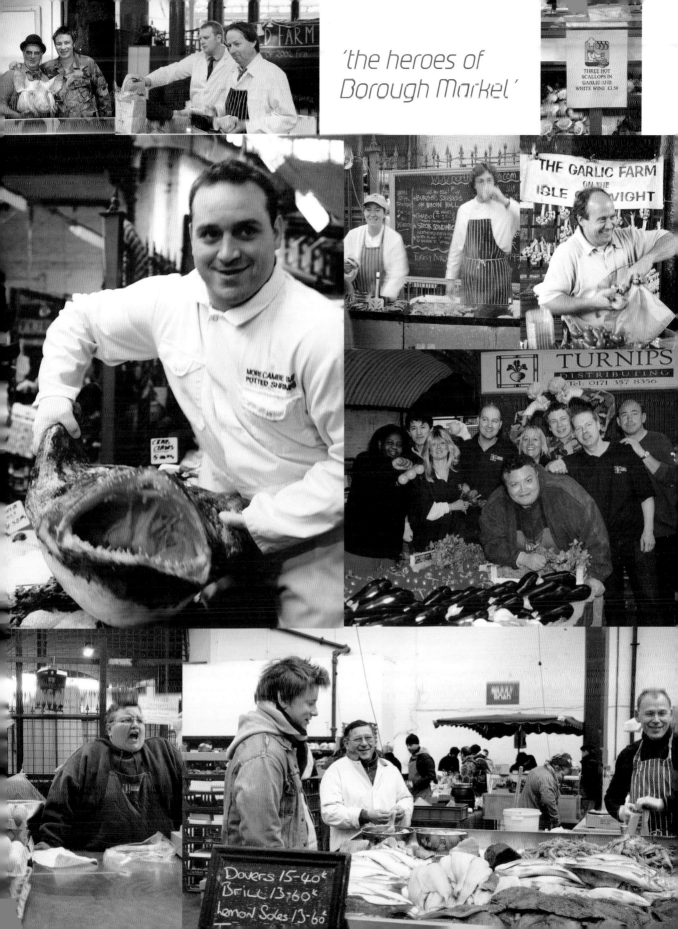

'the heroes of Borough Market'

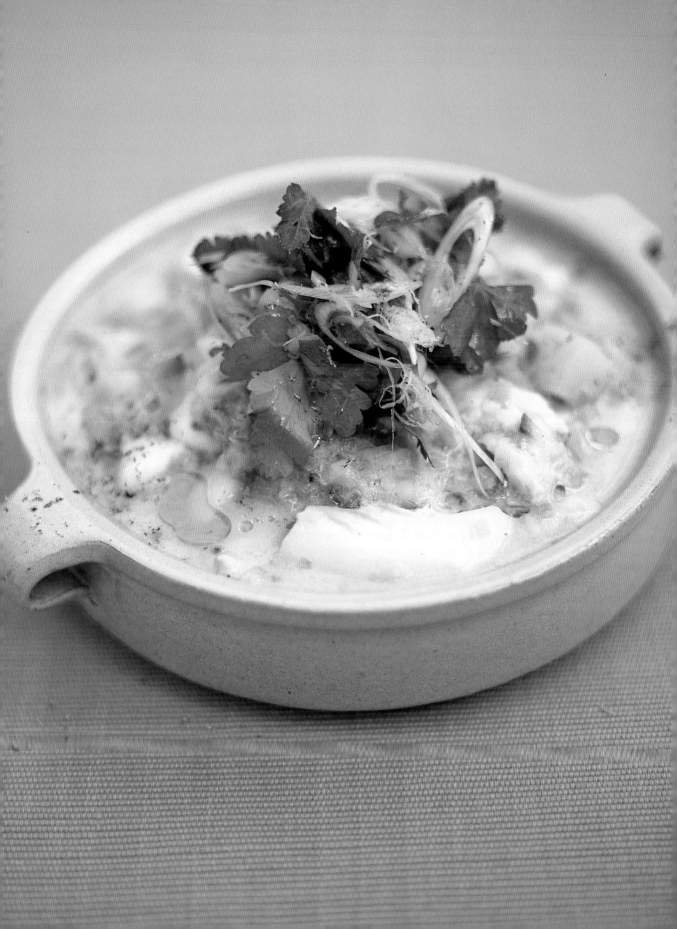

cod, potato and spring onion stew

The inspiration for this one comes from conversations with Icelandic and Danish friends who prize their cod. Traditionally, they prepare it in lots of different ways – pickled, salted, dried or smoked. This stew is similar to the way in which they slowly stew salt cod after soaking it (so that the excess salt seasons the other ingredients in the soup, like the potatoes). Good salt cod is quite hard to find these days, so I've adapted the recipe to use fresh cod, but you can also use hake, bass or halibut.

In an appropriately sized large pan, slowly fry your onion and leek with around 5 tablespoons of olive oil for 5 minutes until soft and tender. With a teaspoon, remove and discard the fluffy tasteless core from the courgettes and grate the rest into the pan. Chop the potatoes into rough 2cm/1 inch dice and add to the pan. Give everything a good stir and then add the anchovies. Turn the heat up and add the white wine. Allow to cook down by half before adding your milk and stock. Bring to the boil and simmer for half an hour until the potatoes are tender. At this point add your cod and simmer for a further 15 minutes until the flesh flakes away – feel free to stir and break up the fish, but it's quite nice to leave some big chunks as well. Season carefully to taste. Divide between your bowls, and serve with a small handful of parsley and spring onion dressed with a little olive oil and lemon juice.

Try this: Sprinkle a little orange zest over the parsley and spring onion. It really works with the cod.

SERVES 4–6

1 onion, peeled and finely chopped

1 leek, washed and finely sliced

extra virgin olive oil

2 medium courgettes, halved lengthways

1kg/2¼lb potatoes, peeled

2 anchovies

1 wineglass white wine

565ml/1 pint milk

565ml/1 pint stock

1kg/2¼lb cod fillet, skinned and pinboned

salt and freshly ground black pepper

1 handful of fresh flat-leaf parsley, roughly chopped

1 bunch of spring onions, finely sliced

juice of ½ a lemon

BONING A CHICKEN

The French call this cutting a chicken for sauté, the principle being that you can stretch a whole chicken a long way, letting everyone taste a bit of white and dark meat.

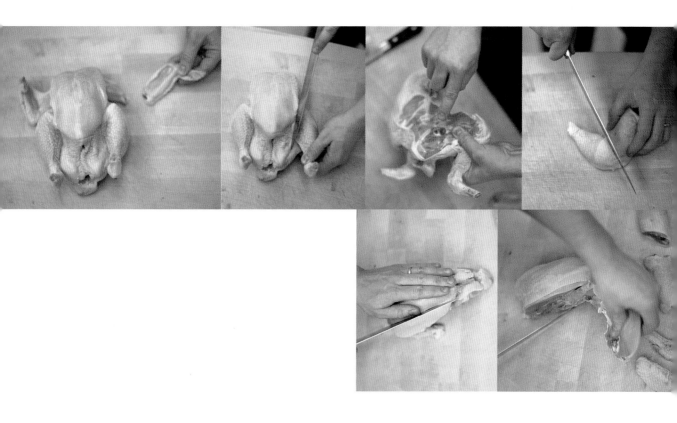

		3. Pop the ball joint out and remove the whole leg, using your knife on both sides.	4. Divide the leg through the joint, into a drumstick and thigh
1. Remove the winglets.	2. Cut round the leg joint.		
		5 and 6. Cut down half-way through the breast on both sides.	

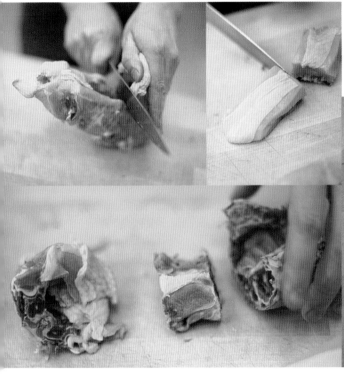

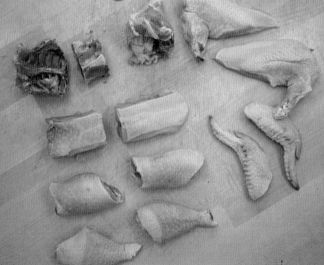

7. Remove the carcass from the remaining breast meat.

8. Cut the breast meat through the bone.

10. A chicken cut for sauté.

9. Cut up the carcass.

lebanese lemon chicken

I've decided to use farika in this Lebanese-style dish that I've been trying out, as it's the authentic wheat grain that would normally be used, but feel free to use bulghur wheat instead. Salted preserved lemons are another Lebanese/North African/Arabic commodity and are absolutely excellent for bringing things like rice dishes, couscous and, in this case, farika to life. If you look around the speciality counters these days you can quite easily come across them. They are slightly salty but with a pungent lemony fragrance – great with some classic Lebanese spices and a nice bit of chicken.

Preheat the oven to 180°C/350°F/gas 4. First, cut your chicken for sauté, then bash all the spices up in a pestle and mortar with the salt until you have a fine powder. Add your flour and mix together well. Rub this intensely flavoured flour all over your chicken and in every crack and cranny. You may have a little flour left over so just reserve this for later.

Heat an appropriately sized casserole-type pan, or a roasting tray, on the hob and add 5 tablespoons of olive oil. Begin to brown your chicken pieces on all sides – you want them to fry in one layer. Once they are nicely coloured, remove to a plate, turn down the heat and then add your fennel, onion, preserved lemons and rosemary to the pan or tray. Fry for around 5 minutes until nice and softened. Then add any excess flavoured flour and your farika or bulghur wheat, and give it a good stir.

Add the tequila, vodka or wine and allow to cook down to leave a fabulous fresh and fragrant taste. Cover with chicken stock or water until it reaches the same level as the grains and the veg. Now you need to make a cartouche (see page 174). Run it under the tap to make it flexible then rub it with olive oil so it doesn't stick. Place the cartouche over the couscous and veg in the pan and put the chicken on top. Place into the preheated oven and cook for 45 minutes until the chicken skin is really crisp. Sometimes the grains catch on the bottom and they get a little bit of colour. I quite like it when this happens, but to prevent it just make sure you place the pan at the top of the oven so it's not getting direct heat from the bottom. Serve straight away with a good dollop of sour cream or crème fraîche and sprinkled with the fennel tops.

SERVES 4

1 large chicken, cut for sautéing (see page 162)

1 teaspoon ground cinnamon

1 teaspoon fennel seeds

½ teaspoon cumin seeds

½ teaspoon chilli powder

1 teaspoon black peppercorns

1 teaspoon sea salt

3 heaped tablespoons flour

extra virgin olive oil

1 large bulb of fennel, roughly chopped, herby tops chopped and reserved

1 red onion, peeled and roughly chopped

2–3 small preserved lemons, chopped

1 small bunch of fresh rosemary, roughly chopped

150g/5½oz farika or bulghur wheat

1 wineglass of tequila, vodka or white wine

565ml/1 pint chicken stock or water

1 small tub of sour cream or crème fraîche

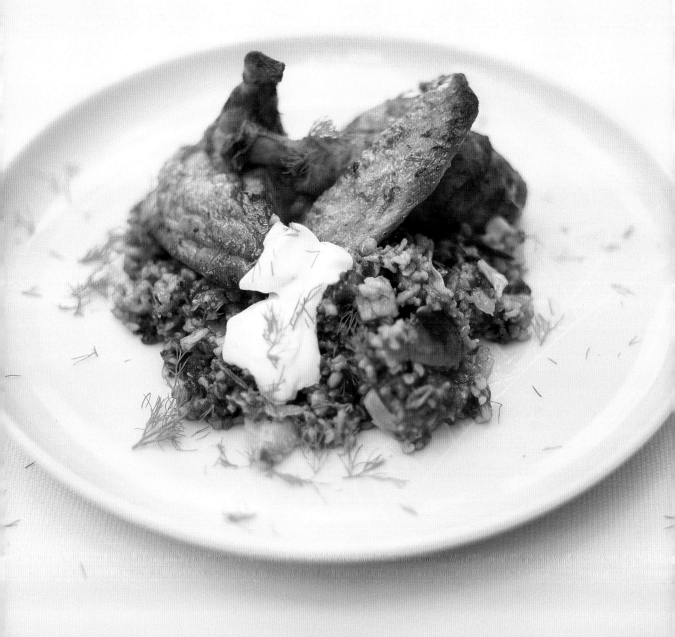

Try this: The chicken can be bulked out with a lot more root vegetables – things like carrots, celery, garlic, other pulses and more grains. This can stretch the dish a lot further.

Or this: If you're a vegetarian, you can make this with nice chunks of vegetables and veg stock.

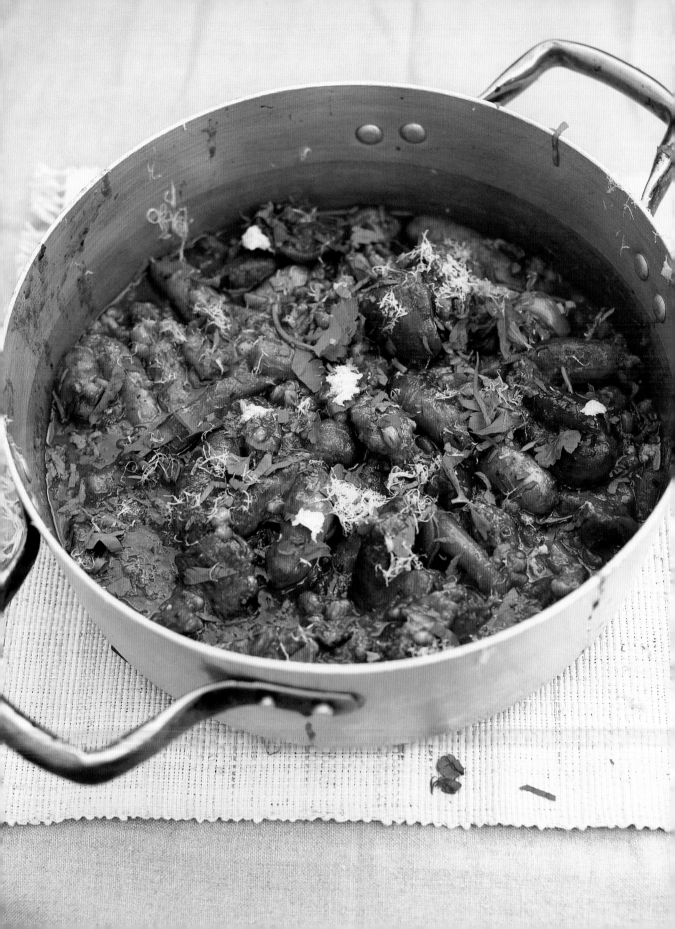

dark, sticky stew

This reminds me of winter days in my youth, when I would come home late completely soaked through and shivering from playing down by the stream in the pouring rain. Mum would give me a rollicking about catching pneumonia, and then she'd give me a big bowl of stew. This dish just makes you feel really happy, and it's also dead cheap to make.

Preheat your oven to 180°C/350°F/gas 4. Put your lamb into a bowl and season well with a good pinch of salt and pepper. Finely chop your rosemary leaves and add to the bowl with the flour. Mix around so that the meat is completely covered. Fry the lamb in a couple of tablespoons of extra virgin olive oil in a hot casserole-type pan – do this in batches so the pieces get a nice bit of colour, then remove from the pan and put to one side.

Turn the heat down, then fry your onion, mushrooms and carrots for about 5 minutes until softened and slightly coloured. Add the lamb back to the pan along with the parsnip, Marmite, pearl barley, ale and stock. Bring to the boil and then simmer for 20 minutes while you skewer 3 chipolatas on to each of the skewers or rosemary sticks. Just before the stew goes in the oven, add the chipolatas to the pan. Then place a lid on or make a cartouche (see page 174), wet it and tuck this over the pan. Cook for around an hour, or until the lamb falls apart. I love to eat it just as it is, almost like a thick soup, with some crusty bread.

Try this: To really get the flavours going, the Italians have something called *gremolata*: finely chop some flat-leaf parsley, a clove of garlic and the zest from 1 or 2 lemons (or try oranges, which are also fantastic). Mix this up, sprinkle over the top of your stew and stir in – it will really give it an amazing kick.

Or this: You can play around with different root veg, or even use different cuts of meat – beef works really well in this stew. Just be aware that you may have to adjust the cooking time. It's ready when the meat is tender and falls apart.

SERVES 6

800g/1¾lb stewing lamb, roughly diced

sea salt and freshly ground black pepper

1 small handful of fresh rosemary, leaves picked

2 heaped tablespoons flour

extra virgin olive oil

1 red onion, peeled and roughly chopped

8 field mushrooms, torn in half

1 handful of baby carrots, scrubbed

1 parsnip, peeled and grated

1 dessertspoon Marmite

2 heaped tablespoons pearl barley

285ml/½ pint rich ale (Guinness, Caffrey's, John Smith's)

565ml/1 pint stock

6 skewers or sticks of fresh rosemary, leaves removed (see page 248)

18 chipolata sausages

quick-time sausage cassoulet

This year I seem to have been working around lots of builders and every time they put a request in for some grub it's been 'sausage this' or 'sausage that'. A foreman called Dusty, who was working next door, kept on talking about a sausage casserole. So I made this one up very quickly, basing it on a French cassoulet-type thing. It's nice and easy to cook for a group as it's all done in one dish. While I was going sausage-mad, I realized that we're fantastically lucky these days to have great sausages available in the supermarkets, farmers' markets and good local butchers. In this dish feel free to use any sausages you like.

Preheat your oven to 220°C/425°F/gas 7. Put your porcini mushrooms into a dish, cover with 565ml/1 pint of boiling water and allow to soak until soft. Heat a large casserole-type pan or roasting tray on the hob. Slice the bacon across into strips – called 'lardons'. Fry in 4 tablespoons of olive oil until crisp and golden. Tie your herbs together with some string and add to the bacon in the pan with your onions, garlic, carrot, celery and bay leaves. Drain the porcini, reserving the soaking liquid, add them to the pan and fry nice and slowly for about 5 minutes. Add the red wine and simmer until the liquid has reduced by half.

Add the tomatoes to the pan, breaking them up with a spoon, then add your strained porcini soaking liquor and the beans. Bring to the boil and simmer for 15 minutes. Lightly season before laying your sausages on top – all higgledy piggledy. Break up your bread into coarse, chunky breadcrumbs, toss with the thyme, a little salt and olive oil and sprinkle on top of the sausages. Place in the oven for around 1 hour until the sausages and breadcrumbs are golden and crisp. Remove the bunch of herbs and serve with something like mashed potato or polenta.

Try this: Any combination of beans and lentils works well in this cassoulet, so feel free to use what you fancy.

And this: Sometimes if I want to make this a bit more healthy and get some greens involved I will stir in a couple of handfuls of fresh spinach right at the end when serving up. The heat from the dish will make the spinach wilt.

SERVES ABOUT 8

2 handfuls of dried porcini mushrooms, broken up

8 thick slices of dry-cured streaky bacon

extra virgin olive oil

1 large bunch of mixed fresh rosemary, thyme and sage

2 red onions, peeled and roughly chopped

2 cloves of garlic, chopped

1 large carrot, peeled and roughly chopped

½ celery heart, finely chopped

2 bay leaves

½ bottle of red wine

3 x 400g/14oz tins of plum tomatoes

2 x 400g/14oz tins of borlotti or cannellini beans, or use a mixture

sea salt and freshly ground black pepper

24 chipolata sausages or 8 larger sausages

1 large, stale loaf, crusts removed

1 small handful of fresh thyme, leaves picked

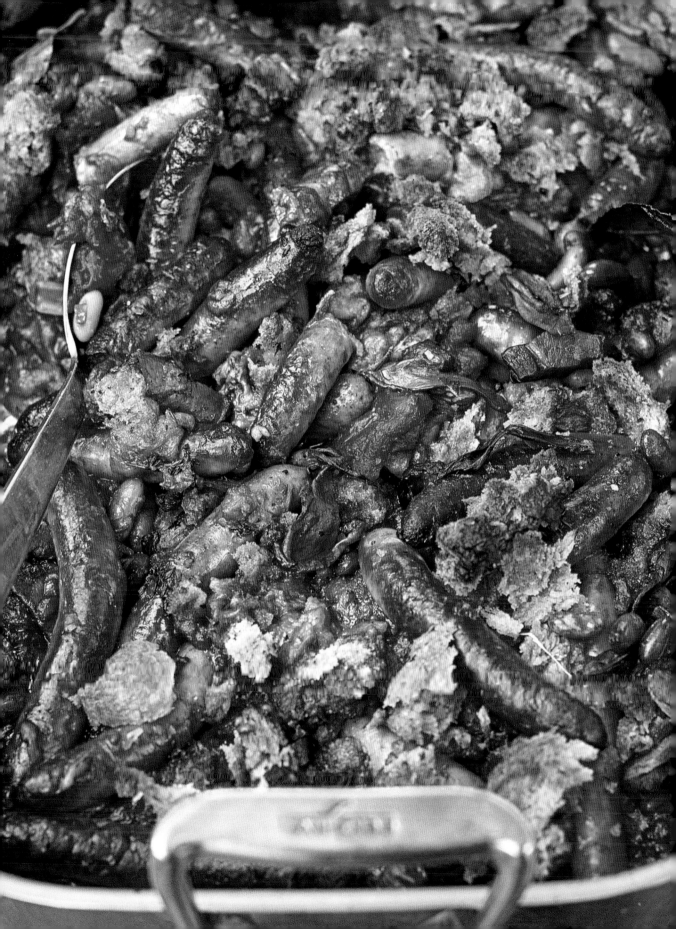

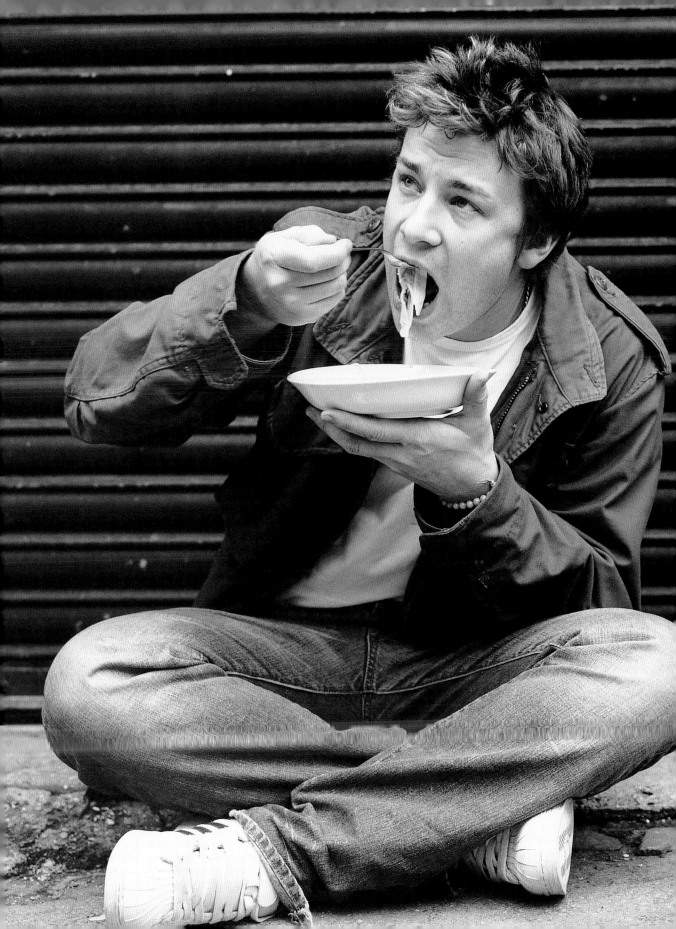

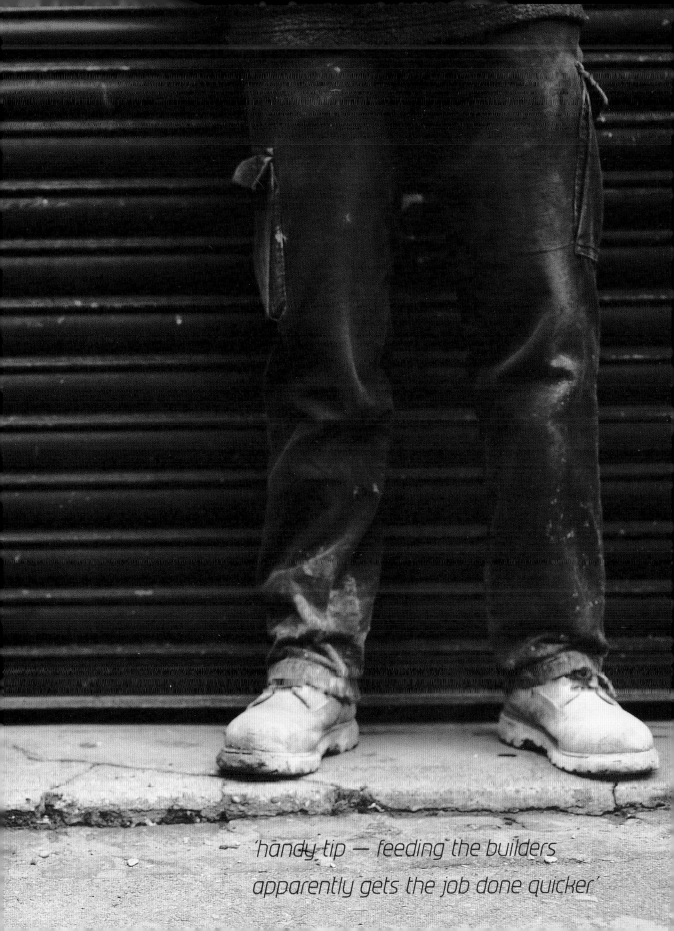

'handy tip — feeding the builders
apparently gets the job done quicker'

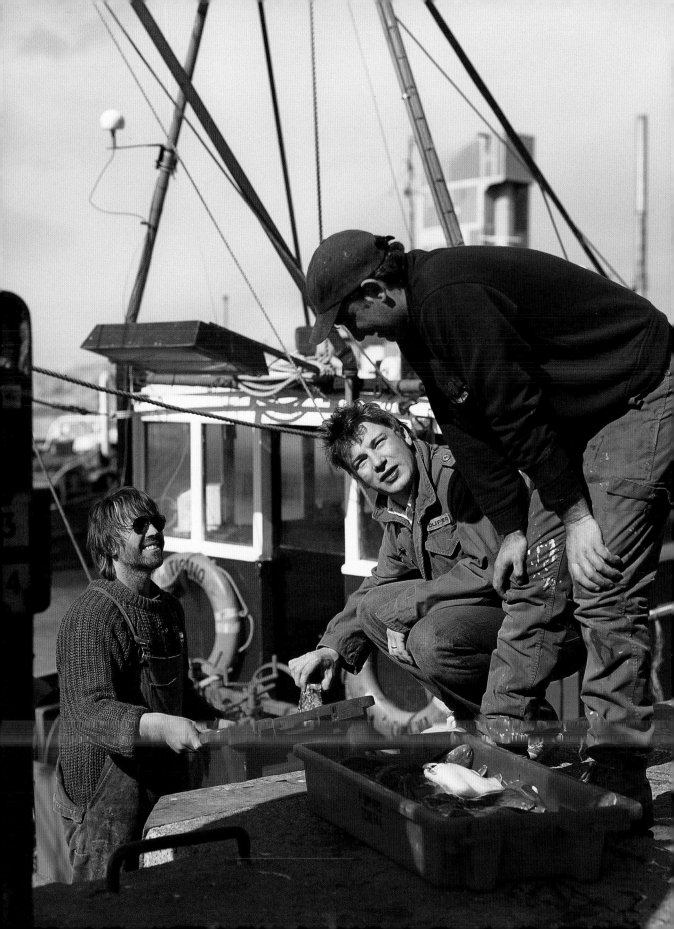

bouillabaisse

A bouillabaisse is a classic fish soup which originates from the South of France, where they use local Mediterranean fish like rascasse and galinette. For my version I've used a mixture of similar British seafood, so feel free to use whatever fish is available and fresh. Ask your fishmonger to scale, gut and clean the fish for you. It's a good idea to cut the fish into similar-sized pieces so that they cook at the same time.

Chop the soup base vegetables roughly, then very slowly fry them with the parsley, fennel seeds and bay leaves in olive oil in a large pan, covered with a cartouche (see page 174), for 40 minutes until really soft. Remove the cartouche, turn the heat up and caramelize gently until coloured. This is when the flavour of the natural sugars will really intensify. Keep stirring to stop the vegetables sticking to the pan. Add the tomatoes, fish stock, saffron and turmeric, then season and bring to the boil. Turn the heat down and simmer very gently for 1 hour.

Meanwhile, prepare the croûtons. Slice a baguette into 0.5cm /¹/₄ inch discs, brush each side with melted butter, and place on a baking tray. Bake at 180°C/350°F/gas 4 for about 15 minutes or until crisp and golden brown.

For the rouille, make a batch of aïoli but add a pinch of saffron and 1 teaspoon of cayenne pepper to the garlic when it's in the pestle and mortar. It should be bright yellow, with a good, hot, garlicky, saffrony taste.

When the soup is ready, pour it into a food processor and pulse gently – you don't want it to be completely smooth. Correct the seasoning, then pour into a deep roasting tray and place it on the hob to bubble gently. Season the fish, then add to the soup, making sure they are covered with the liquid. It shouldn't be too thick, so add boiling water or stock to thin it down if necessary. Now slowly stew the fish gently in the soup for about 10 minutes, or until cooked. Traditionally the soup is eaten first, with the rouille and croûtons, followed by the fish, which can be eaten straight from the roasting tray. Lovely washed down with a good chilled Provençal rosé wine.

Try this: You can use any mixture of fish – try cod steaks, whole gurnard, red or grey mullet, hake, monkfish, bream, John Dory, skate, halibut, turbot, eel, lobster, crab or whole large prawns – but don't use salmon, or oily fish like mackerel.

SERVES 6

2 x 400g/14oz tins of tomatoes

1 litre/1³/₄ pints fish stock or water

a pinch of saffron

a pinch of turmeric

sea salt and freshly ground black pepper

2kg/4¹/₂lb mixed seafood, scaled, gutted and prepared

for the soup base

1 bulb of fennel

1 head of celery, trimmed

1 bulb of garlic, peeled

2 large onions, peeled

2 large carrots, peeled

1 handful of fresh parsley, roughly chopped

1 teaspoon ground fennel seeds

2 bay leaves

extra virgin olive oil

for the rouille

1 x aïoli recipe (see page 203)

a pinch of saffron

1 teaspoon cayenne pepper

for the croûtons

1 baguette or ciabatta loaf

butter

173

MAKING A CARTOUCHE

A cartouche is a French term which basically means 'scroll' or 'packet'. Basically, in cooking terms, it's a paper lid that is used to slow down the reduction of moisture in cooking. A lid only lets a little moisture escape whereas using no lid lets lots of moisture escape. Using a cartouche is a half-way house between the two and also stops things from colouring too much.

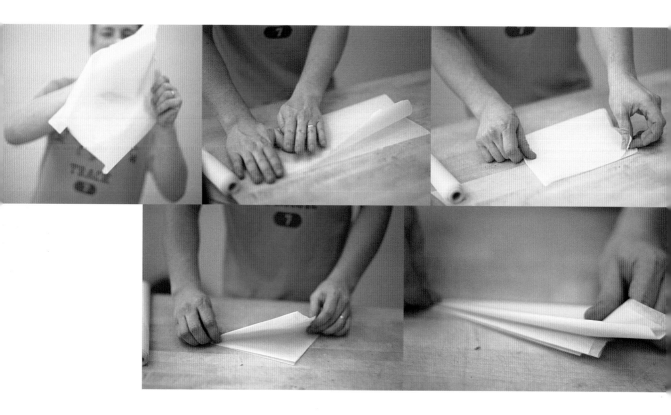

1. Get yourself a piece of greaseproof paper and tear off a square.

2. Fold the square in half . . .

3. . . . and in half again.

4. Keep folding the same way so that the tip becomes the centre.

5. When it's pretty pointy you're ready to measure up.

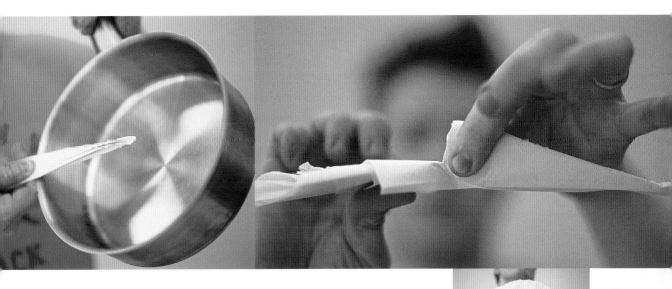

6. Hold the tip of the cartouche against the pan to estimate its size, using your thumb as a measure.

7. Tear or cut off the excess.

8. Open out to a circle, perfect for the job. P.S. You can get away with the cartouche being a little larger than the pan, so don't worry if you make it a bit too big.

tender braised leeks with wine and thyme

I always love new things to do with vegetables. Sometimes in my search for doing things a little differently I try too hard but this is the kind of recipe that brings me straight back down to earth – simple, tasty and great with just about anything.

Tear back and discard the first two layers of skin on your leeks, leaving the tender whiter flesh. Wash well and slice into 2.5cm/1 inch pieces. Finely slice the dark green ends of the leeks.

    You really only want one layer of leeks, so you need to use a wide, shallow casserole-type pan, or even a roasting tray. On the hob on a low heat, slowly fry the garlic and thyme in the butter with the dark green leek tops until the garlic is softened but not coloured. Add the pieces of white leek and toss them in the flavoured butter, then pour over your wine and stock and cover with a cartouche (see page 174). Cook in the oven at 180°C/350°F/gas 4 for 35 minutes or on the hob until tender and tasty. The butter should emulsify with the stock and wine to create a slightly shiny broth. If for some reason the butter splits from the pan juices, just jiggle the pan about for 30 seconds and that's normally enough to get it back before you season and serve.

Try this: Use baby leeks if you like. They will be a little sweeter and will take less time to cook.

Or this: Add a little cream to the leeks and toss with some cooked tagliatelle and a couple of handfuls of grated Parmesan cheese. Really tasty.

SERVES 4

4 big leeks, ends trimmed and dark green tops reserved

2 cloves of garlic, peeled and finely sliced

1 bunch of fresh thyme, washed and picked

115g/4oz butter

2 wineglasses of Chardonnay

285ml/½ pint vegetable stock

sea salt and freshly ground black pepper

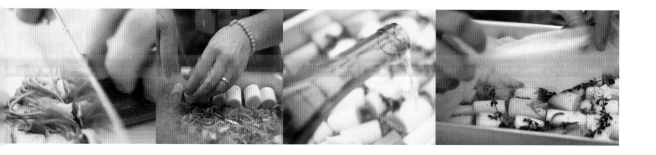

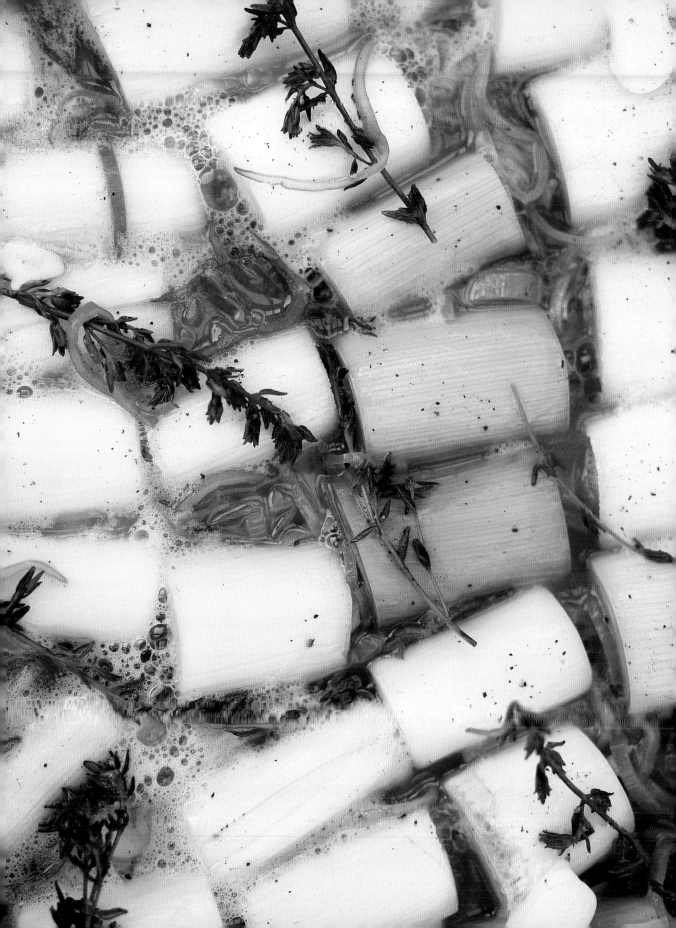

FRYING

SHALLOW-FRYING

This is a fantastic way to cook, using a shallow hot pan with a little fat: oil, butter, animal fat like lard and dripping, even things like coconut oil and avocado oil, can be used. Apart from being quick and direct, frying caramelizes the natural sugars in food, which gives an amazing golden colour and a lovely sticky sweetness you can only get from pan-frying and roasting. The best thing is that you're in constant contact with the pan. You smell it, you see it, you hear it – all your senses are going. It's a very exciting way of cooking. Remember, you're in control – if it's too hot then turn it down, too cold then turn it up. Generally for shallow-frying you use thin first-class cuts of meat or fish that will cook through fast. If the cuts are any bigger you may want to slow down the frying process or finish them off in the oven – this is called pan-roasting (see page 211).

DEEP-FRYING

This method of cooking requires good clean oil, a consistently hot temperature (180°C), and generally coating fish or vegetables in some kind of batter, flour or breadcrumbs – apart from the good old chip, of course. Batters were originally developed to encase meat or fish so that they could be cooked quickly, having been steamed inside. People soon cottoned on to the idea that a crispy outside and a steamed centre were a delicious combination.

pan-seared venison loin with blueberries, shallots and red wine

It's not often that I cook a nice bit of venison, but it's definitely worth a try. I think you'll be surprised how much you'll like it – the meat tastes like a well-hung steak and can be very juicy. It goes so well with the fruit in this dish, and is great served with some steamed purple sprouting broccoli. Mashed potato, parsnip or celeriac go well with this too.

Bash up the thyme and juniper berries in a pestle and mortar with a really good pinch of salt and pepper. If you haven't got a pestle and mortar, use the end of a rolling pin and a metal bowl. Loosen with 3 good lugs of olive oil. Pat the venison dry with some kitchen paper, and rub the oil mixture all over it. Sear the meat in a hot pan on all sides turning it every minute – roughly 6 minutes for medium rare, 7–8 minutes for medium, and you'd have to be a nutter if you wanted to cook it for any longer than that! Depending on the thickness of the meat and the heat of the pan, it may need a little less or more time to cook – so don't look at the clock, look at the meat. This is the time when you want to try to be instinctive with your meat. Remove it from the pan when it's cooked to your liking and allow it to rest on a plate for 4 minutes, covered with tinfoil.

Reduce the heat under the pan and add a good lug of oil. Add the shallots and the garlic and fry gently for around 3 minutes until translucent and tender. Turn up the heat again, add the wine, and let it reduce by half. Add the blueberries and simmer slowly for 4 minutes, then remove the pan from the heat, add the butter, and jiggle and shake the pan around so the sauce goes slightly opaque and shiny. Season to taste.

Slice the venison into 2cm/³/₄ inch slices and serve with steamed purple sprouting broccoli or some other good greens. Add the meat's resting juices to the sauce and spoon over the venison. Absolutely fantastic.

SERVES 4

1 small handful of fresh thyme, leaves picked

5 dried juniper berries

sea salt and freshly ground black pepper

extra virgin olive oil

1 x 800g/1³/₄lb venison loin, trimmed

4 shallots, peeled and finely sliced

1 clove of garlic, peeled and finely sliced

1 glass of robust red wine

200g/7oz fresh blueberries

2 large knobs of butter

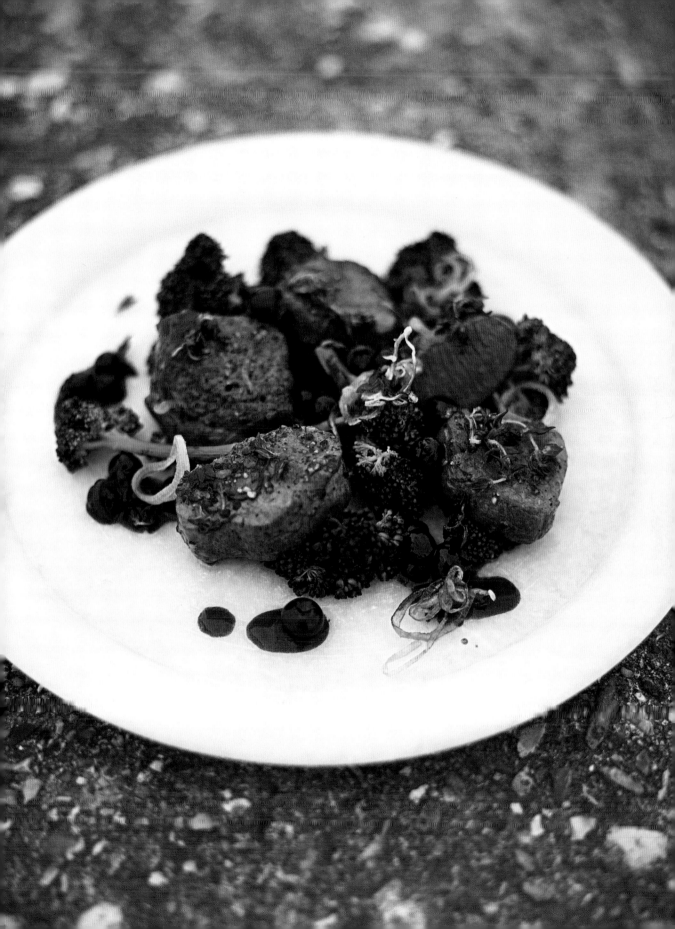

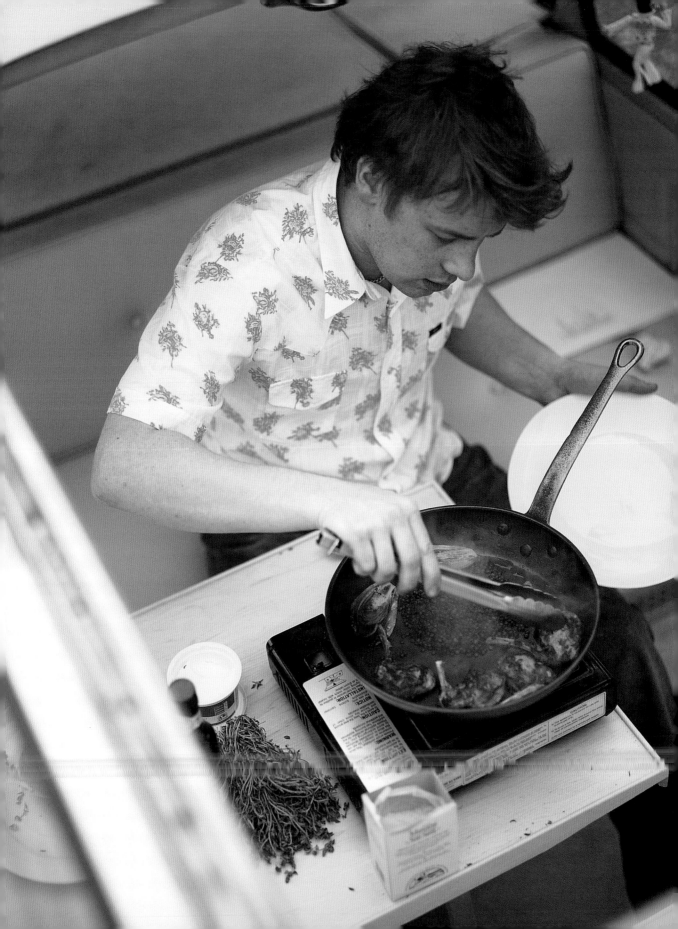

pan-fried lamb chops with puy lentils, loadsa herbs, balsamic vinegar and crème fraîche

This is a great way of cooking lamb really quickly and bashing in some good flavour using brute force! Instead of Puy lentils you can use cannellini, borlotti or butter beans.

First of all, put your lentils in a saucepan, then cover with water and add the tomato (this will help to soften the skins). Bring to the boil and cook gently for around 15–25 minutes until the lentils are tender but still holding their shape, then remove from the heat. Bash up your fresh thyme and garlic in a pestle and mortar (or use a metal bowl and the end of a rolling pin). Add a good lug of olive oil and then rub this over both sides of the lamb chops. Season them with salt and pepper then place them between 2 pieces of clingfilm and bat them out to around 1cm/½ inch thick by using the bottom of a small saucepan, or a rolling pin. This will improve their flavour and texture as well as making them quick to cook.

Heat a frying pan, add a couple of tablespoons of extra virgin olive oil, and fry the lamb chops on each side until golden. You can use an extra pan if you prefer, or cook the lamb in 2 batches. When the chops are cooked, remove from the pan and allow them to rest on a large plate for a minute. Remove any fat from the pan.

Drain your lentils and discard the tomato. Add the balsamic vinegar to the frying pan, bring it to the boil, scraping all the goodness from the bottom of the pan, and add the lentils, parsley and basil. Heat through until the herbs have wilted down, then season to taste with salt, pepper and extra virgin olive oil. Divide the lentils between 4 plates and place the lamb on top, with any resting juices from the meat poured over the top. Serve with a dollop of crème fraîche.

Try this: I like to serve this with the roasted radicchio on page 214.

Or this: Try dressing the lentils with a little extra vinegar and oil, and toss with a load of salad leaves to make a beautiful salad.

SERVES 4

150g/5½oz Puy lentils

1 plum tomato

1 small handful of fresh thyme, leaves picked

1 clove of garlic, peeled and finely sliced

extra virgin olive oil

12 lamb chops

sea salt and freshly ground black pepper

4 tablespoons balsamic vinegar

1 handful of fresh parsley, leaves picked

1 handful of fresh basil, leaves picked

4 tablespoons crème fraîche

FRYING

183

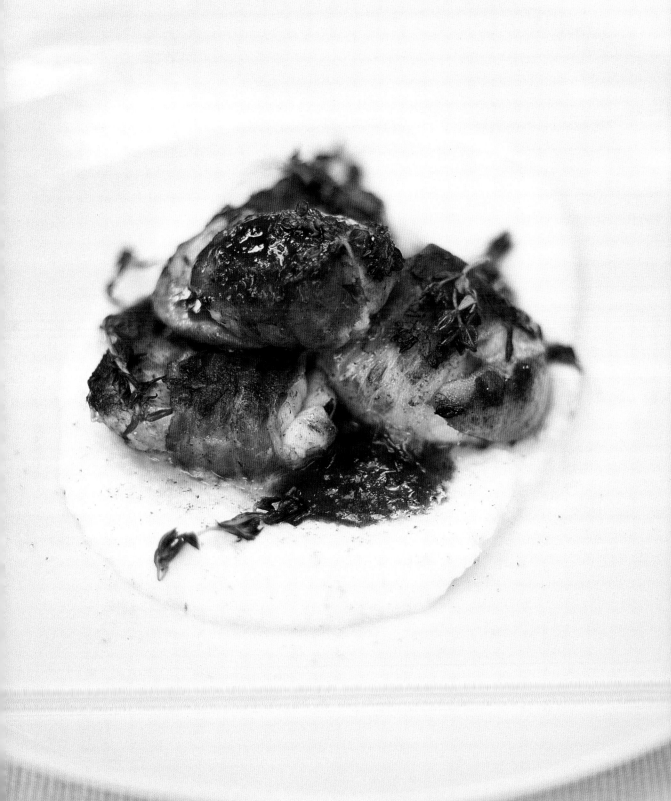

pan-seared scallops wrapped in pancetta with creamed celeriac

This is one of those simple recipes you'll never forget. Look for nice big scallops, preferably in the shell, and ask your fishmonger to trim them up for you. In Italy pork belly fat is heavily salted, cured with herbs and spices and called lardo. It can be eaten raw as an antipasto with bresaola and prosciutto or can be wrapped around fish and meat before roasting to protect and give flavour. I've slightly modified the recipe using pancetta or smoked streaky bacon, as they're more accessible, but if you come across lardo do buy some.

First of all, cut your peeled celeriac into rough chunks and put them into a pan of boiling salted water. Cook until tender, then drain. While the celeriac's cooking, bash up half the thyme in a pestle and mortar (or in a metal bowl using the end of a rolling pin) and stir in 6 table-spoons of olive oil. Rub this over the scallops and the pancetta before wrapping each scallop in a slice of pancetta. Secure each one with a rosemary stalk or a cocktail stick and place in the fridge.

When your celeriac is cooked, drain and put it into a food processor and whizz it up until really fine (or simply mash it). Loosen with 4 or 5 tablespoons of extra virgin olive oil and season well to taste. Get a non-stick pan hot (you don't need to add any oil). Put the scallops in and cook them for just 2 minutes on each side until the pancetta is nice and crisp, by which time the scallops should be perfect inside. When you turn the scallops over to cook them on the second side, get your plates ready and divide the celeriac between them.

Just as the scallops are finishing sprinkle in the remaining thyme – it'll crisp up in 20 seconds. Remove the scallops and thyme then divide on to the celeriac. Allow the pan to cool a little, then squeeze in the lemon juice and a couple of tablespoons of olive oil. Stir in any sticky goodness stuck to the bottom of the pan, then drizzle this dressing all over your scallops, while it's warm. Nice served with a green salad and a bottle of wine.

Try this: If you like your mash to be nice and smooth, then a good tip is to push it through a sieve with a spatula after you've mashed it.

SERVES 4

2 celeriacs, peeled

sea salt and freshly ground black pepper

1 handful of fresh lemon thyme, leaves picked

extra virgin olive oil

3 or 4 scallops per person

6–8 rashers of pancetta

optional: sticks of fresh rosemary (see page 248)

juice of 2 lemons

FRYING

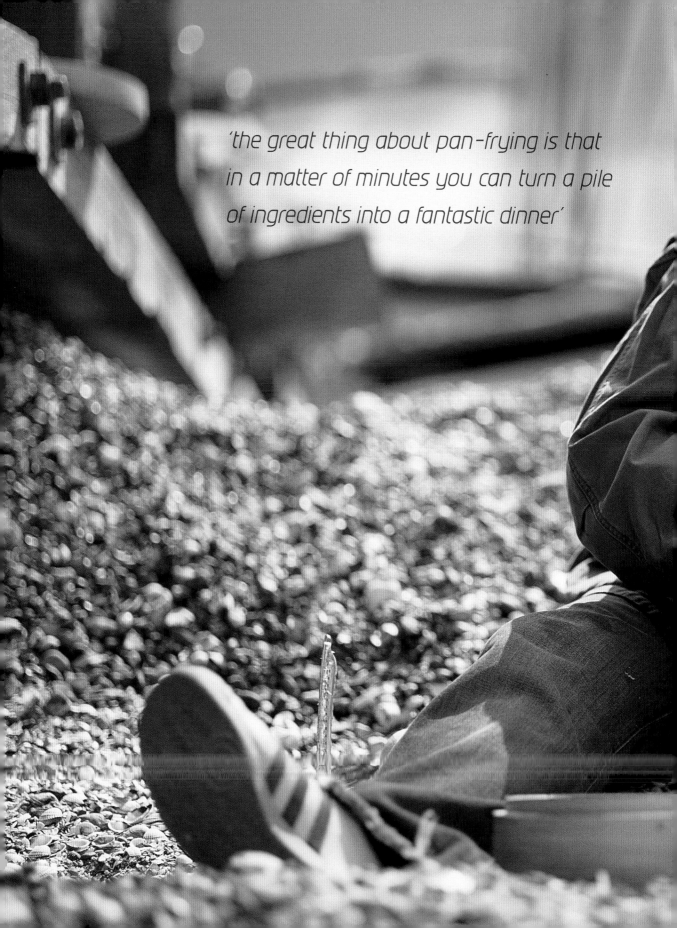

'the great thing about pan-frying is that in a matter of minutes you can turn a pile of ingredients into a fantastic dinner'

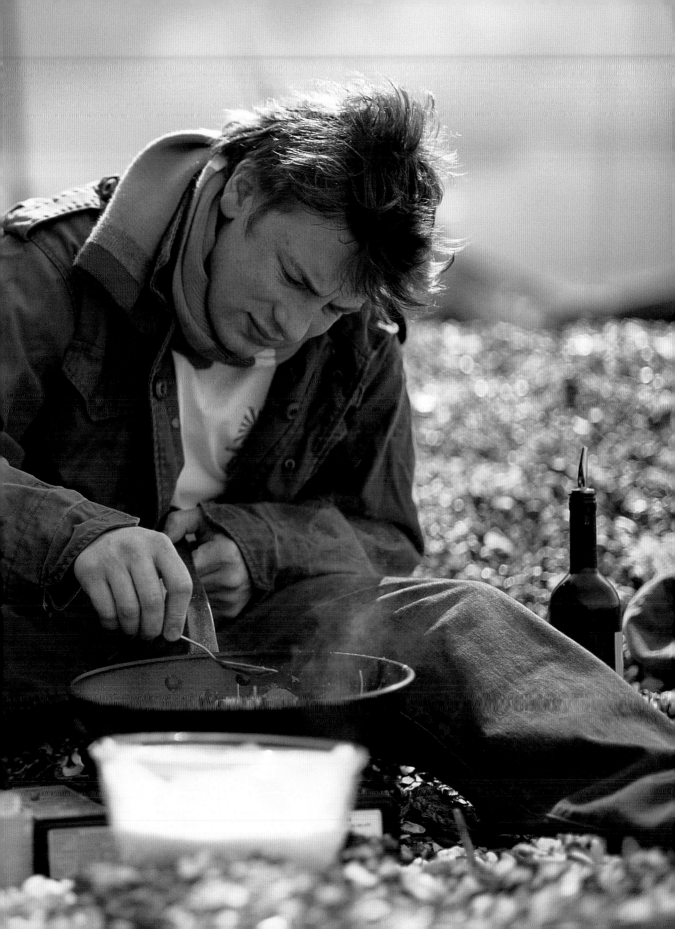

pan-seared sole fillets with loadsa herbs, capers, butter and wet polenta

This is a great dish – it's light, comforting and really quick to cook. I love the combination – Italians go mad for fish with wet polenta, which looks a bit like porridge (you can also make a thicker polenta and grill it). You can buy polenta in just about every supermarket these days, and using this method it tastes fantastic. I've noticed that supermarkets sell ready-made polenta, which is the most disgusting thing, so make sure that you get the authentic dried version. P.S. Depending on how your fishmonger filleted the lemon sole, you may have 2 double fillets or 4 single ones per fish – either way it doesn't really matter.

Put 1 litre/1¾ pints of water in a large high-sided pan over a high heat. As soon as it starts to boil, whisk in the polenta, reduce the heat to a low simmer and place the lid on – if it boils too hard it sometimes bubbles up and spits like a volcano. Stir it every 2 or 3 minutes if you can. After 25 minutes the polenta should have a porridge-like consistency – if it's too thick, loosen it with a little extra boiling water from the kettle. Remove from the heat and season well to taste with salt, pepper, the Parmesan and two-thirds of the butter. Whisk hard until the polenta is smooth, then place a lid on top (it can sit happily for 20 minutes).

Preheat a large non-stick frying pan so it's nice and hot. Season the fish fillets on both sides with salt and pepper and lemon zest. Add a couple of tablespoons of olive oil to the hot pan then add your fish fillets – you may have to cook them in batches. After a minute have a look underneath one of the fish. If it's golden, lower the heat, add the remaining butter, flip the fillets over, sprinkle in the capers, marjoram, chervil and celery leaves, and cook until lightly golden on the other side. Remove from the heat and squeeze the lemon juice into the pan. This should foam with the butter, giving you a light sauce. Just before you serve, check the consistency of the polenta and give it a stir. If it has thickened up then just add a little water to it. Divide the polenta between your plates, put the fish on top and drizzle over the pan juices. Sprinkle with the capers and herbs.

Try this: In place of lemon sole you could use plaice, Dover sole or dabs, which are often called a poor man's lemon sole. Scallops and nice fresh prawns are also really good with it.

SERVES 4

150g/5½oz polenta

sea salt and freshly ground black pepper

2 handfuls of freshly grated Parmesan cheese

150g/5½oz butter

4 lemon soles, filleted and skinned

zest and juice of 2 lemons

extra virgin olive oil

2 heaped tablespoons small capers

1 small handful of fresh marjoram, leaves picked

1 small handful of fresh chervil, leaves picked

yellow leaves from 1 celery heart

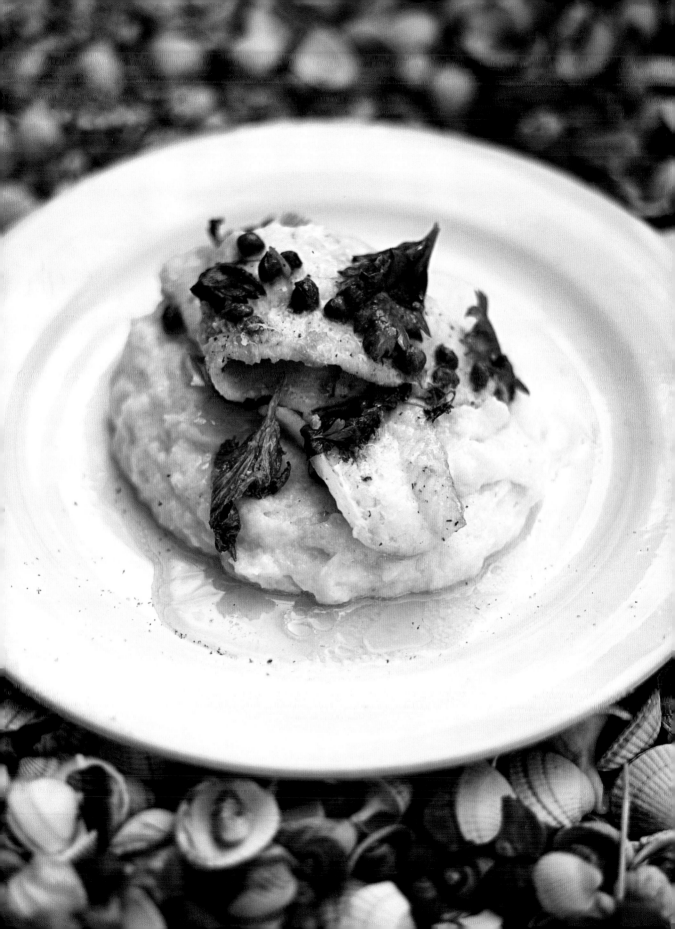

FILLETING A FLAT FISH

Here are some pictures to show you how to go about filleting a flat fish. You can do the same to any flat fish like brill, turbot or halibut.

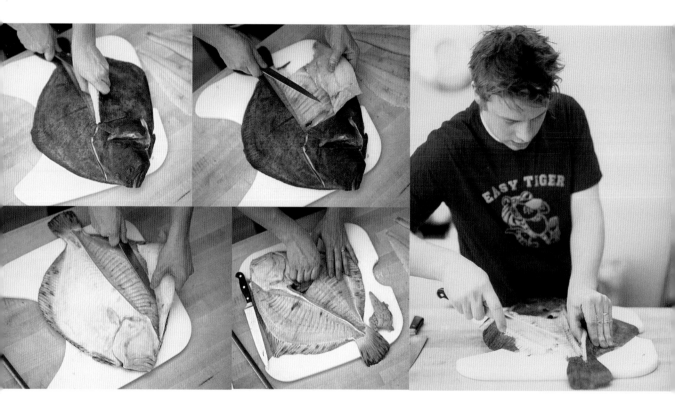

1. Score down the natural line of the fish along the spine.

2. Using a flexible filleting knife allows you to push the knife against the bone so you don't cut into the fish.

3. Make clean slices to loosen and remove the fillet.

4. Do this on all sides to give you a lovely filleted fish.

5. Easy Tiger!

TRANCHING A FLAT FISH

To cut a fish into 'tranches' means to cut it into steaks. It involves cutting through the bone, which can be slightly tricky, but give it a go.

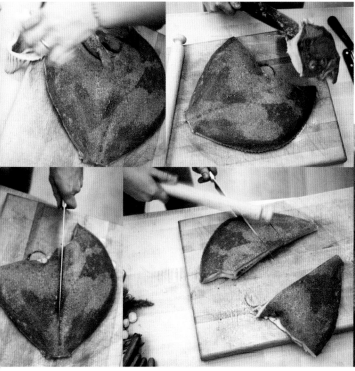

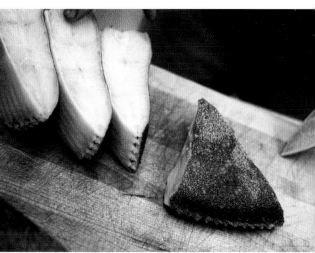

1. Remove the 'skirt' of the fish – follow the natural line of the body.

2. Cut around the head. Try not to cut away too much of the flesh.

3. Using a large knife, cut down the backbone. Simply follow the natural line.

4. Cut into 'tranches' and bash the heel of the knife with a rolling pin to help cut through.

5. Lovely fish steaks.

the best tempura lobster with dipping sauce

Tempura is a crisp batter which originates from Portuguese settlers in Japan and has become a part of Japanese culture. It's great for battering fish, shellfish and vegetables. In Japan there are lots of tempura restaurants where everyone sits behind a bar and you get given the most amazing tempura for over two hours by a chef and his 'master', who does a lot of shouting.

To kill the lobsters take a sharp knife, place it at the crown of the head, and cut straight down – this will kill them straight away. Twist off the tail and both claws and discard the rest of the body and the legs (or keep to make soup or stock). Cut the tail in half lengthways and each tail half into 3. Chop the claws into 3 and place, in a bowl, with the tail pieces.

Mix the dipping sauce ingredients together in a bowl and set aside.

I suggest you use a deep-fat fryer as it's easier to control. Heat it to 170°C/325°F. You can use a wok half-filled with sunflower oil, safely positioned on a stove with a thermometer, but be aware of other people (curious kids) and of possibly knocking things over if doing it this way. To make the batter, whisk the egg yolks and iced water together, add the cornflour and flour, and stir together using chopsticks – this helps to keep the batter a bit lumpy, which is what you want. Add the okra, chillies and lobster pieces to the batter. Once battered, pick up the lobster and veg, shake off any excess batter and carefully put them into the oil.

Don't try to cook the tempura all at once – do them in 4 or 5 batches. Cook them until light golden and crisp on both sides. Remove them using a slotted spoon, drain on some kitchen paper and then put them on to a plate. Serve the tempura with the dipping sauce and a dish of flavoured salt – I would suggest either jasmine tea salt or citrus salt (see page 244).

Try this: I once worked in a Japanese restaurant and when the chefs put the veg into the oil, they dripped extra batter from a height on to them. This gave the tempura a really crunchy, spiky look and feel. You don't have to do this but it's a good little trick.

Or this: Tempura other veggies like fine slices of sweet potato, whole spring onions, coriander stalks and baby courgettes.

SERVES 4

2 x 1.3kg/2lb 14oz live lobsters

sunflower oil

1 handful of okra, left whole

4 fresh red chillies, left whole

optional: edible flowers, such as viola, borage, courgette

for the tempura batter

2 egg yolks

350ml/12fl oz iced water

1 teaspoon cornflour

175g/6oz self-raising flour

for the dipping sauce

12 tablespoons rice wine vinegar

4 tablespoons sugar

2 tablespoons soy sauce

2 teaspoons grated fresh ginger

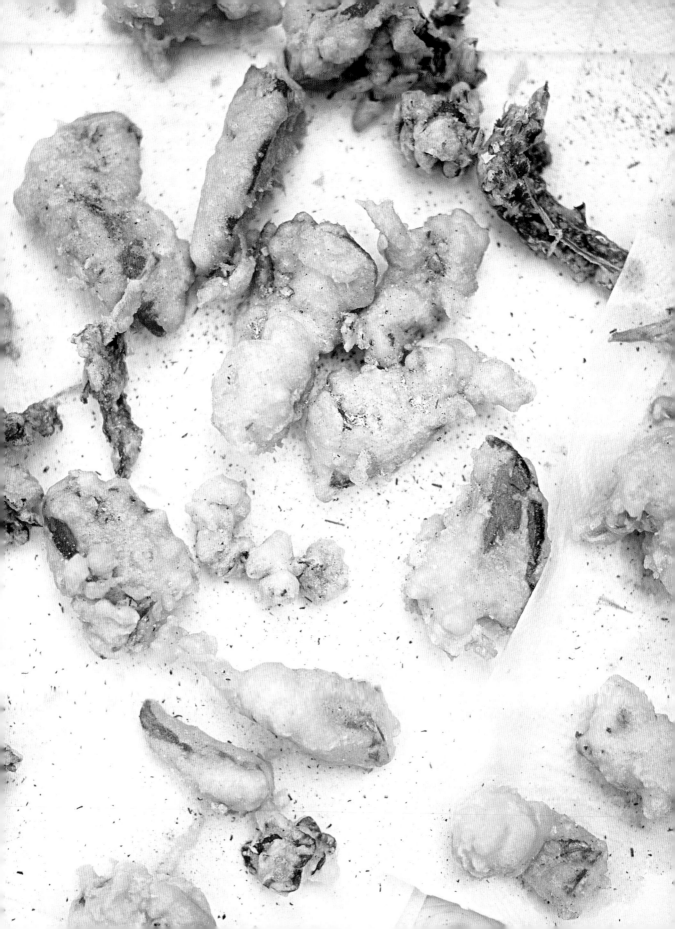

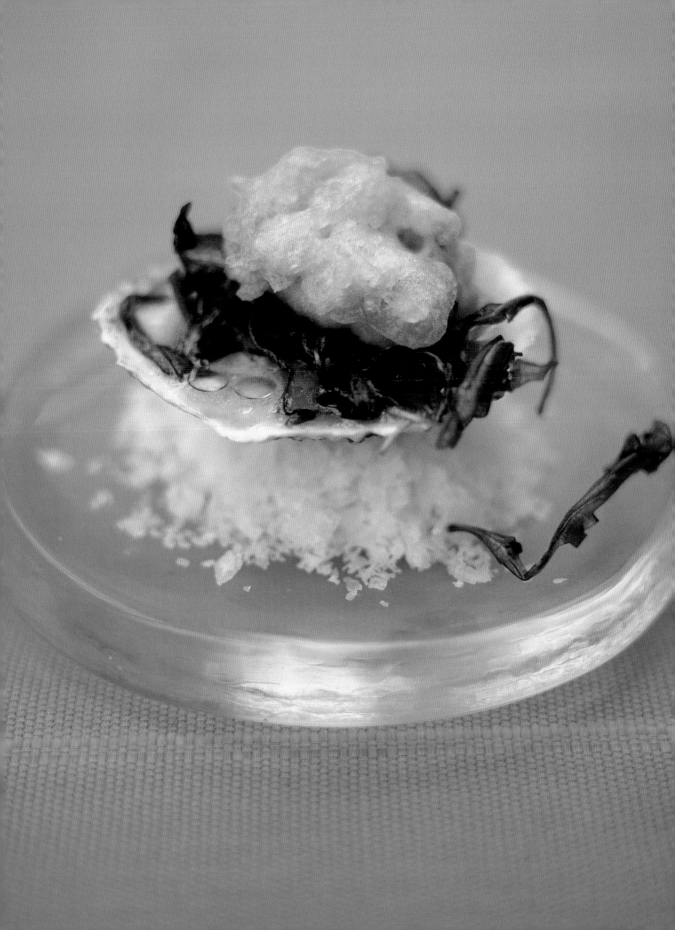

deep-fried oysters with fried rocket and tomato dressing

I first put these oysters on the menu at Monte's – they were served raw with the tomato dressing. One day we tempuraed them to serve as canapés and they went down so well I thought I'd give you the recipe. When picking the kids for the new restaurant I served these to them as a bit of a taste test and asked for their reaction. They're such an experience to eat as they're crunchy, soft, sour, sweet and salty. You can serve these as a starter, or as canapés.

Open the oysters and clean the shells or ask your fishmonger to do this for you. To make the batter, whisk the flour with the cold water and fold in the stiff whisked egg whites and a tablespoon of olive oil. To make the dressing, whizz the tomatoes in a blender with the horseradish, garlic and vinegar. Add the Tabasco and season with salt and pepper. Tweak the amounts of Tabasco and vinegar to taste – you want it to be hot and tangy. Pass the mixture through a fine sieve to remove any chunky bits. This will give you a nice smooth dressing. Check the seasoning.

Heat the oil in a deep-fat fryer to 180°C/350°F and fry the rocket in small batches for about 25 seconds until nice and crisp. Remove and place on some kitchen paper. Drop each oyster into the batter, then remove with a spoon and fry for around 2 minutes until crisp and golden. Serve each oyster in its shell on a little fried rocket, drizzled with the tangy tomato dressing.

Try this: You can place the shells on some cracked ice or a bed of coarse sea salt, as I have done in the picture.

SERVES 4 ·

24 native oysters

100g/3½oz flour

170ml/6fl oz cold water

1 egg white, whisked

olive oil

1 litre/1¾ pints vegetable oil

2 bags of rocket

for the dressing

12 ripe plum tomatoes

2 tablespoons of horseradish, creamed or freshly grated

¼ of a clove of garlic, peeled

2 tablespoons white wine vinegar

a couple of drops of Tabasco

sea salt and freshly ground black pepper

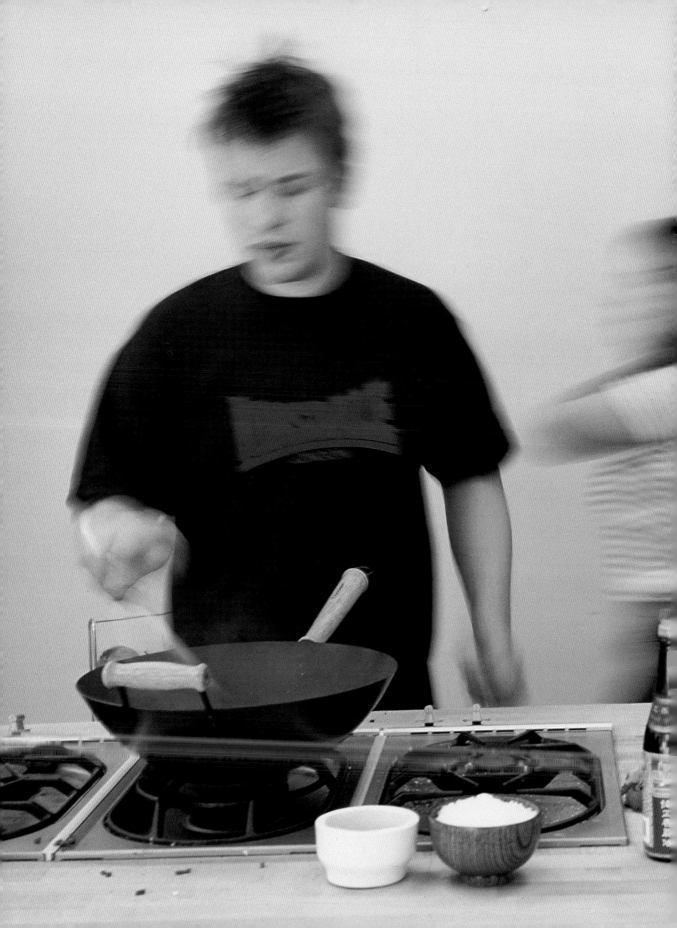

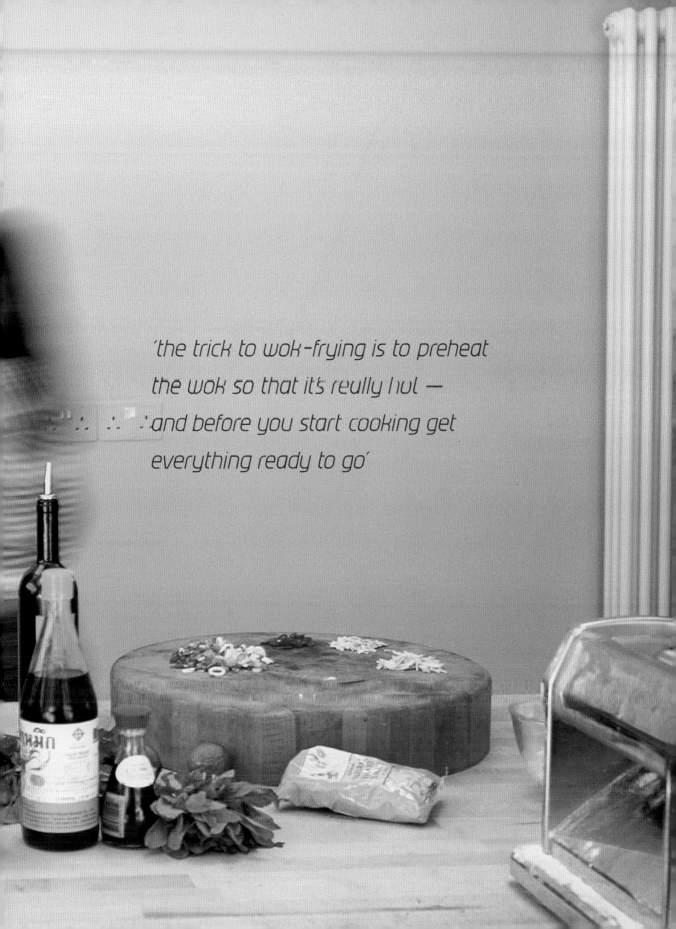

'the trick to wok-frying is to preheat
the wok so that it's really hot —
and before you start cooking get
everything ready to go'

FILLETING A ROUND FISH

You can ask your fishmonger to do this for you, but if you want to have a go yourself, this is how it's done. These basic steps show how to prep all round fish, like bass, trout, haddock or red mullet. It might be an idea to ask your fishmonger to scale and gut the fish for you first, as this can be quite a messy job.

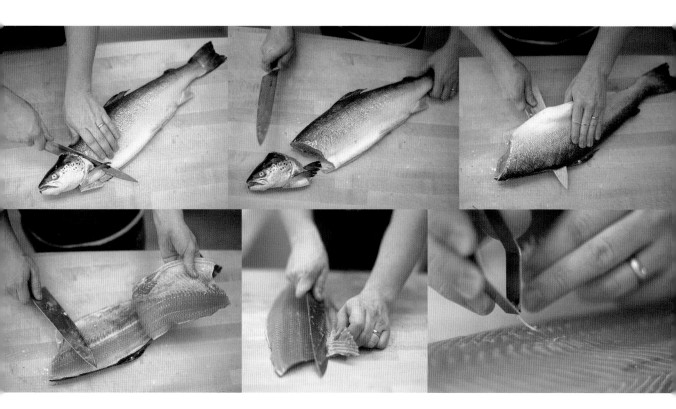

1. Score towards the head at the end of the fillet.

2. Do this on both sides of the fish and then cut through to detach the head.

3. Using a sturdy knife, slice down the length of the fish close to the spine bone.

4. Once you've cut through you can remove the fillet.

5. Skim off the rib bones.

6. Remove the pinbones with some fish tweezers.

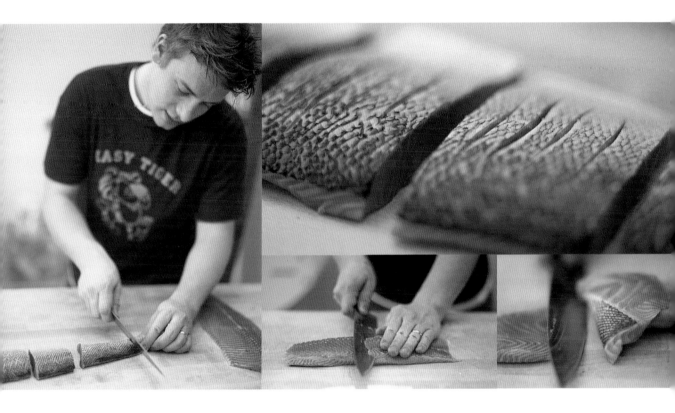

7. Place the fillets skin side up then divide them into 200-225g/7-8oz fillet portions (sometimes called supremes or steaks).

8. Score through the skin about 1cm/½ inch deep – you can season or push herbs into the score marks.

9. Cut the portions at an angle to give you escalopes.

10. You can leave the skin on the fish when you cook it and simply remove it before eating if you prefer.

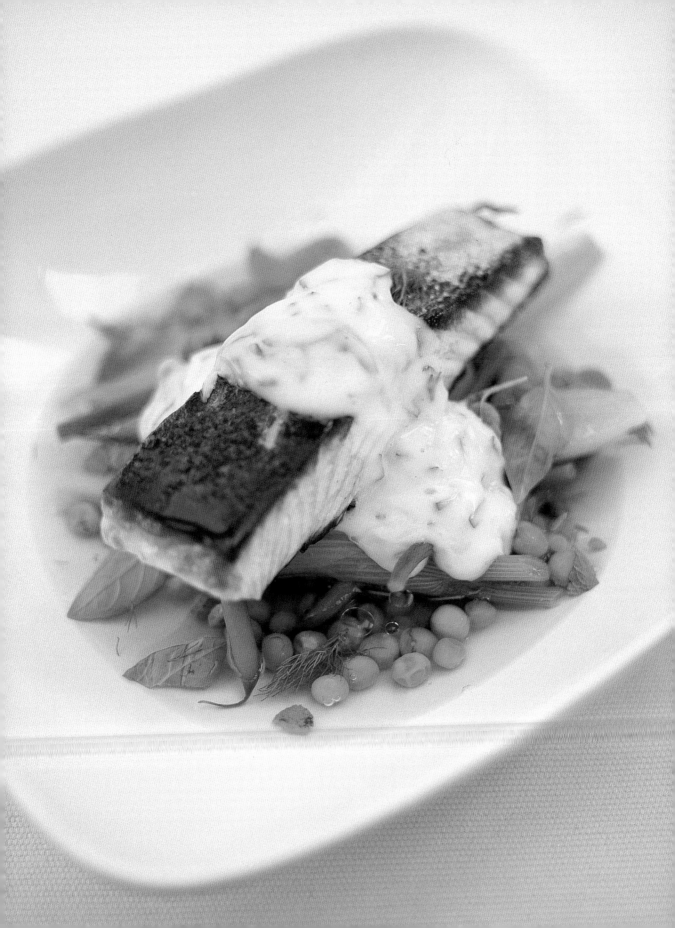

crispy fried salmon with spring vegetable broth

There's nothing like a piece of perfectly cooked salmon with a crispy, crunchy skin, perfectly complemented by a spring veg broth. In the markets and supermarkets these days you can get some fantastic spring vegetables: baby carrots with tops, baby fennel with its herby leaves, baby turnips, peas and broad beans, fine green and yellow French beans, all really colourful and easy to cook with. Here's a nice little combination – it's all cooked in the same pot and gives you a lovely broth. The only thing you have to do is control the cooking times by adding the veg that need longer in the pot first.

First, make the aïoli. When you've done that, bring your stock to the boil in a large pan then add your fennel and allow this to boil for 4 minutes while you heat up a non-stick frying pan. Take your salmon steaks and, if you fancy it, you could finely slice a little of your mint and basil and push this into the score marks. Pat the salmon steaks with a little olive oil, season and place skin-side down in the frying pan. Leave them for 2 minutes to get really crispy then check how they're doing. They'll want around 4 minutes on the skin side and 1 minute on the other. You'll get an idea of how they're cooking as you'll see the salmon change colour.

When the fennel has had 4 minutes, add the green beans and the broad beans. Give them a further 2 minutes. By this time you will probably want to turn over the salmon steaks for their last minute. Add the peas to the other veg and cook for a final 2 minutes. Don't be tempted to overcook the salmon – remove it from the heat. Divide the vegetables between 4 bowls, rip over the mint and basil, ladle over some of your hot cooking stock and place the salmon on top. Serve with a dollop of aïoli. Fantastic!

SERVES 4

1 x aïoli recipe (see page 203)

850ml/1½ pints chicken or vegetable stock, lightly seasoned

8 baby bulbs of fennel, stalks removed and herby tops reserved

4 x 170–225g/6–8oz salmon steaks, scored (see page 199)

1 small handful of fresh mint, ripped

1 small handful of fresh basil, leaves picked

extra virgin olive oil

sea salt and freshly ground black pepper

around 100g/3½oz green beans, finely trimmed

around 100g/3½oz podded broad beans

around 100g/3½oz podded peas

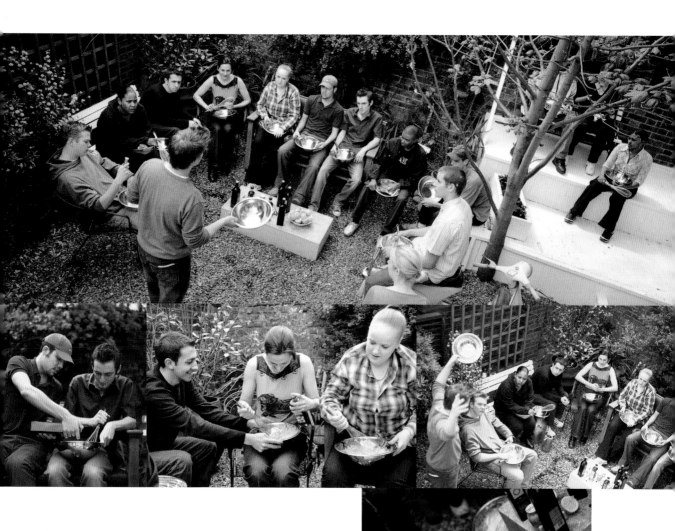

'after I'd talked them through it, my guys made aïoli with no problems at all'

aïoli

Aïoli is a lovely fragrant and pungent type of mayonnaise – and the great thing is that you can take the flavour in any direction – try adding some pounded or chopped basil, fennel tops, dill or roasted nuts. Also great flavoured with lemon zest and juice. It's normally seasoned well and is used to enhance things like fish stew in order to give them a real kick. You might wonder why I suggest using 2 types of olive oil to make this. By blending a strong peppery one with a mellower one you achieve a lovely rounded flavour.

Smash up the garlic with 1 teaspoon of salt in a pestle and mortar (or use the end of a rolling pin and a metal bowl). Place the egg yolk and mustard in a bowl and whisk together, then start to add your olive oils bit by bit. Once you've blended in a quarter of the oil you can start to add the rest in larger amounts. When it's all gone in, add the garlic and lemon juice and any extra flavours (see above). To finish it off, season to taste with salt, pepper and a bit more lemon juice if needed.

Try this: Lemon- or basil-flavoured aïoli are good with salads, all types of fish, and in seafood soups. Also great with roasted fish, chicken or pork, and classic with salmon.

SERVES 8

½ a small clove of garlic, peeled

sea salt and freshly ground black pepper

1 large egg yolk

1 teaspoon Dijon mustard

285ml/½ pint extra virgin olive oil

285ml/½ pint olive oil

lemon juice, to taste

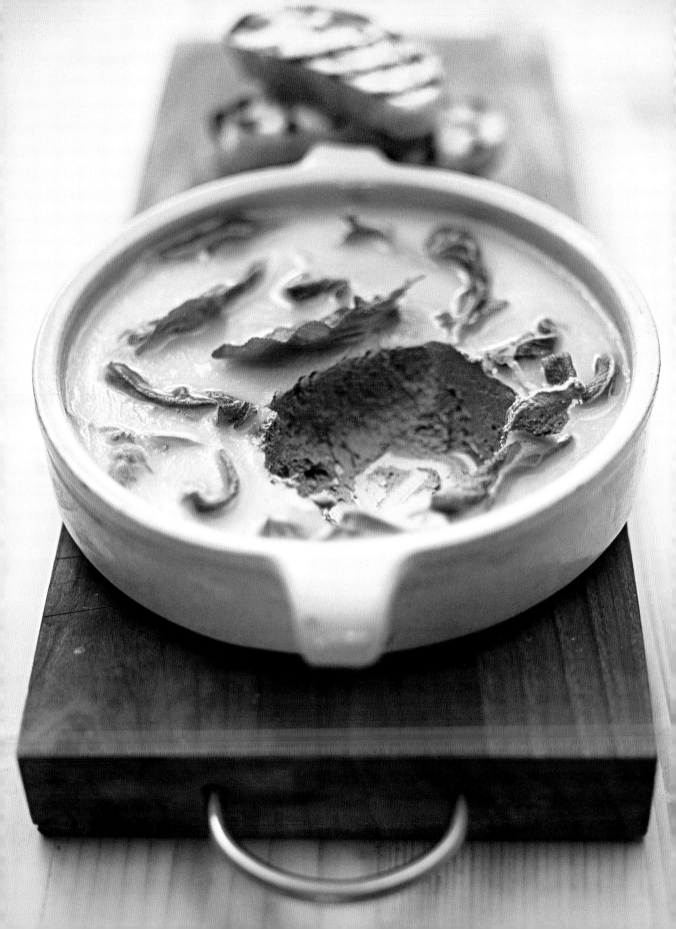

chicken liver parfait

This is quite an old-school dish, but it's so quick, cheap and simple to do. Have a go at making it.

First put 150g/5½oz of butter in a bowl and melt slowly in the oven at 110°C/225°F/gas ¼ until it has separated. Strain off the yellow clarified butter into another bowl and set aside. Throw away the milky liquid.

Get yourself a frying pan and heat a little olive oil in it. Slowly fry the onion and garlic for 5 minutes until soft and tender then remove to a plate. Wipe the pan clean then turn up the heat, add a little lug of olive oil and throw in your livers and thyme. Cook the livers in one layer until lightly coloured but still a little pink in the middle – if you overcook them they will become grainy rather than having a smooth texture. Pour in the brandy – if you're using a gas hob you can flame it until the alcohol cooks off but watch your hair! Simmer for a minute, then take the livers off the heat and tip into a food processor with the cooked onion and garlic. Blitz until you have a smooth purée. Add the rest of the butter and continue to blitz, then season the mixture well. I like to push it through a sieve twice before dividing it into serving bowls.

Fry the sage leaves in a little hot oil until crisp and drain on kitchen paper. Sprinkle over the parfaits. Spoon the clarified butter over the sage leaves. Leave the parfaits to set in the fridge for 1 hour. They will taste beautiful straight away but even better if the flavours are left to develop for a couple of days – they never tend to last that long in my house though! They will keep for at least 2 weeks if you make sure that the butter seal is not disturbed and so is kept airtight.

Try this: You can make this parfait using duck or rabbit livers, and try flavouring it with different herbs or a different kind of booze.

SERVES 6

400g/14oz softened butter

olive oil

1 onion, peeled and finely chopped

2 cloves of garlic, finely chopped

455g/1lb chicken livers, trimmed

1 small bunch of fresh thyme, leaves picked and chopped

1 large wineglass of brandy

sea salt and freshly ground black pepper

a few fresh sage leaves

polenta-encrusted fried chicken with sweetcorn mash, fried bananas and green tomato relish

I was thinking about green tomatoes, corn and yams the other day and was inspired to come up with this cracking little dinner – a sort of cross between the food from New Orleans and the West Indies.

Carefully cut each fresh corn cob in half and strip the kernels off by sitting each cob on its end and slicing down the sides. To make the mash, boil the potatoes in salted water until cooked. Drain and return them to the hot pan with the milk, corn kernels and some salt and pepper. Bring back to the boil, then turn off the heat. Throw in the spring onions. Mash up with a masher, season and keep warm.

To make the relish, put the vinegar, sugar and sliced shallots in a saucepan. Bring to the boil and cook until reduced by half. Add the chopped tomatoes and warm through. Remove from the heat, season with salt and pepper, and add the olive oil. The herbs are added just before serving.

Take each chicken breast and make 2 slices into the meat lengthways so that the breast fans out into 3 'prongs'. Mix the flour with the spices and salt and pepper and spread it out on a plate. Now beat the egg in a bowl with a fork, and pour the polenta on to another plate. Place the 2 plates and the bowl next to each other. Dip the chicken breasts in the flour first, shaking off any excess, then in the egg, and finally in the polenta. This will give you a lovely polenta crust.

Heat a large frying pan and gently fry the chicken in 2 tablespoons of the butter for about 5 minutes on each side, turning it half-way through. When the chicken is cooked and golden brown, remove it from the pan and keep it warm. Peel the bananas and cut it in half lengthways. Fry in a little more butter until tender and golden.

To serve, spoon a mound of mash on to each serving plate with a piece of banana on top. Place a piece of crispy chicken on top. Stir the parsley and mint into the relish and put a big dollop on top of the chicken.

SERVES 4

4 skinless chicken breast fillets

200g/7oz flour

1 tablespoon allspice

1 teaspoon cinnamon

1 teaspoon chilli powder

2 eggs

200g/7oz polenta

2–3 tablespoons butter

2 bananas

for the mash

8 medium potatoes

sea salt and freshly ground black pepper

255ml/9fl oz milk

4 cobs of corn

1 bunch of finely sliced spring onions

for the relish

100ml/3³/₄fl oz vinegar

2 teaspoons sugar

2 shallots, peeled and sliced

400g/14oz green or red tomatoes, chopped

6 tablespoons extra virgin olive oil

2 handfuls of fresh flat-leaf parsley, chopped

2 handfuls of fresh mint, chopped

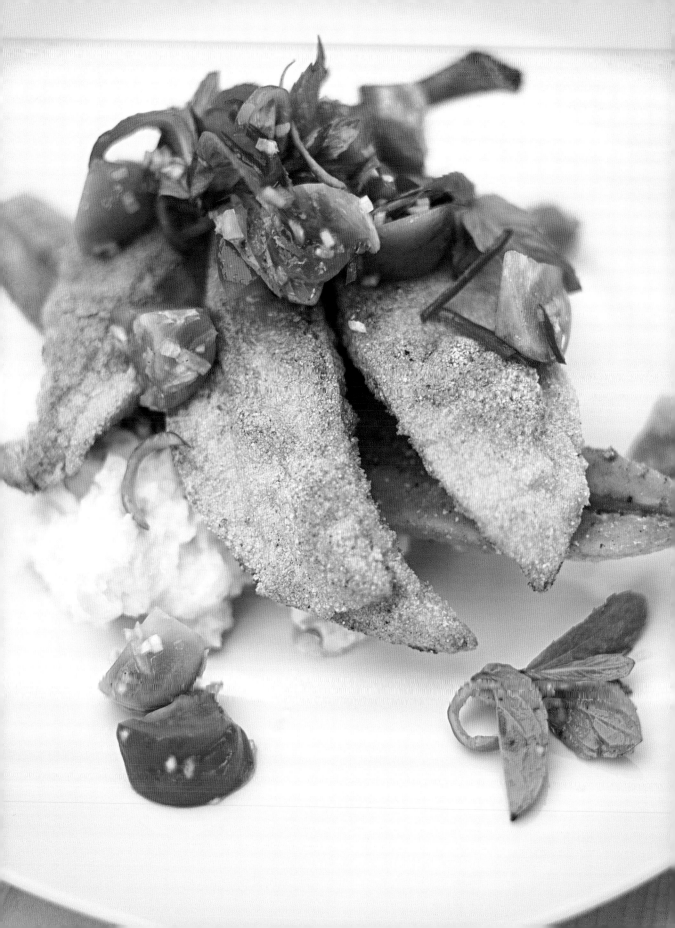

chips

I'm putting chips in the book because if they're cooked properly they're one of the tastiest things in the world. That crunch and fluffy softness inside is absolutely irresistible – especially if they're someone else's!

A good chip requires control and vigilance when cooking. Get yourself a nice spud – Maris Piper, Desirée and King Edward are all good. You can peel them or leave the skin on – either way, slice them up 1cm/$\frac{1}{2}$ inch thick and then 1 cm/$\frac{1}{2}$ inch across into chips. I remember when I was 7 years old and my first job in the kitchen after being promoted from cleaning the bins, washing up and cleaning the vegetables was chipping. I used to have to stand on a pale ale beer crate so that I was high enough to chip. After 3 sacks of potatoes you get quite fast at chipping! But from a safety point of view, it's important that you get yourself a nice flat edge on your potato before starting to slice fast. So, first of all, cut a 1cm/$\frac{1}{2}$inch slice off the potato, then roll it on to that flat edge so it doesn't wobble about and continue to slice up all your spuds. Wash them in water, so they don't stick to each other, and dry them well on some kitchen paper.

Half fill your fryer or chip pan with clean sunflower oil. Heat it to 150°C/300°F – if you haven't got a thermometer, test the oil by putting one chip into the basket. It's hot enough when it sizzles at a moderate speed. Make sure that the chips are nice and dry, then put them into the basket in small batches and gently lower into the oil. Be aware of whether the temperature is too hot or too cold. Continue to cook the chips without letting them colour until they feel softened when you poke them. Drain well, and if you're eating them later, scatter them on to greaseproof paper, then put them to one side on a tray until you are ready to fry them again before eating them.

If you're eating them straight away, turn the heat up to 180°C/350°F (or when a chip fries fast). Carefully place the basket back into the oil and cook until the chips are crisp and golden. Drain well and season with sea salt. Even better is to use one of the flavoured salts on page 244. This will make them absolutely fantastic. It's really only worth cooking chips for a small number of people, otherwise you may as well go down the chippie, but the best ones can be made at home.

PS: other parsnips, sweet potatoes and butternut squash can all be deep fried as chips. They won't be quite as crisp as potato chips, but they will be damn fine.

opposite: 'today's headline, tomorrow's chip wrapper'

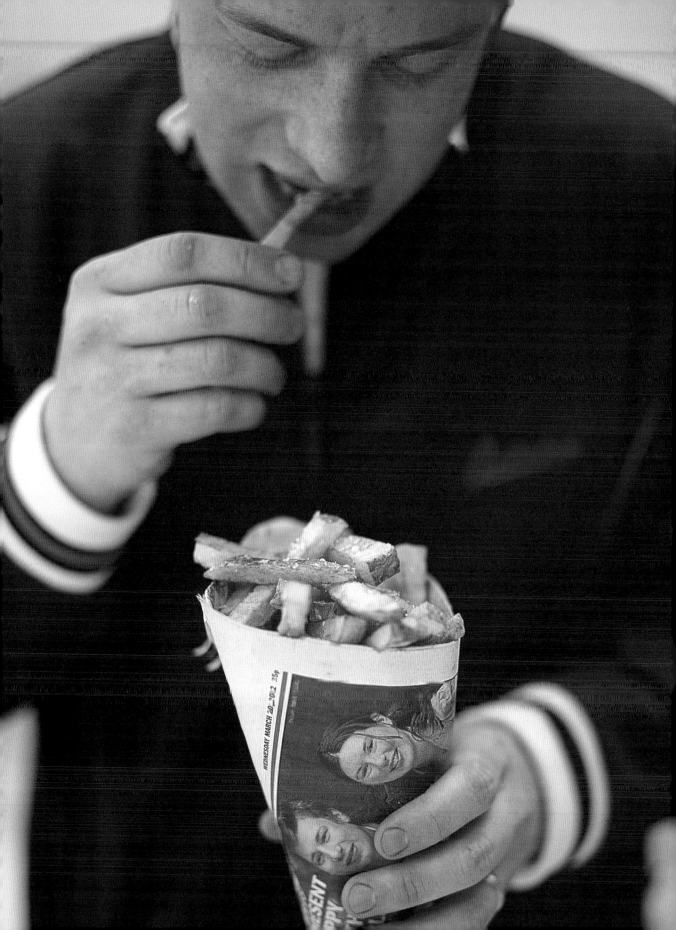

ROASTING,
POT-ROASTING
AND
PAN-ROASTING

ROASTING

I think roasting is my favourite way of cooking. It uses dry oven heat, radiated from above and below, sometimes with a convection fan. Using different oils and flavourings rubbed over food before cooking, roasting gives meat, fish and vegetables a beautiful, succulent flavour. It's convenient, because you can cook a single pork chop, a whole loin of pork for a big family or do a whole chicken or a rack of lamb. You might even want to try roasting a whole suckling pig (see page 236).

Roasting doesn't have to use expensive cuts of meat like fillets and loins – you can very successfully roast shoulders and bellies of pork and lamb, which usually get stewed or made into sausages and mince. With longer cooking and slightly less heat these can be just as good as more expensive cuts.

POT-ROASTING

Pot-roasting is a cross between roasting and braising. You can pot-roast anything you like but traditionally it was used for cooking tougher cuts of meat for a long time. However, any cut of meat or fish can be pot-roasted for a shorter length of time, with great results. Stick to quite large cuts – enough to feed about 8 people. The idea is that you get a snug-fitting, high-sided pan or roasting tray, cover the bottom with a mixture of roughly chopped vegetables, put your browned meat on top, seasoned in any way you like, add a little stock or booze and then cover it with a lid and roast it, basting the meat a couple of times during cooking. This maximizes the flavour of everything in the pan, resulting in tasty succulent meat and the potential for a fantastic sauce.

PAN-ROASTING

With pan-roasting you start things off in a hot pan on the hob – game birds and whole fish are both good cooked like this. Once the meat is lightly coloured it goes into the oven to finish off for the rest of the cooking time.

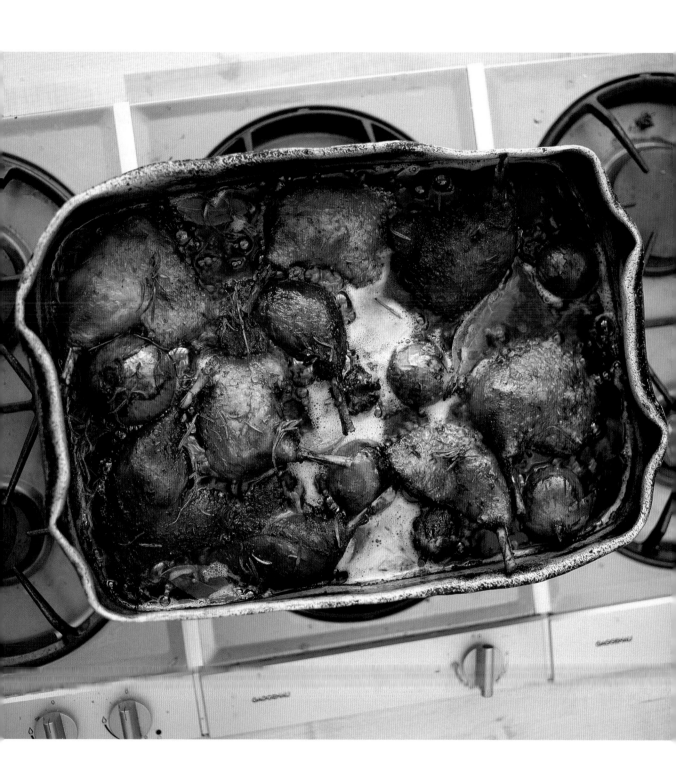

italian-style confit of duck

This is a great way to cook as the meat becomes so moist and sticky, and the skin becomes dead crispy. Confit of duck is traditionally duck legs which have been preserved after simmering in their own fat. It can be stored for 3 or 4 months in the larder or fridge. It's best kept in a sterilized jar, but to be honest I've used plastic Tupperware containers quite successfully and kept them in the fridge for a couple of months. Duck or goose fat is available from supermarkets or good butchers.

In a pestle and mortar (or in a metal bowl using the end of a rolling pin) bash up the marinade ingredients. Rub this over the duck legs and leave overnight to let the flavours penetrate and any moisture drip out.

Preheat the oven to about 170°C/325°F/gas 3. Brush the marinade off the duck legs and put them into a small heavy-bottomed roasting tray that they can fit into tightly. Add your duck or goose fat. Put the tray into the preheated oven and cook for about 2 hours, spooning the fat over the duck legs every so often, until the skin of the duck is crisp and the meat is tender. Five minutes before the end, add the rosemary, bay leaves, juniper berries and peppercorns to the tray to crisp up.

Take the tray out of the oven and allow the duck legs to cool a little. Put them into a sterilized container or Tupperware tub with the thyme, bay leaves, juniper berries and peppercorns. Pour over the fat from the roasting tray – you may want to sieve it. Cover and allow to cool. The confit is now ready to store in the fridge.

When you want to eat some, just remove the number of duck legs you need. Put them on a roasting tray in a hot oven at 250°C/450°F/ gas 8 for about 20 minutes, until the skin is really crisp and the meat is so tender it will fall off the bone.

Try this: Lovely served with roasted radicchio (see page 214).

Or this: Whole onions can be added to the tray with the duck legs. They roast really well, especially like this on a low heat for a couple of hours. Cook until soft.

SERVES 8

8 large duck legs

2kg/4½lb duck or goose fat

1 handful of fresh rosemary, leaves picked

10 fresh bay leaves

1 tablespoon dried juniper berries

1 tablespoon peppercorns

for the marinade

8 tablespoons coarse sea salt

1 small bunch of fresh thyme, leaves picked

10 fresh bay leaves

1 small handful of dried juniper berries

zest of 2 oranges

roasted radicchio

In England we never really think about roasting radicchio as a vegetable. In fact, most people don't like it that much – it has a slight bitterness to it. But in Italy and France they cook radicchio and its slightly slimmer brother, which the Italians call treviso, as well as other relatives called cicoria and Belgian endive. By adding various herbs and spices to radicchio so many different flavours can be experienced – sweet, sour or smoky, for example. Here's a great way of cooking with radicchio – it can be made into a warm salad with other fresh salad leaves, served alongside fish and meat, or chopped up and used in risottos or pasta dishes.

Preheat your oven to 190°C/375°F/gas 5. Carefully cut the radicchio into quarters – try to keep the core intact so all the leaves stay together. Bash the garlic and thyme to a pulp in a pestle and mortar (or in a metal bowl with a rolling pin). Stir in about 6 tablespoons of extra virgin olive oil and season lightly, then drizzle this flavoured oil over the quartered radicchio so the flavour gets right into it. Wrap a rasher of bacon around each radicchio quarter, leaving the core exposed to the heat. The bacon will protect the delicate leaves and give it a fantastic smoky flavour. Place the radicchio quarters in an ovenproof dish in which they will fit snugly, and sprinkle over the balsamic vinegar. Roast in the preheated oven for 25–30 minutes, until the leaves have softened and the bacon is crisp.

SERVES 4

2 radicchio, outer leaves trimmed back

1 clove of garlic, peeled

1 small bunch of fresh thyme

extra virgin olive oil

sea salt and freshly ground black pepper

8 rashers of dry-cured smoky bacon, or pancetta

10 tablespoons cheap balsamic vinegar

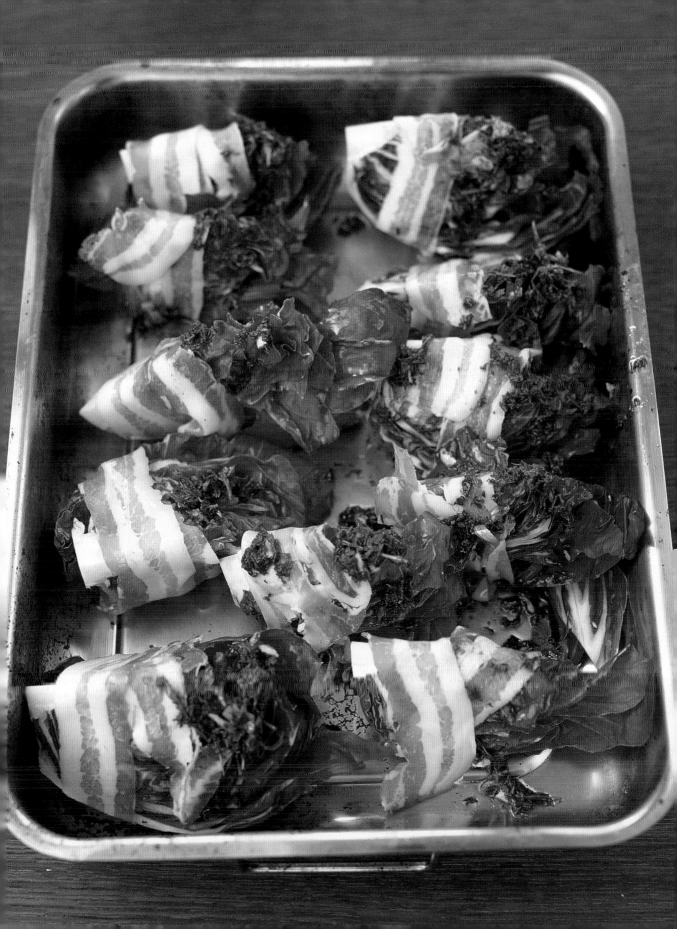

roasted trout and artichokes with almonds, breadcrumbs and mint

I used to go trout-fishing with Grandad when I was a kid. We would catch them, then go straight back to his pub and grill them with a little bit of butter. I liked to eat them with fried potatoes with onions – so good – and a nice squeeze of lemon juice. I came up with this recipe using preserved artichoke hearts from my local deli. In the picture opposite I've used one large 8lb trout, but it works just as well if you use individual trout fillets. Salmon trout or salmon are both good too. Ask your fishmonger to scale, gut and fillet the fish for you.

Preheat the oven to 220°C/425°F/gas 7 and rub a roasting tray with a little olive oil. Lay 4 of the trout fillets, skin side down, on the tray, with a few bits of string under each fillet. Lightly toast the almonds in the oven for a couple of minutes – watch them carefully as they don't take long – then bash them up using a pestle and mortar (or a metal bowl and a rolling pin). Try to get some powdery and some chunks. Put the almonds into a bowl and rip in the mint. Take the crusts off the ciabatta and whizz it up in a food processor or chop up. Add the lemon zest, chopped garlic, artichoke hearts, and 5 tablespoons of olive oil to the bowl with a good pinch of salt and pepper. Mix it up well and sprinkle a good handful of the mix over each trout fillet. Place the other 4 fillets on top of the breadcrumb mix, skin side up, laying a bacon rasher along the top of each one, and secure with the string (see picture below). Sprinkle the thyme over the top and any excess filling around the tray.

Place in the middle of the preheated oven and cook for about 15 minutes, until the trout is golden and crisp. Season the crème fraîche generously with salt and pepper and add a little lemon juice.

When the fish is ready, cut the string and serve the fillets with a nice drizzle of crème fraîche and a green salad. Give everyone a lemon half on their plate so they can squeeze the juice over their fish.

SERVES 4
extra virgin olive oil
8 x 200g/7oz trout fillets
1 good handful of almonds, blanched
1 bunch of fresh mint, leaves picked
1 ciabatta, preferably stale
zest and juice of 2 lemons
1 clove of garlic, peeled and finely chopped
16 marinated artichoke hearts, drained and sliced
4 rashers of smoked streaky bacon
sea salt and freshly ground black pepper
1 small handful of fresh thyme, leaves picked
5 tablespoons crème fraîche or fromage frais

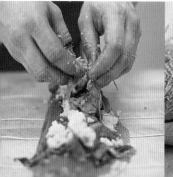
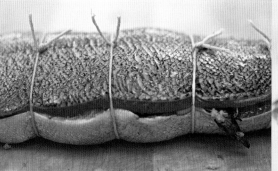
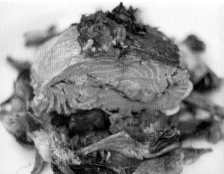

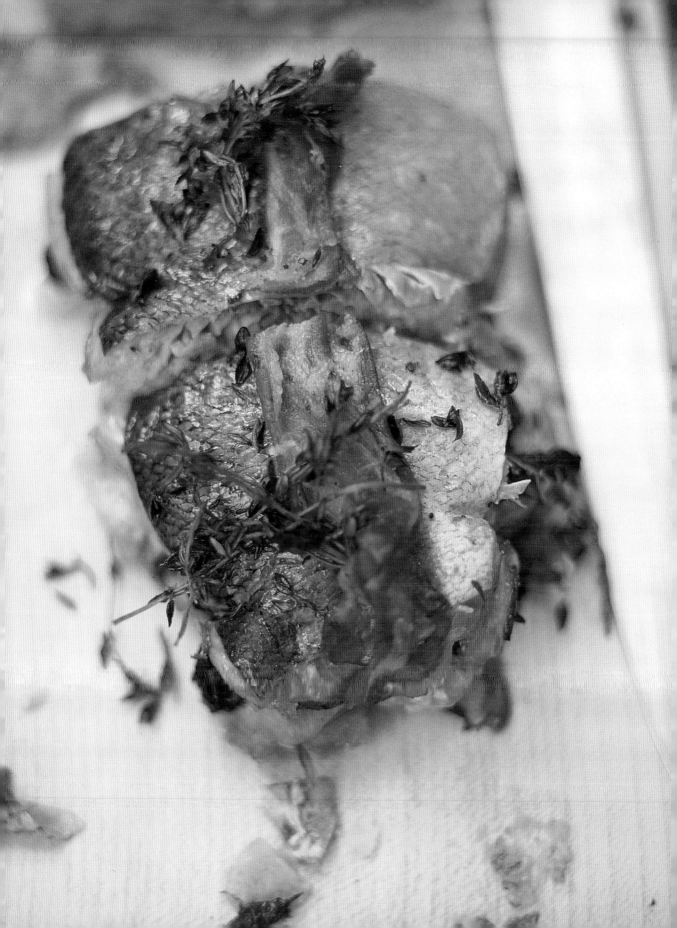

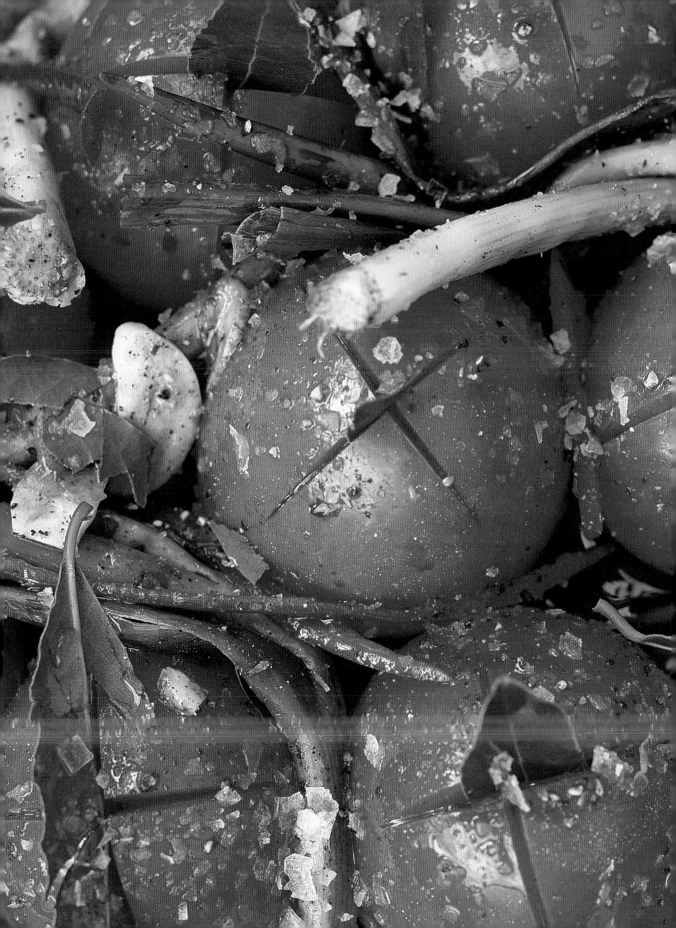

slow-roasted balsamic tomatoes with baby leeks and basil

This is one of those recipes that, apart from being damn tasty, is kind of slapdash but so easy to make and consistently good. You can really get some mileage out of it. The key things are to get yourself some best-quality plum tomatoes and buy some cheap balsamic vinegar, as you'll be using a lot of it.

Preheat the oven to 170°C/325°F/gas 3.

Score the tops of the tomatoes with a cross. Take an earthenware dish that the tomatoes will fit snugly into, and sprinkle the garlic and basil all over the bottom of it. Stand the tomatoes next to each other in the tray, on top of the garlic and basil, then push the bay leaves well into the scores in the tomatoes and season well. Lay the leeks on a board and sprinkle generously with salt and pepper. Using a rolling pin, press down on top of the leeks to really squeeze the seasoning into them. This will also loosen their texture. Weave the leeks in and around the tomatoes. Pour over the balsamic vinegar, drizzle over the olive oil, and bake in the preheated oven for an hour. Before serving, remove the bay leaves.

Try this: These tomatoes are great served as a vegetable dish, or as part of a warm salad. Also good as a base for soup, puréed to make a sauce or served over pasta.

SERVES 6

12 plum tomatoes

4 cloves of garlic, peeled and finely sliced

1 handful of fresh basil, leaves picked and torn up

12 fresh bay leaves

12 baby leeks, trimmed and washed

sea salt and freshly ground black pepper

200ml/7fl oz cheap balsamic vinegar

2 tablespoons extra virgin olive oil

roasted chicken stuffed with fragrant couscous and cooked on a sweet potato stovie

I made this up the other night when the mother-in-law came round for dinner. I wasn't too sure about it beforehand, but it worked really well. I bought a big organic chicken and treated the couscous like a stuffing. And I'd managed to get hold of some really interesting dried fruit, so I decided to use sour berries, blueberries, strawberries and cherries. Just a small handful of each, but what an amazing result. The sweet potato stovie is mushy and moreish and rather like a Moroccan bubble and squeak.

Preheat your oven to 190°C/375°F/gas 5.

Put your couscous, orange and lemon zest and juice, dried fruits, nuts and fresh herbs into a bowl. Add a couple of tablespoons of extra virgin olive oil and a wineglass of warm water and mix everything together. Coarsely grate your potatoes and sweet potatoes into a bowl and set aside. In a pestle and mortar, pound up all the spices with the salt until you have a fine powder.

Stuff the chicken cavity with all the flavoured couscous. Really push it in, and if there's any left over you can mix it with the grated potatoes. Block the cavity with one of the lemon halves that you have squeezed the juice from – this will keep the couscous inside the chicken while it cooks. Rub the chicken with a little olive oil and half the spice mix, adding the rest of it to the potatoes. Rub a couple of tablespoons of olive oil into a roasting tray or casserole-type pan, then add your potato mixture and press down on it. Put the chicken on top of the potato and place in the preheated oven for 1½ hours, turning the heat down to 170°C/325°F/gas 3 after half an hour.

When the chicken is cooked, discard the lemon half from the cavity, remove the tray from the oven and check that the couscous is thoroughly hot. Leave the chicken to rest for about 5 minutes, then put it on a carving board. Remove some of the excess fat from the potatoes with a little kitchen paper – just lay it over the top to let it soak up the fat, then throw it away. To serve, carve the meat and divide it between the serving plates, giving each one a nice spoonful of the potato stovie, then scrape out your fantastically flavoured couscous. Sprinkle the extra mint and parsley over the top, and serve with some crème fraîche or sour cream.

SERVES 4

150g/5½oz couscous

zest and juice of 1 orange

zest and juice of 1 lemon, reserving 1 of the lemon halves

2 good handfuls of mixed dried fruit (bilberries, blueberries, redcurrants, wild strawberries, dates, cherries or apricots)

2 handfuls of mixed nuts (almonds, pistachios, pinenuts or walnuts), crushed

1 large handful of mixed fresh mint and parsley, plus a little extra to serve, roughly chopped

extra virgin olive oil

2 large potatoes, peeled

3 large sweet potatoes, peeled

1 teaspoon fennel seeds

1 teaspoon coriander seeds

½ teaspoon ground cinnamon

½ teaspoon cumin seeds

2 cardamom seeds

1 teaspoon black peppercorns

1 teaspoon sea salt

1 x 1.4kg/3¼lb organic chicken

crème fraîche or sour cream

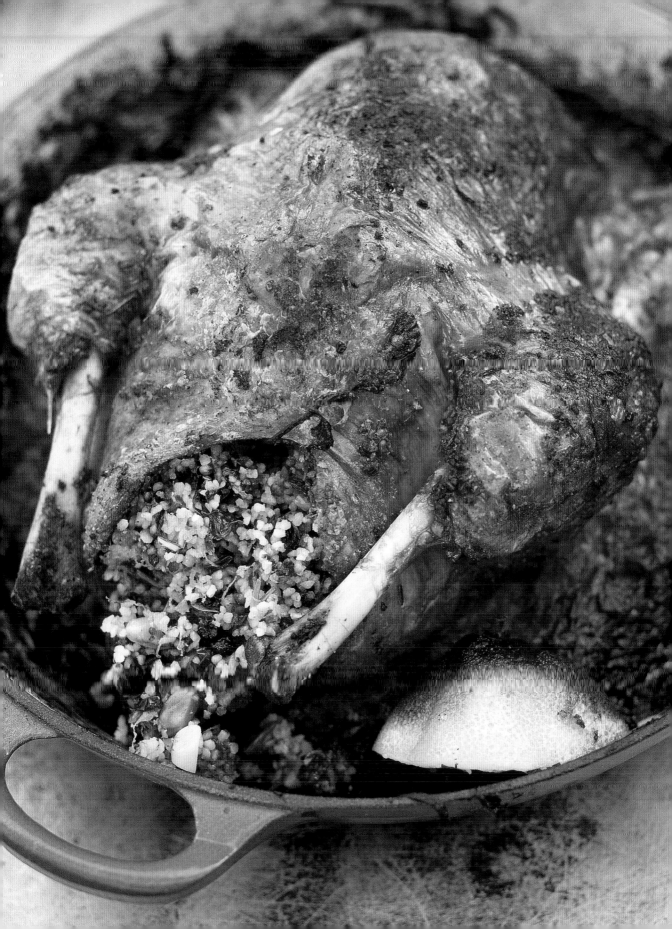

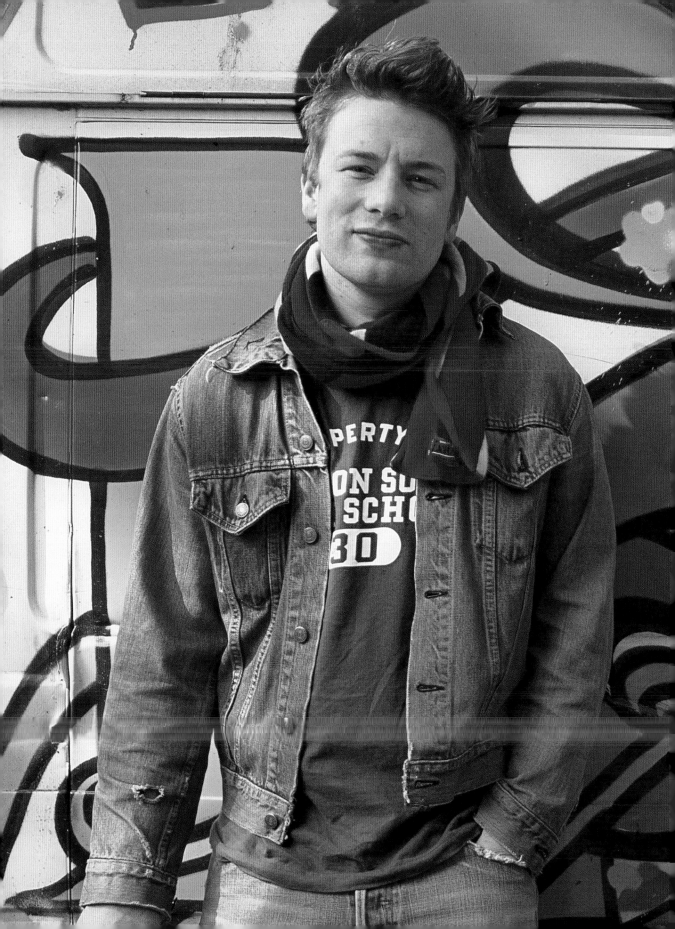

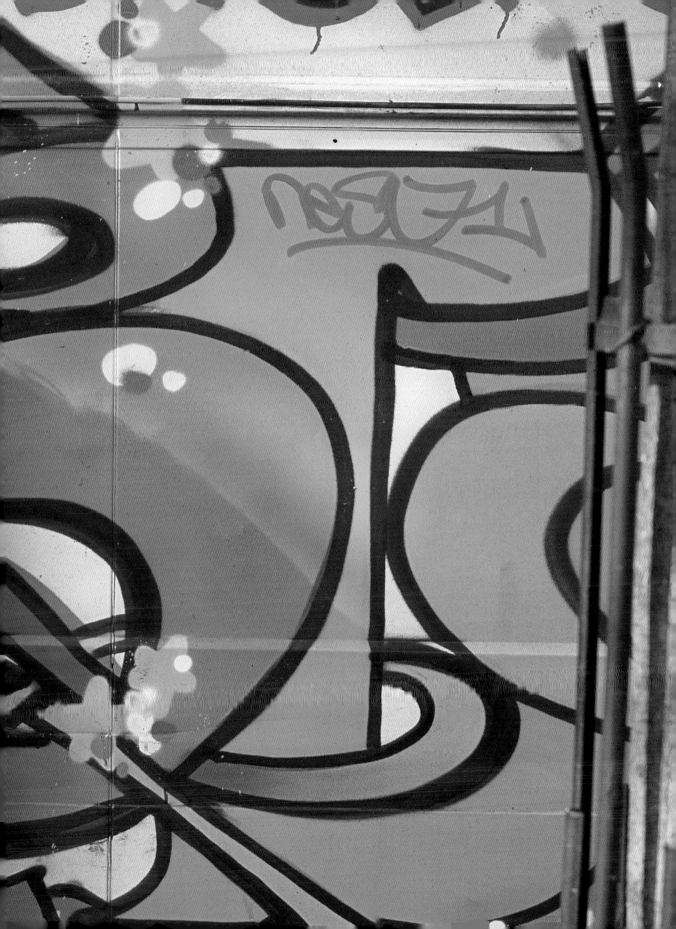

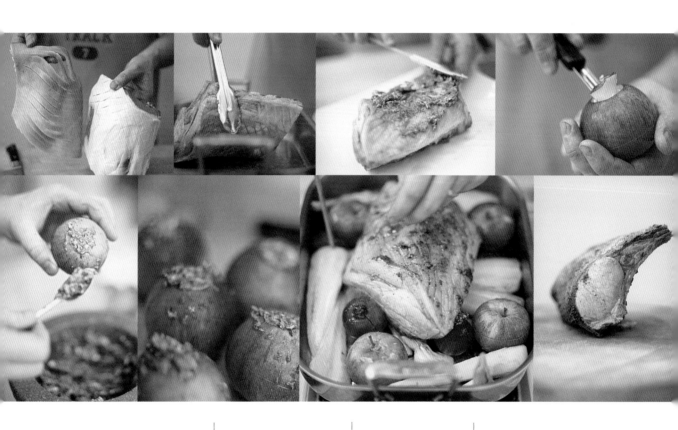

1. Remove the skin and score it

2. Brown the meat.

3. Smear on your flavoured butter.

4. Remove the core from the apples and score around the outside of the skin.

5. Stuff the apples . . .

6. . . . until they're all filled.

7. Add your veg to the tray and place the pork on top.

8. After cooking, allow the meat to rest for 10 minutes before serving.

unbelievable roast pork with stuffed apples and parsnips

As usual I was mucking about, trying to reinvent the apple sauce and roast pork story. I roasted everything in the pan together, and the flavours were absolutely amazing. What a brilliant way to eat apples with pork rather than having boring old apple sauce.

Preheat your oven to 220ºC/425ºF/gas 7. Sometimes the fat in pork can be too thick and never goes crisp. So ask your butcher to score through the skin about 1cm/½ inch apart then remove it from the loin. You want to try to leave about 0.5cm/¼ inch of fat on the loin, and score this across so it goes nice and crisp when you cook it. Season the skin well and place on a tray in the oven to start crackling – this will take around 15–20 minutes, depending on how moist the skin is. Remove when golden and crisp and put to one side. Meanwhile parboil your parsnips and red onions in boiling, salted water for about 5 minutes.

In a pestle and mortar (or in a metal bowl using the end of a rolling pin) bash up the sage, allspice, nutmeg, garlic and orange zest with a good pinch of salt and pepper until you have a fine powder. Put the mixture into a bowl with your butter, then mix it all up well. Run a knife around the middle of each apple – this will stop them bursting when they cook. Remove the core with a peeler without piercing right through the apple (see picture opposite) and discard. Pack your flavoured butter into the cavity of each apple where the core was – any excess butter can be smeared all over the pork loin. Place the apples in the tray, butter side facing down, with the parboiled parsnips and red onions. Put the pork on top and place in the oven for 1 hour. After half an hour, take the tray out of the oven, remove the pork to a plate, and carefully toss the onion and parsnips in all the lovely cooking juices, trying not to disrupt the apples. Put the pork back on top and continue cooking for half an hour at 180ºC/350ºF/gas 4 until nice and golden. When done, remove the pork from the oven and allow to rest for 5 minutes before slicing. Turn the oven off, but keep the veggies and crackling warm in the oven until you're ready to serve.

Carve the pork and divide between your 6 plates with the veggies and an apple each.

Try this: Steam yourself some nice greens, toss them in the buttery juices from the roasting tray and serve alongside the pork.

SERVES 6

½ a pork loin, rib-end

6 large parsnips, peeled and cut lengthways

6 small red onions, peeled

sea salt and freshly ground black pepper

2 handfuls of fresh sage, leaves picked

1 heaped teaspoon ground allspice

½ a nutmeg, grated

2 cloves of garlic, peeled

zest of 1 orange

150g/5½oz butter, softened

6 good eating apples

roast duck with bubble and squeak and stir-fried greens

You may think that duck is fatty . . . and, yes, sometimes it can be. But this method of cooking actually cooks out about 95% of the fat (which can be kept for making the best roast spuds another day).

Preheat the oven to 200°C/400°F/gas 6.

Bash up the thyme with the salt in a pestle and mortar (or in a metal bowl with a rolling pin). Rub this over the duck inside and out then tie it up (see page 228). Place the duck in a roasting pan, prick the skin to allow the fat to come out and cook in the preheated oven for about 2½ hours, draining the fat off 2 or 3 times so you are left with just meat juices.

Meanwhile, bring some salted water to the boil in a large pan and cook the swede for 10 minutes. Add the carrot and potatoes to the pan and continue to cook until they are all tender, then drain. Allow the veg to steam off some of their moisture before mashing them all together.

Heat some olive oil in a pan, add the onion, garlic and thyme and fry for about 3 minutes until softened. Pour in the brandy – if you're using a gas hob you can flame it until the alcohol has cooked off. Add the tomatoes and cook for 20 minutes until you have a thick sauce. Finally, add a dash of white wine vinegar and season to taste.

Check to see if the duck is ready by pinching the thigh meat – it should feel tender and the skin should be crisp. If it's cooked, remove it to a plate and leave it to rest in a warm place for half an hour. Remove any excess fat from the pan, add a little water, then scrape up the sticky goodness. Pour this into your sauce and then correct the seasoning. While the sauce is simmering, heat the butter in a non-stick pan and fry the Brussels sprouts for 3 minutes. Add the mashed veg, pat together, season to taste and fry, stirring every minute, until golden brown.

To serve, divide the bubble and squeak between your plates, carve the duck and give everybody a bit of leg and breast. Spoon over the sauce. Lovely!

SERVES 4, WITH LEFTOVERS

1 good handful of fresh thyme, leaves picked

2 tablespoons sea salt

1 x 2kg/4½lb duck

300g/11oz swede, peeled and diced

300g/11oz carrots, peeled and diced

600g/1lb 6oz potatoes, peeled and diced

100g/3½oz butter

400g/14oz finely chopped Brussels sprouts or Savoy cabbage

for the sauce

olive oil

1 medium onion, chopped

2 cloves of garlic, finely chopped

1 small handful of fresh thyme, leaves picked

1 wineglass of brandy

1 x 400g/14oz tin of plum tomatoes

dash of white wine vinegar

sea salt and freshly ground black pepper

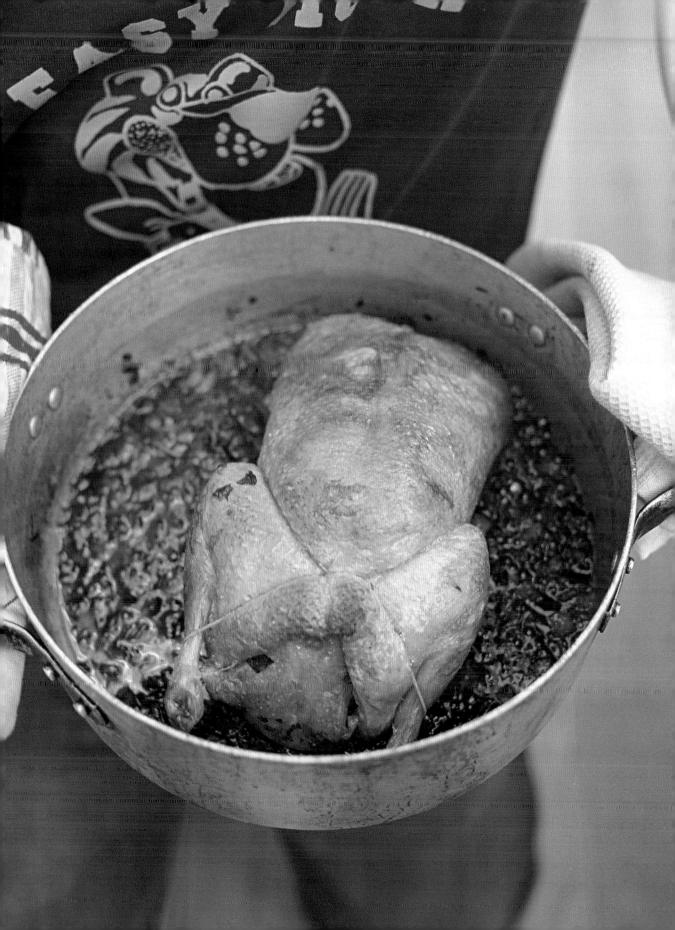

TYING UP A BIRD

The principle of tying or trussing up birds is to keep them nice and secure.

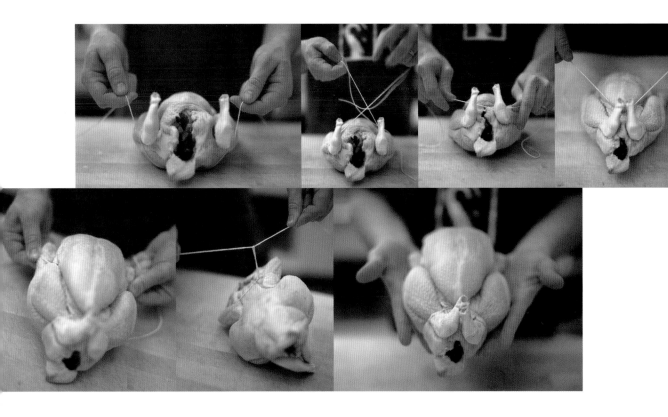

1. Place the string under the front of the bird.	2. Tie a double knot.	3. Pull tight.	4. Guide the string to the back of the bird, following the line of the breast.
5. Pull underneath.	6. Tie a knot twice.	7. All nice and cosy and in place!	

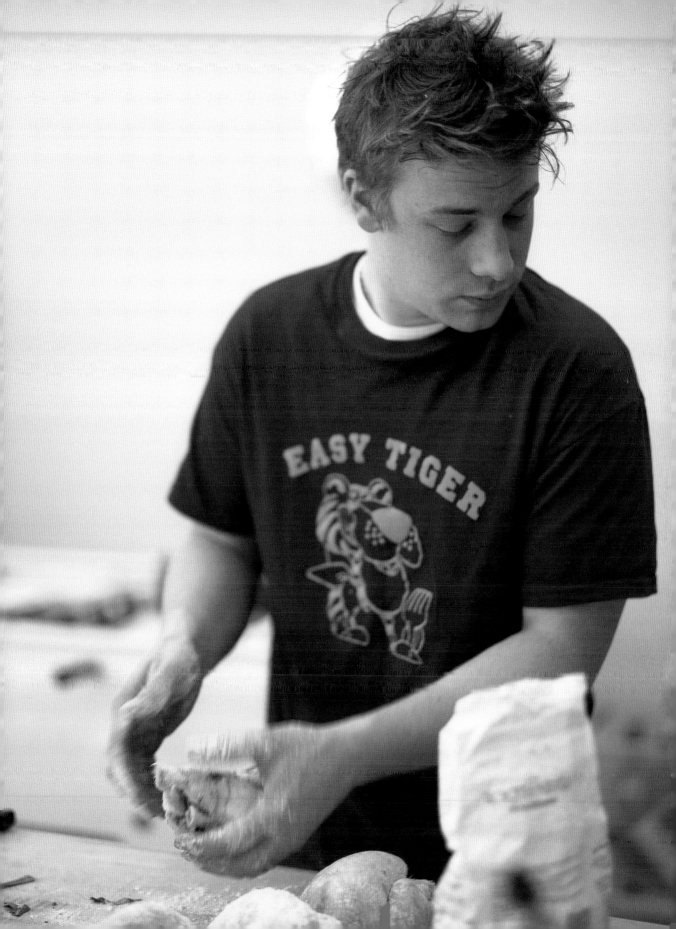

pot-roasted guinea-fowl with fennel, potatoes and blood orange

In this recipe you could use chicken or pheasant instead of guinea-fowl. If you can't get hold of any blood oranges then normal ones will do, or try using mandarin oranges.

Cut the guinea-fowl legs away from the breast meat. This is because they take different times to cook, and you want to get it perfect. (See the pictures opposite.)

To make the marinade, bash up the fennel seeds, half the rosemary, half the thyme and the garlic in a pestle and mortar. Mix in the gin and the zest and juice of the oranges with 5 tablespoons of extra virgin olive oil. Season with black pepper only.

Now get yourself a small clean bin liner as they're nice and tough, but you can use sandwich bags as well. Make sure there are no holes in it. Push the guinea-fowl legs and breasts down into one corner of the bag, then add the marinade. Squeeze out all the air you can and tie a knot in the bag. Put it in a bowl or on a large plate and keep it in the fridge for a day, turning the bag over when you remember.

When you're ready to cook, preheat your oven to 250°C/450°F/gas 8. Parboil your potatoes in boiling salted water for about 5 minutes, then add the fennel, continue to boil for 5 minutes more and drain. Remove the guinea-fowl from the fridge, drain away the marinade, and place the meat on a board. Use a piece of kitchen towel to blot off any excess moisture from the meat. Put the legs into a big roasting tray and roast in the preheated oven for 20 minutes. Take the tray out of the oven – you should have a nice bit of fat in the bottom. Remove the legs to a plate. Put the potatoes, fennel and the rest of the thyme and rosemary into the tray and give it a really good shake about. Then put the legs back in the tray, along with the breast meat, which should be skin side up. Place in the oven for about 30 minutes, until both the skin of the breast meat and the potatoes are nice and golden. Remove from the oven, sprinkle with olives and allow to rest for 5 minutes.

To serve, cut the guinea-fowl into chunks. Divide a bit of everything between your plates and sprinkle with the herby fennel tops.

Try this: Make a blood orange dressing with the juice of an orange and the same amount of olive oil. Season and drizzle it over everything.

SERVES 4

2 x 1.2kg/2¹/₂lb guinea-fowl, pheasants or small chickens

1 wineglass of gin

1 tablespoon fennel seeds

1 small handful of fresh rosemary, leaves picked

1 small handful of fresh thyme, leaves picked

1 bulb of garlic, crushed

zest and juice of 5 blood oranges

extra virgin olive oil

sea salt and freshly ground black pepper

2kg/4¹/₂lb potatoes, peeled and halved

2 large bulbs of fennel, trimmed and each cut into 8 pieces, herby tops reserved

1 large handful of black olives, destoned

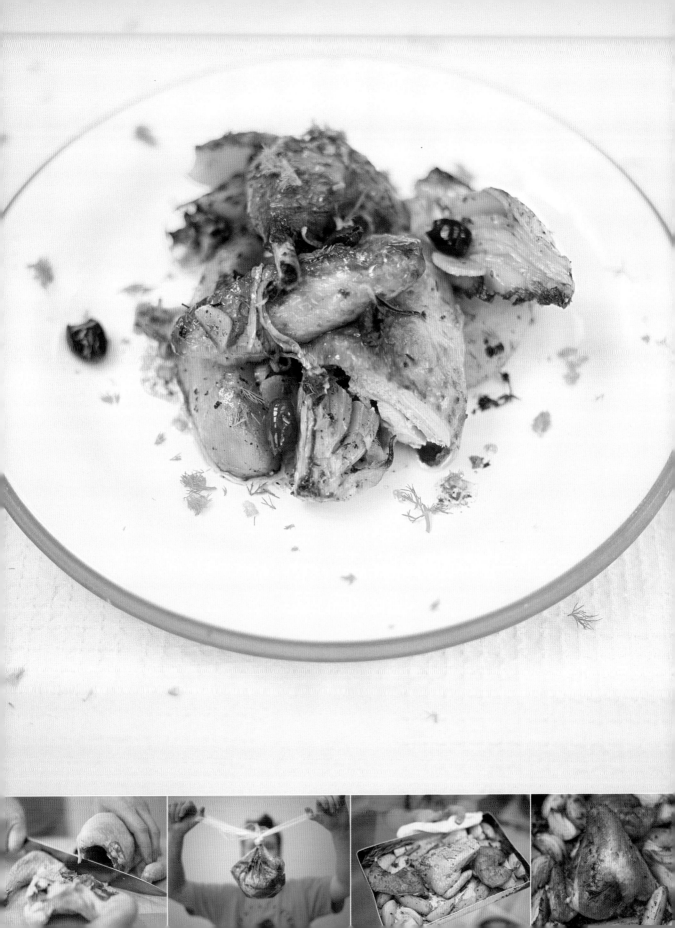

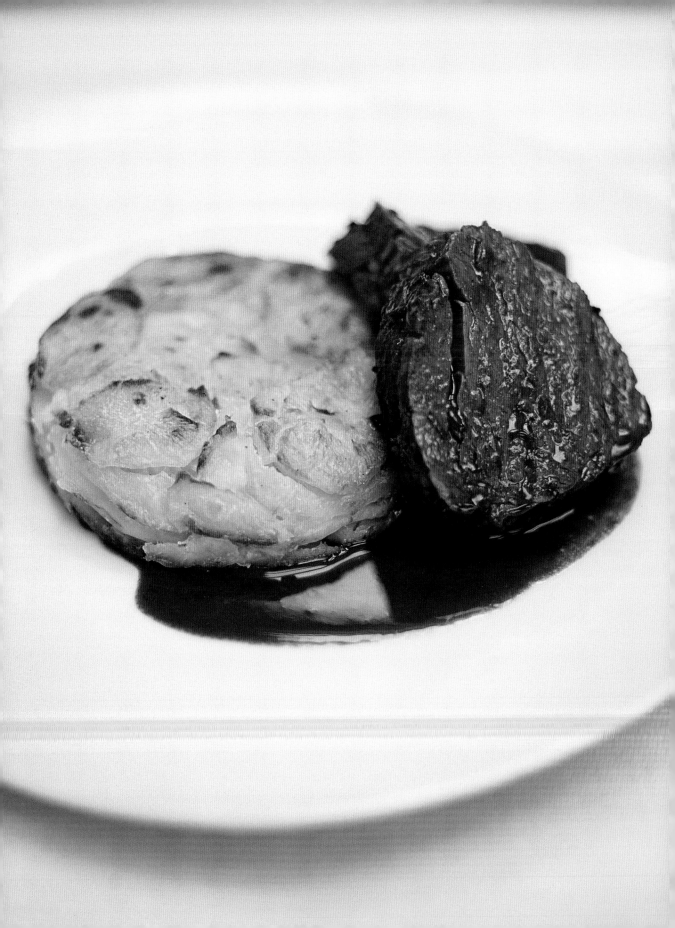

marinated and pot-roasted beef fillet with a brilliant potato and horseradish cake

Generously season the beef fillet with salt and pepper. In a pestle and mortar bash up about a quarter of the rosemary with a clove of garlic to make a paste. Loosen with 5 tablespoons of olive oil and then rub this all over the beef. Tie the beef up with 4 pieces of string then poke the remaining rosemary sprigs under the string. This way the beef is almost protected by the herb during the cooking and it will also give great flavour.

Preheat the oven to 250°C/450°F/gas 8. Parboil your sliced potatoes in boiling salted water for around 5 minutes. Drain in a colander, and transfer to a bowl with just enough olive oil to coat them. Season well. I like to make the potato cake in a round greased or nonstick cake tin, but you can use a non-stick frying pan with a metal handle if you have one. Or you can even make small individual ones. Place half the potatoes into the tin or pan, smearing the creamed horseradish over the top. Place the rest of the potatoes on top then pat down and put to one side.

Brown off the beef in a snug-fitting roasting tray until all sides are coloured. Add the garlic cloves to the tray, place the beef on top of them and put in the oven with the potatoes on a shelf below. Cook for 20 minutes, then turn the beef over, baste it and add the red wine and butter to the tray. Remove the potato dish then carefully place a clean tea towel over it and push down to compact the spuds into a nice tight cake. Put the potatoes back into the oven for another 15–20 minutes.

I serve the beef cooked medium, but you can cook it more or less to your preference. Remove the beef from the oven and while it is resting continue browning the potato cake for 5 minutes if it needs it. When you're ready to serve, remove the string and the rosemary sprigs from the beef and carve it into nice slices.

Turn the potato cake out on to a board, or just scoop it out of the pan with a spoon if it's stuck and divide between your 4 serving plates beside the meat. Save any juices from the rested meat and return them to the tray, where the red wine and butter and all the goodness from the meat will have made a very simple but tasty cooking sauce. Finish by mushing up the garlic cloves, then pass the sauce through a sieve on to the meat. Lovely served with some dressed watercress.

Try this: You could do the same recipe with a pork loin or venison.

SERVES 4

1 x 900g/2lb whole fillet of beef, trimmed

sea salt and freshly ground black pepper

2 handfuls of fresh rosemary sprigs

1 bulb of garlic, broken up, cloves left whole with skins on

extra virgin olive oil

2kg/4½lb Desirée or Maris Piper potatoes, peeled and sliced 0.5cm/¼ inch thick

3 heaped tablespoons creamed horseradish

½ bottle of red wine

70g/2½oz butter

pot-roasted shoulder of lamb with roasted butternut squash and sweet red onions

This is a recipe inspired by my having a shoulder of lamb, butternut squash and some red onions all waiting to be used! No quaint story to tell but it did taste bloomin' lovely.

Preheat the oven to 190°C/375°F/gas 5.

Lay out your shoulder of lamb. What you want to do is delicately flavour the meat, so pound up the coriander seeds with the rosemary and a pinch of salt in a pestle and mortar (or use a metal bowl and a rolling pin) until nice and fine. Take half this mixture and rub it over the inside of the lamb. Season it well with salt and pepper, then roll up the lamb and secure it with 4 or 5 pieces of string. The reason for doing this is to make the meat a consistent thickness – don't worry about doing it neatly, as long as it holds together it's fine.

Put a high-sided roasting tray on the hob and brown the lamb on all sides in a little olive oil. Remove from the heat, allow the lamb to cool a little, then add the red onions to the tray. Lift up the lamb, stir the onions around to cover them in all the flavoursome juices, then sit the lamb back on top and cook in the preheated oven for around 2 hours, adding the cranberry juice after the first half an hour and turning the heat down to 170°C/325°F/gas 3.

Turn the meat in its cooking juices when you can. By the end of the 2 hours you want the meat to be nice and crisp on the outside but really melt-in-your-mouth and tender. Sometimes the lamb may need a little longer, depending on the age of the animal. You'll also want enough juice left in the bottom of the tray to give everyone a nice spoonful – if it looks as if the liquid is going to cook away too quickly, add a little water and place a cartouche on top (see page 174). Skim off any fat that cooks out of the meat.

While the lamb is cooking, rub the butternut squash with the rest of the spice mix and a drizzle of olive oil. Lay it in another roasting tray, season well and put it in the oven when the lamb's been cooking for just over an hour. Cook for around 45 minutes, until sweet and tender.

When the lamb's cooked, let it rest for 10 minutes, then remove the string. In a bowl mix together the coriander leaves, spring onions, lemon juice, 4 tablespoons of olive oil and seasoning. Toss together.

To serve, divide the squash between your plates, cut up the lamb into irregular sized slices, spoon over some tray juices, and sprinkle on the herb salad. A dollop of crème fraîche on top is lovely.

SERVES 4–6

1 shoulder of lamb, deboned and untied

1 dessertspoon coriander seeds

1 small handful of fresh rosemary, leaves picked

sea salt and freshly ground black pepper

extra virgin olive oil

3 red onions, peeled and quartered

565ml/1 pint cranberry juice

2 butternut squash, quartered

1 small handful of fresh coriander, leaves picked

4 spring onions, trimmed and finely sliced

juice of 1 lemon

6 tablespoons crème fraîche

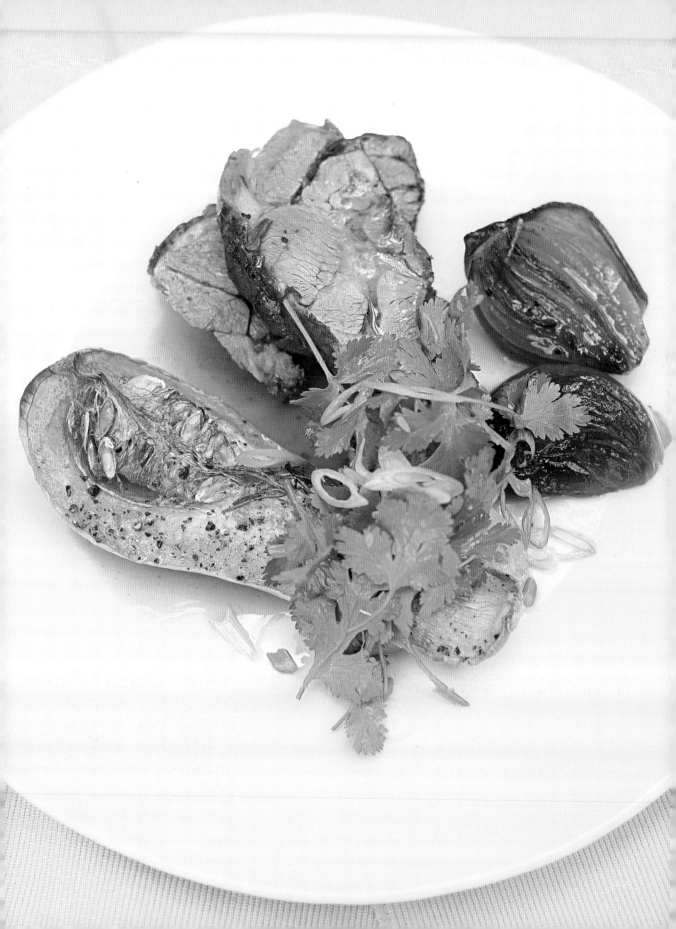

pork loin with a great herby stuffing

This recipe for pork is great. You can serve it as a conventional roast, or let it cool and either serve it as part of a buffet, or in sandwiches as they do in Italy. On my first trip there we stopped at a caravan by the side of the road where we had lovely big porchetta (pork sandwiches) filled with salad leaves, mustard and some very bready salsa verde.

If you're feeling adventurous then try out this recipe using a whole suckling pig. It's one of the most special things you can cook – great for weddings and parties. Good butchers will normally be able to get hold of a suckling pig if you order in advance – you should expect to pay between £70 and £100 for a whole one, which will feed about 12 people. If you do decide to use a suckling pig, then double the stuffing recipe, stuff the cavity, secure it and allow it a couple of extra hours to cook. It will be ready when the leg and shoulder meat falls off the bone.

Preheat your oven to 200°C/400°F/gas 6.

Place your pork loin in front of you and score across the skin with a sharp knife, or a Stanley knife, about 1cm/¹⁄₂ inch deep and about 1cm/¹⁄₂ inch apart. Pound up the rosemary and fennel seeds with a tablespoon of salt – bash the mixture up until really fine and then rub it into all the score marks on the pork. Remove the crusts from the bread and slice it up. I like to toast the bread in a toaster or on a griddle until lightly golden, as this gives the stuffing a really fantastic smoky flavour. While the bread is toasting, slowly fry the onions, garlic, sage and pinenuts in a little olive oil for 10 minutes until the onions are sweet and soft. Season with salt and pepper, add the balsamic vinegar and put the mixture in a bowl. Rip your bread into pieces and add to the bowl. Squash everything together, really squeezing the onions into the bread. Have a taste – it may need a little more seasoning. Put to one side and allow to cool.

Insert your knife into the eye meat of the pork loin and make a cavity for your stuffing (see the pictures opposite). Pack in the stuffing, then roll the pork over and tie it with a few pieces of string. Place the pork on a roasting tray and cook in the preheated oven for just over an hour until crisp and golden.

¹⁄₂ a pork loin, preferably the rib end, off the bone

1 small handful of fresh rosemary, leaves picked

3 heaped tablespoons fennel seeds

sea salt and freshly ground black pepper

500g/1lb 2oz sourdough or rustic bread

2 red onions, peeled and finely sliced

3 cloves of garlic, peeled and finely sliced

1 small handful fresh sage leaves, ripped up

1 handful of pinenuts

extra virgin olive oil

4 tablespoons balsamic vinegar

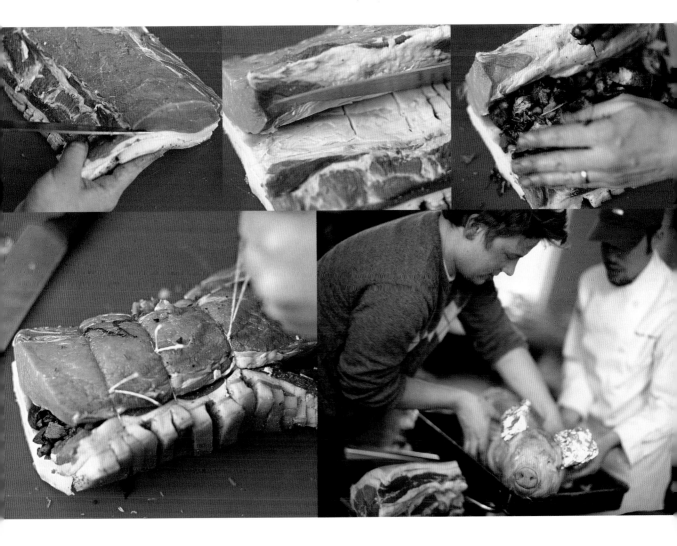

1. Stick the knife in at the edge of the eye meat.

2. Partly remove the meat.

3. Pack the gap tightly with your stuffing.

4. Tie up to secure.

5. Try this with a whole suckling pig one day – it's great for a party!

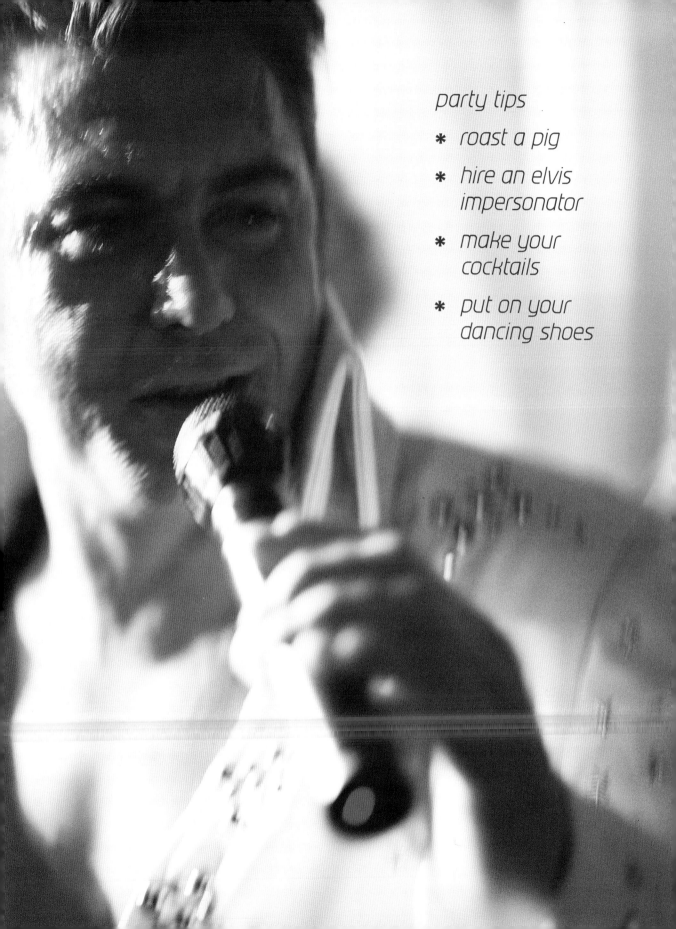

party tips

* roast a pig

* hire an elvis
  impersonator

* make your
  cocktails

* put on your
  dancing shoes

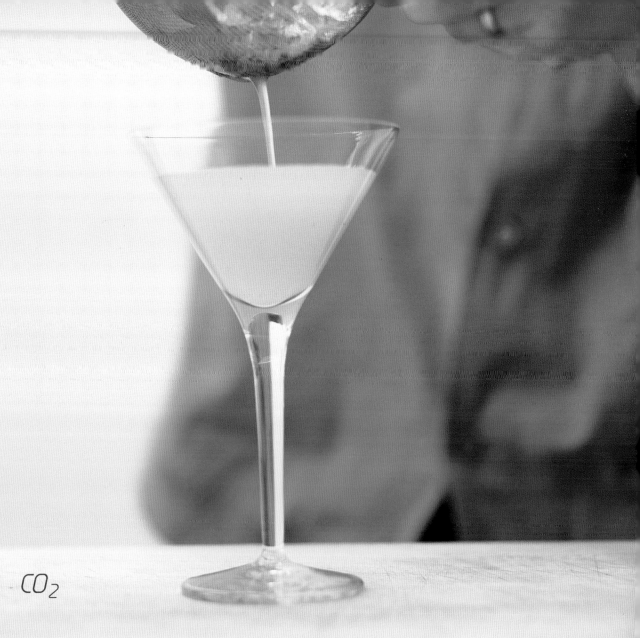

CO_2

This is a cocktail that I invented with Giancarlo d'Urso, the barman from Hakkasan in London.

Drop the lemongrass, chilli slices, coriander and pepper into your cocktail shaker. Bash them up a bit using a pestle to get all the lovely flavours out. Add the tequila and ice. Squeeze in the lime juice and add the pineapple. Shake, strain and pour into a chilled Martini glass.

SERVES 1

1 stick of lemongrass, peeled back

a couple of slices of fresh red chilli, to taste

4 sprigs of fresh coriander, leaves picked

freshly ground black pepper

juice of 1/2 a fresh lime

2 shots of tequila

3 shots of pineapple juice

2 handfuls of ice

GRILLING AND CHARGRILLING

GRILLING

Grilling uses heat from above. It's good for gratinating, toasting, caramelizing and cooking small cuts of meat or fish. It's a pretty handy method because it's almost a dry heat so you can get things very crunchy and crispy, depending on the temperature.

CHARGRILLING

Chargrilling is a sexy way to cook and basically stems from what we would call a barbecue. These days we have ridged griddle pans that can go on a gas hob, and In restaurants we have chargrills which are gas-fired with coals underneath – these retain the heat. They give great colour and flavour, but the real genius way of chargrilling is how they cook over hot coals in Turkey using wood chippings, which is like our way of barbecuing. I know it's a classic that when a bloke barbecues he burns everything and it's still raw in the middle. However, the flavours that the coals give are absolutely sublime when you learn to gauge the heat – i.e. having a high pile of coals at one side for searing heat and colour and then just a few coals on the other side to slow down the heat, so that everything cooks in the centre. Chargrilling is fast and effective and is generally used to cook first-class quality cuts of meat and fish – even whole fish if they're small enough. The thing to remember Is to always get your griddle pan really hot before cooking on it, and never add any oil to the pan otherwise it will smoke you out of the house!

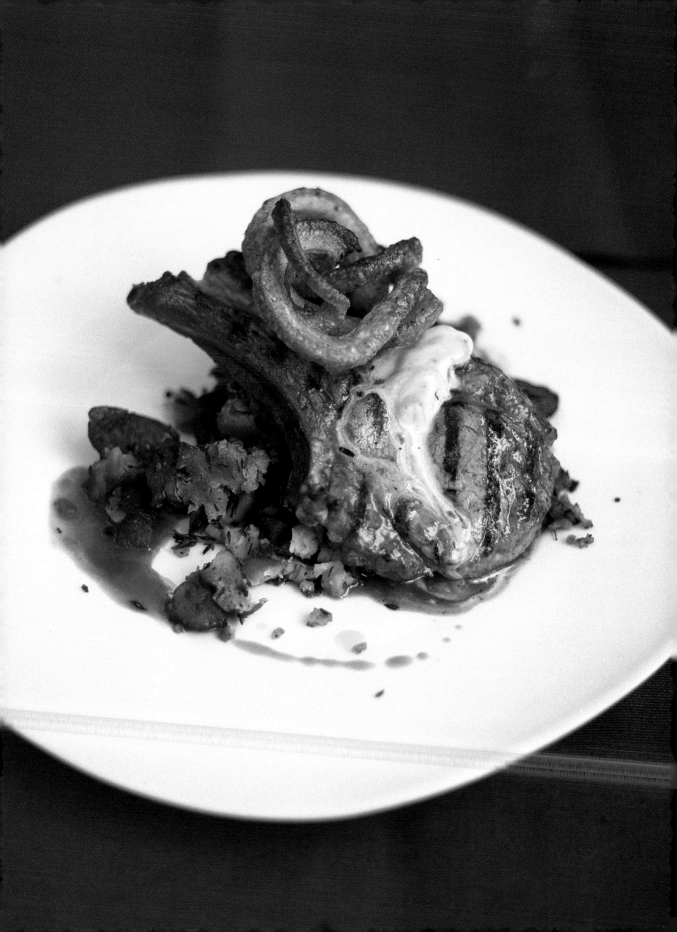

the best pork chop with fresh bay salt, crackling and squashed purple potatoes

I have to be honest – once you've eaten pork in Italy you have to really look around for anything as fine over here. You see, we've become attracted to breeds of pigs that grow very fast to be butchered and sold on a.s.a.p., whereas our old farming methods used breeds that are now considered rare. They take longer to grow to maturity, which gives the meat a fantastic depth of flavour and plenty of snowy white, waxy fat that just melts in the pan. Once you've tried that, everything else comes second best. But at Borough Market the other week I bought two of the most remarkable chops from a Long Lop pig. I cooked up a great meal that night with things I picked up on my shopping trip, like the purple spuds (often called 'truffle potatoes') and the cider.

Preheat the oven to 200°C/400°F/gas 6. Parboil your potatoes in salted boiling water for around 15 minutes until tender, then drain. Score the pork skin, season it and put it in a hot roasting tray with a drizzle of olive oil. As it begins to crisp up, add your potatoes and thyme. Toss once or twice (making sure the crackling ends up on top of the potatoes so it crisps up even more) and put in the oven for around 15 minutes until cooked.

Meanwhile, pound up your fennel seeds and bay leaves in a pestle and mortar with 2 tablespoons of salt until you have a fine green moist paste. Shake this through a sieve into a bowl – this will stop it from sticking together in lumps. Pat your pork chops with a little oil – this will stop them sticking to the pan. Season the pork chops on both sides with the herb salt and keep any excess to use another day. Preheat your griddle pan until really hot. Don't add any extra oil to the pan – if you do it will start to smoke. Add your pork chops, and cook for around 3–4 minutes on each side, depending on the thickness of the pork. Try to avoid the temptation to overcook them. Once cooked allow to rest for about 4 minutes.

Heat a little pan and add the cider and mustard. Bring to the boil, then reduce by half and add the crème fraîche. Bring back to the boil and reduce again until the sauce thickens, then remove from the heat. Add the butter and shake the pan around a bit so the sauce thickens and shines. Season to taste.

Serve up the potatoes – I like to bash up half of them so they kind of smash and crumble – with the pork, a lovely piece of crackling and any resting juices from the meat. Drizzle over the cider sauce and eat – what a pleasure. Nice with a simple green salad and a pint of cider.

SERVES 4

1kg/2¼lb purple or Desirée potatoes, peeled and halved

sea salt and freshly ground black pepper

4 pork chops, skin removed but kept

extra virgin olive oil

1 small handful of fresh thyme, leaves picked

1 teaspoon fennel seeds

10 bay leaves

285ml/½ pint cider

1 tablespoon wholegrain mustard

4 tablespoons crème fraîche

2 knobs of butter

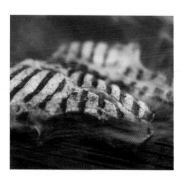

flavoured salt

A flavoured salt is one of the simplest and most basic ways of finishing a dish – it's so easy and tasty, yet hardly anyone does it. When I was growing up, celery salt seemed very uninspiring, but actually sprinkled over a tomato salad or used to season a beef stew it was gorgeous. Flavoured salts can give some really fragrant and shocking results to your palate. Things like jasmine tea salt have traditionally been used in Japanese and Chinese cooking for flavouring things like tempura. Even a simple portion of chips can be taken in a different direction by sprinkling them with flavoured salt – using, for example, Mexican or English herbs to flavour.

There's nothing better than trying things out for yourself, but if you start off with a good mineral salt which is not too strong, and fresh ingredients, you'll get amazing results. Garlic and citrus, and soft herbs like coriander, mint and basil, will gradually lose the real flavour qualities you're after, i.e. the aroma and freshness, so they are best made to order – but they only take a few seconds, so that's cool. I prefer to make them as I need them, or a day in advance, so that they'll taste amazing, but if you want to make them ahead of time they'll happily sit on the shelf for months in an airtight container, though they won't be quite as vibrant.

Get your chosen flavours together and bash them up in a pestle and mortar until you have a powder or pulp. If you are using ginger, lemongrass or fresh chillies, these need to be sliced and warmed in the oven before pounding to dry them out, otherwise they will make the salt wet. Add 3 times their weight in salt, pound together and then either leave the mixture coarse or pass it through a sieve. You can also use a food processor. The moisture in your flavouring will probably cause your salt to dry into a block after a day or two, which is fine, because you can just bash it up when you need it. Alternatively, once the salt's been flavoured, you can lay it out on a tray and put it in the oven at its lowest temperature overnight. Doing this means that the salt will stay granular.

Feel free to make up your own combinations of flavours, or try one of the five I've suggested here. As long as the combination works, these salts can complement just about anything – meats, vegetables, fish, savoury pastries . . . you name it.

Here are a few of my favourite flavourings for salt:

jasmine tea

fennel seed, lemon zest and vanilla

lavender, rosemary and thyme

lime zest, lemongrass, chilli and ginger

Szechuan peppercorns, chilli and ginger

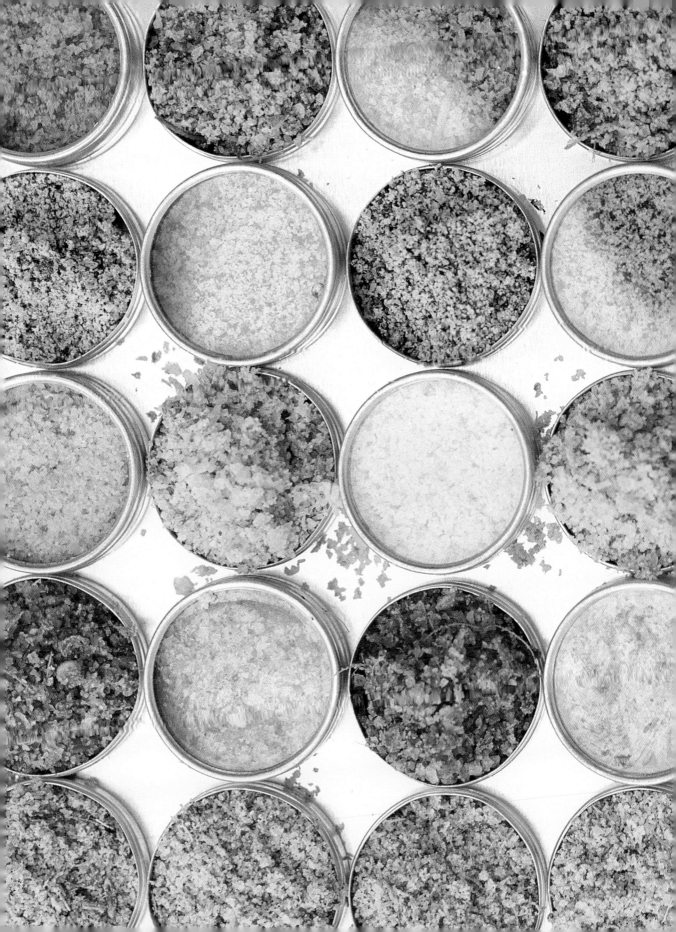

the best marinated kebabs

If you're cooking for a load of friends, or for a party, these kebabs will do the trick. They are so easy to make and damn tasty. I've marinated each type in a different blend of spices, so choose your favourite and tuck in. They can all be grilled, chargrilled or cooked on the barbie.

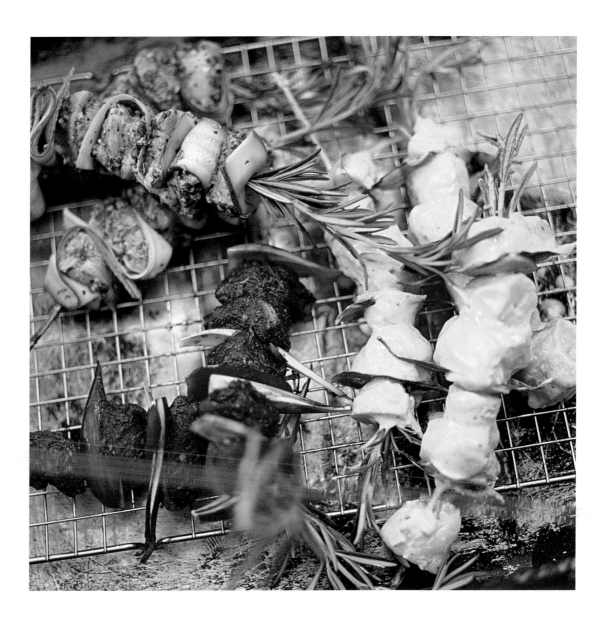

LAMB KEBABS

SERVES 6–8 500g/1lb 2oz lamb, trimmed and cut into 2.5cm/1 inch cubes ∗ 6–8 skewers or sticks of fresh rosemary, lower leaves removed, tips kept on (see page 248) ∗ 2 red onions, peeled and quartered ∗ 2 red peppers, deseeded and cut into 2.5cm/1 inch pieces

for the marinade *1 tablespoon smoked paprika ∗ 2 cloves ∗ ½ teaspoon cumin seeds ∗ 2 teaspoons coriander seeds ∗ sea salt and freshly ground black pepper ∗ olive oil*

First bash up all the spices in a pestle and mortar until fine, then mix with the oil to make a thick marinade paste. Put the lamb pieces into a bowl and cover with the marinade. Let them sit there for half an hour to an hour. Then, using the rosemary sticks or skewers, spike each piece of meat alternately with red onion and peppers. Grill for around 5 minutes, turning regularly, to give you nicely charred meat on the outside with juicy pink on the inside. Allow to rest for a few minutes – that is, if you can stop yourself eating them straight away!

CHICKEN KEBABS

SERVES 6–8 500g/1lb 2oz free-range boneless chicken breasts ∗ 4 courgettes, sliced very thinly lengthways ∗ 6–8 skewers or sticks of fresh rosemary, lower leaves removed, tips kept on (see page 248)

for the marinade *1 handful of fresh coriander ∗ 1 handful of fresh mint ∗ 3 cloves of garlic ∗ 6 spring onions ∗ 1 red chilli ∗ zest and juice of 1 lemon ∗ sea salt and freshly ground black pepper ∗ olive oil*

Cut the chicken into 2.5cm/1 inch cubes and place in a bowl. Blanch the courgette strips in salted boiling water for 30 seconds then drain and allow to cool. Blitz all the marinade ingredients (except the olive oil) in a food processor, then loosen to a paste with a little olive oil. Add the marinade to the chicken pieces and mix well. Allow to sit for up to an hour. Then weave the courgette strips in between the chicken pieces on the rosemary sticks or skewers. Grill for around 5 minutes, turning regularly, until cooked. Feel free to cut a piece open to check if they're done.

FISH KEBABS

SERVES 6–8 500g/1lb 2oz monkfish tail (or cod or haddock), trimmed of all skin and bone and cut into 2.5cm/1 inch cubes ∗ 6–8 skewers or sticks of fresh rosemary, lower leaves removed, tips kept on (see page 248) ∗ 255g/9oz boiled new potatoes, halved

for the marinade *2 thumb-sized pieces of fresh ginger, thinly sliced ∗ juice and zest of 1 lemon ∗ 1 teaspoon turmeric ∗ 2 cloves of garlic ∗ 2 dried chillies, crumbled ∗ 1 handful of fresh mint ∗ 4 tablespoons natural yoghurt*

Put all the marinade ingredients except the yoghurt into a food processor and blitz until smooth. Stir in the yoghurt. Using the skewers or rosemary sticks, skewer the fish alternately with the new potatoes. Drizzle with the marinade and grill for 2 minutes each side.

TURNING ROSEMARY STICKS INTO SKEWERS

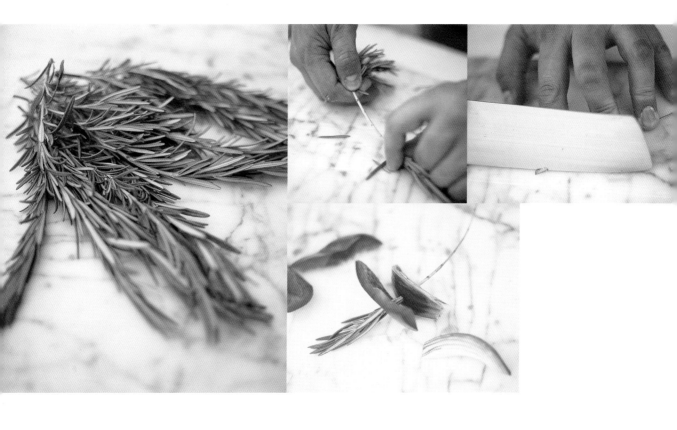

1. Get yourself a bunch of rosemary.

2. Keeping the leafy tops on, run your fingers down the stalk to remove the rest of the leaves.

3. Sharpen the tip of each stalk by cutting across at an angle.

4. Your rosemary stick is ready to use as a skewer.

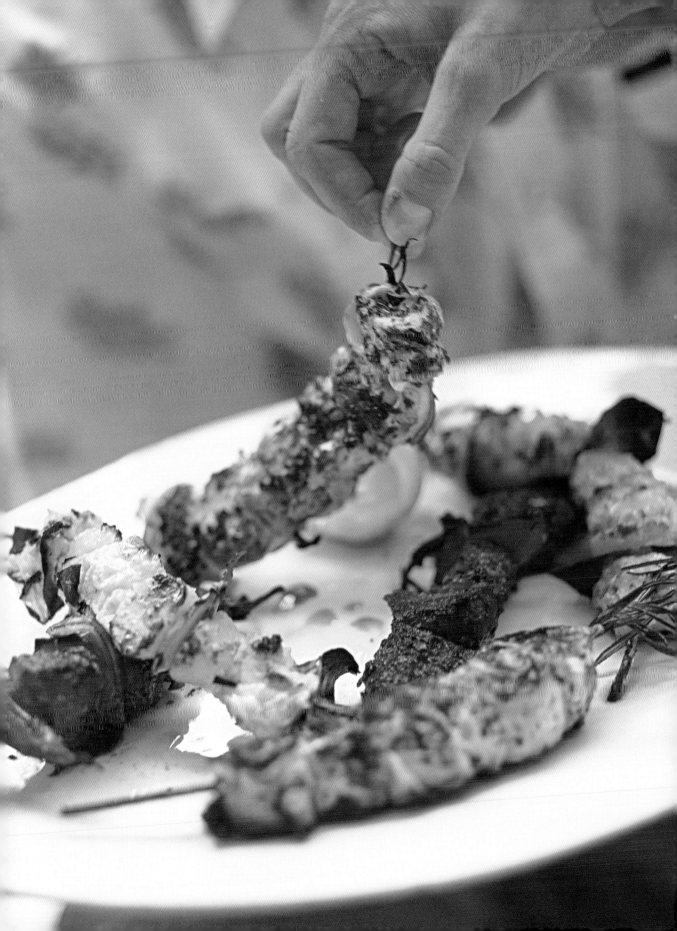

"anyone can train to be a chef, but to be really good you
need to live and breathe food"

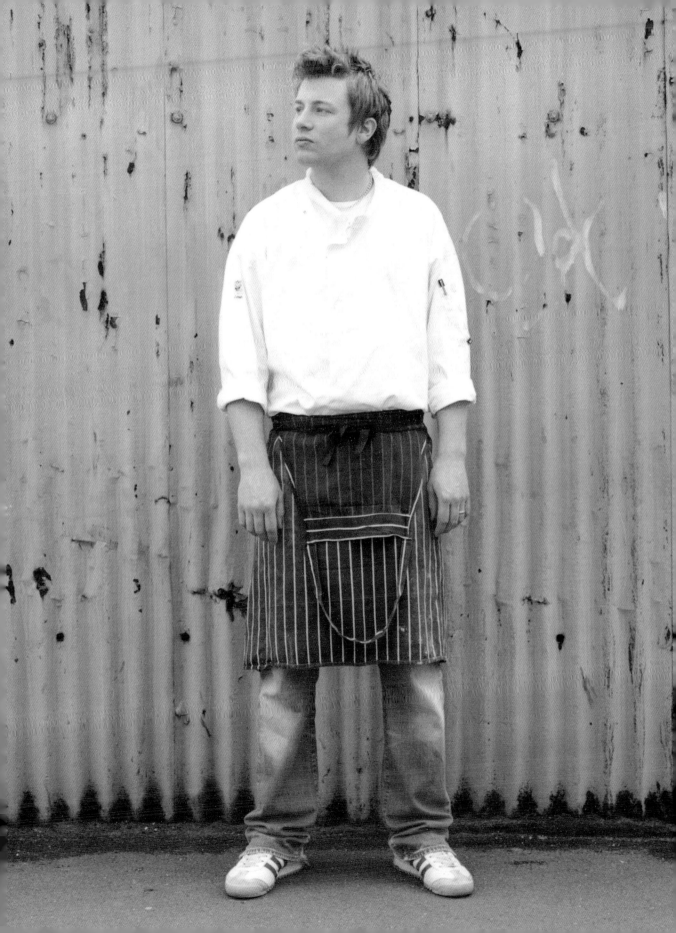

seafood mixed grill

As a child I made so many mixed grills in my parents' restaurant that I thought it would be really great to reinvent it. The thing that makes all the difference here is that I've flavoured each fish with the herb or spice which I think best complements it. I'll talk you through the seafood that I like to include. All you have to bear in mind is that the fish will all be cooked at the same time, so having your pieces the same thickness is important.

FOR AROUND 4 PEOPLE

First off, get yourself a large tray that fits under the grill and rub it with a little olive oil.

Prawns: Run a knife down the back of 8 large peeled prawns and remove the vein. In a pestle and mortar, bash up a little fresh coriander, a little grated lime zest, 1 teaspoon of grated ginger and a drizzle of olive oil. Rub this all over the prawns and place on the tray.

Red mullet: Cut it through the bone, as this will give it extra flavour and succulence when cooking. Bash up a little rosemary with some extra virgin olive oil in a pestle and mortar and rub this all over the fish. Put the red mullet on the tray.

Salmon: Bash up some basil leaves in a pestle and mortar with a little extra virgin olive oil and rub this all over some thin slices of salmon fillet, then fold the slices over a few olives and more basil leaves. Use a cocktail stick to secure and add these to the tray.

Plaice, Dover sole or lemon sole: Get your fillets, grate over some lemon zest, roll the fillets up and wrap a piece of pancetta around each one. Use a cocktail stick to secure and put on the tray.

Mussels, clams and razor clams: These are great scattered among the fish.

Cherry vine tomatoes: Rub these with oil and a little oregano and place on the tray.

A lemon: Cut this into quarters. When cooked they will become juicy and jammy and it's nice to squeeze the juice over the fish once it's cooked.

To cook, sprinkle over some finely chopped garlic, some seasoning and some small knobs of butter. Whack the tray under a hot grill for around 4 minutes until the fish is golden and sizzling and all the shells have opened. Once cooked, divide between 4 plates, giving everyone a little bit of everything. Squeeze the jammy lemon juice into the tray, scraping any goodness off the bottom, and drizzle over the fish. I love this served with new potatoes and a green salad and definitely a nice bottle of white. Give it a bash – you'll love it too.

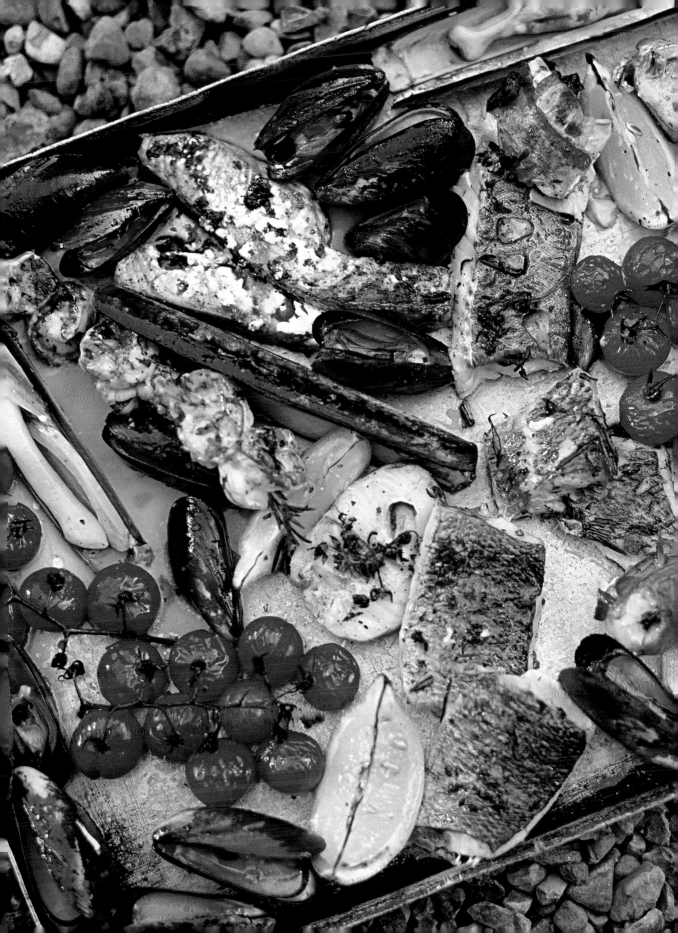

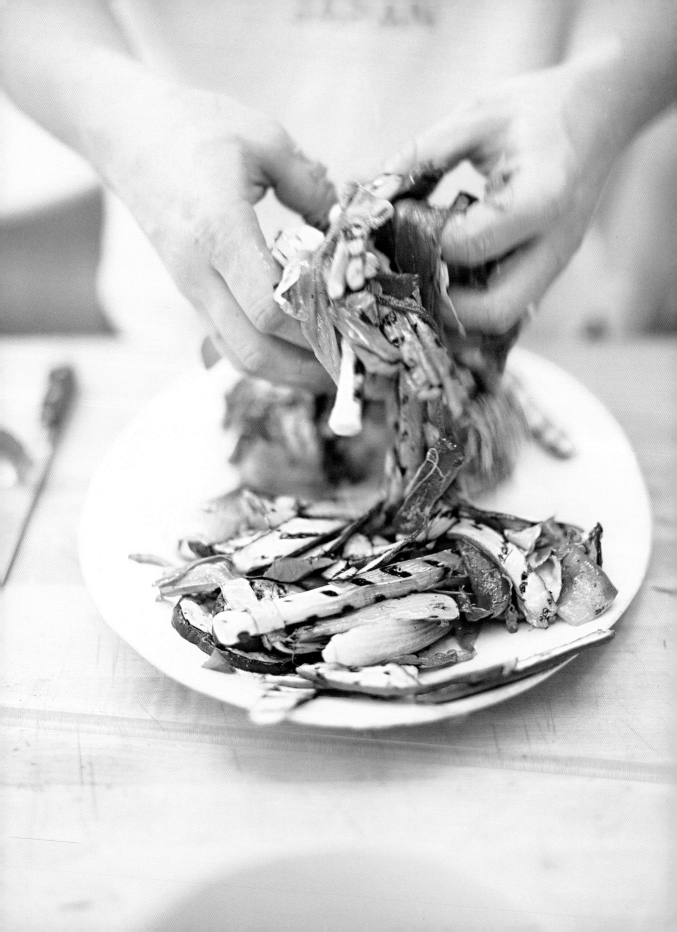

chargrilled marinated vegetables

The first time I ever made this was at the Neal Street Restaurant, and about two years later, when I was at the River Café, Rose Gray showed me her way of doing it. She inspired me to think of grilling as a really exciting way to prepare vegetables.

Wash all your vegetables. Heat the barbecue or a griddle pan, put your whole peppers on it, and get them really black on all sides. While still hot, put them in a bowl, cover with clingfilm and leave to cool.

Slice your courgettes lengthways about 0.5cm/¼ inch thick and do the same with your fennel, reserving the herby tops. Grill the courgette and fennel together on the griddle pan for about a minute on each side or until nicely charred. You don't want them too black or too raw. Remove to a clean tea towel in one layer, making sure they don't sit on top of each other, otherwise they will steam and go soggy.

Cut the aubergine across into slices 1cm/½ inch thick. Every now and again you get an aubergine that is really seedy – if this happens, it will be bitter and no good, so throw it away and get yourself another one. Chargrill the aubergine slices, turning them 4 times until nicely marked, then remove to the tea towel.

Boil the baby leeks in salted water until they're just cooked. Then drain, rub with a little olive oil, and chargrill them quickly until lightly marked.

Peel the peppers but don't hold them under the tap as all the sweet fantastic flavour will go down the drain. Carefully rub off the black skin, then remove the stalk and pips and tear the peppers up into large strips. Now put all the vegetables into a large bowl.

Take about a quarter of your basil leaves and bash them in a pestle and mortar with a good pinch of seasoning until you have a smooth pulp. Add about 8 tablespoons of extra virgin olive oil and the vinegar, to taste. Pour this over the vegetables and toss quickly so that everything gets coated in the lovely basil oil, then throw in the remaining whole basil leaves. Slice the garlic really thinly to give you a delicate flavour and add to the bowl with the fennel tops. Mix everything together, and serve on a large plate at room temperature. Great with any grilled fish or meat, or as part of an antipasti plate with some toasted bruschetta and some fresh buffalo mozzarella.

SERVES 4–6

2 red peppers

2 yellow peppers

2 medium courgettes

1 bulb of fennel

1 aubergine

8 baby leeks

sea salt and freshly ground black pepper

extra virgin olive oil

1 large bunch of fresh basil, leaves picked

2 tablespoons herb or white wine vinegar

1 clove of garlic

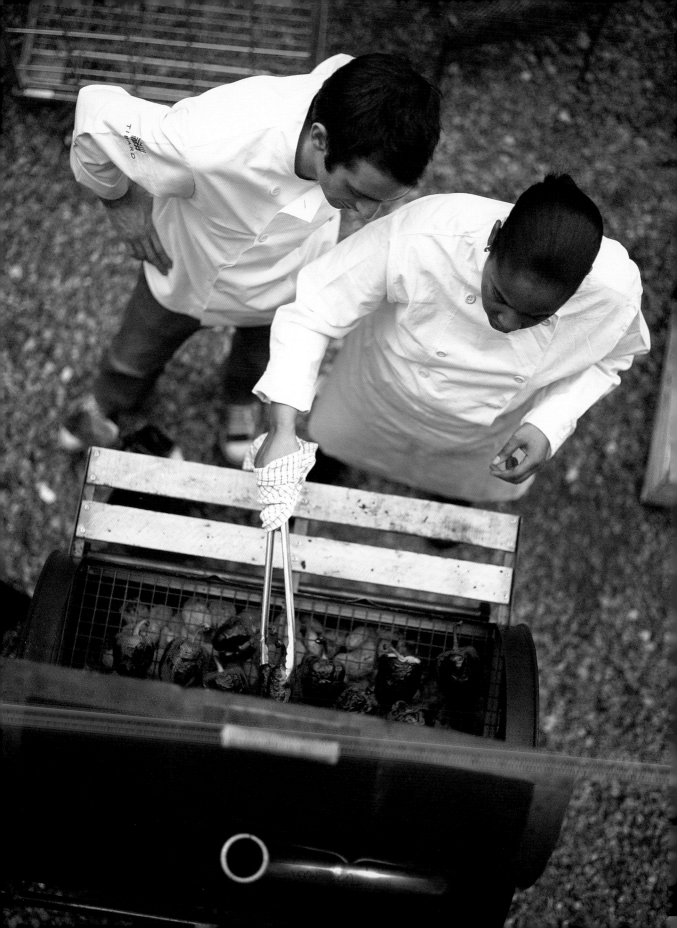

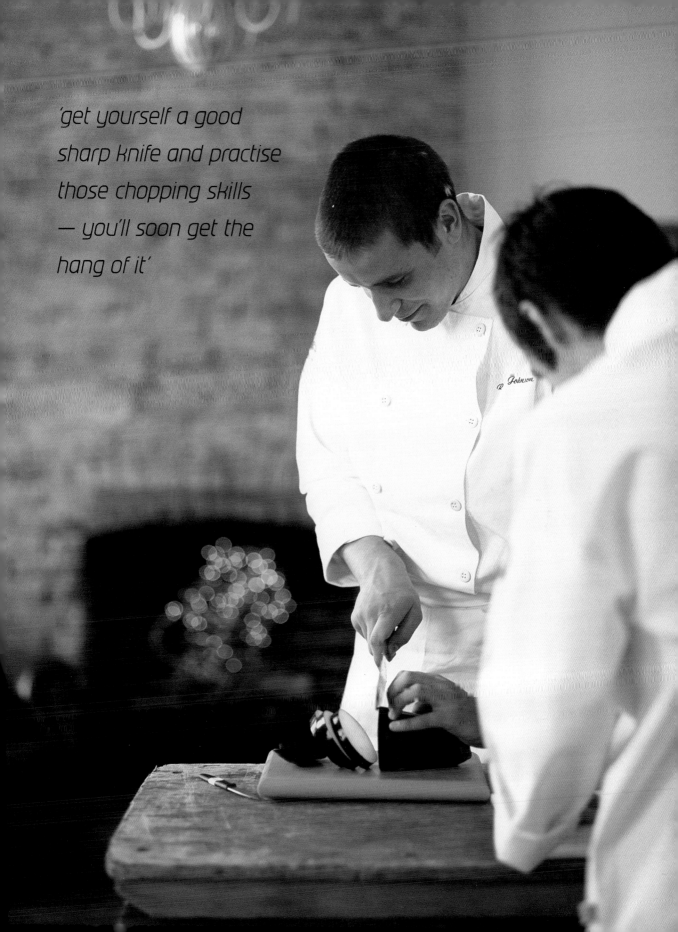

'get yourself a good
sharp knife and practise
those chopping skills
— you'll soon get the
hang of it'

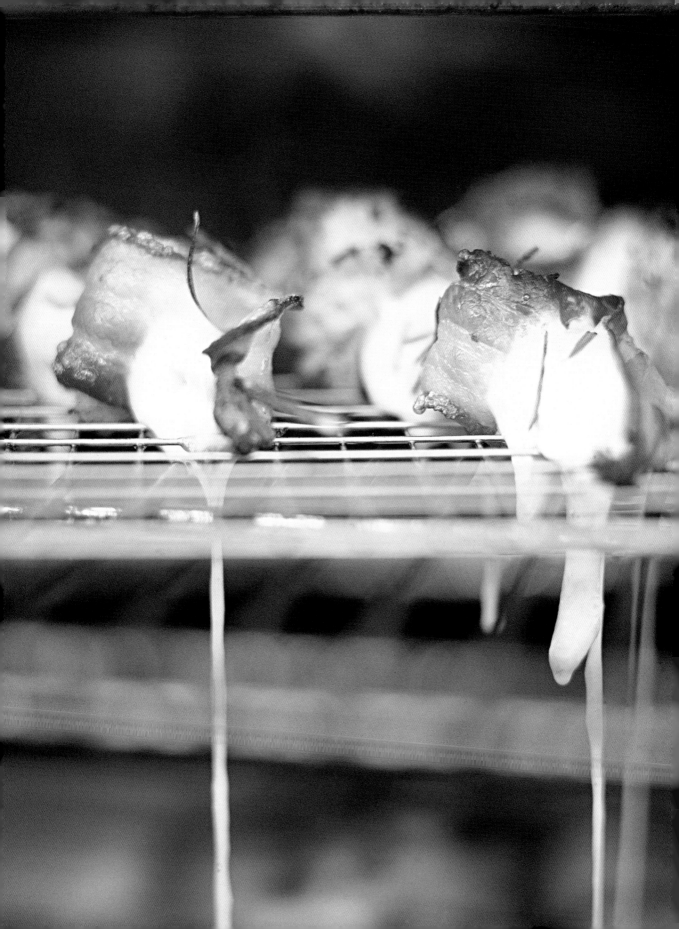

grilled marinated mozzarella with crunchy bread, smoked bacon and a black olive and lemon dressing

This is an absolutely genius combination. It's not very often that mozzarella gets cooked in a credible way but this is one time it does. I love the whole idea of putting the bread, mozzarella and smoky bacon together because when cooked they complement each other so well – the bread goes really crisp and soaks up all the lovely juices, the milky mozzarella starts to melt and go really gooey, and served with a fresh herb salad it's lovely. Great for a starter or a snack, and I've even made little mini ones as canapés (dare I say that word?!).

Remove the crusts from the ciabatta and tear up into rough 2.5cm/1 inch pieces. Throw into a bowl with the bacon and lemon zest. Divide each mozzarella into 8 similar-sized pieces and add to the bowl. Keeping the leaf tips on the rosemary sticks, remove the lower leaves (see page 248) and then smash these up in a pestle and mortar with the garlic. Stir in 8 tablespoons of olive oil, then pour this mixture over the bread, cheese and bacon. Marinate for anything from 15 minutes to an hour.

Thread your mozzarella and bread on to your rosemary sticks, weaving the bacon in and around. Line up the kebabs on a wire rack and place under the grill on a very high heat until the bread and bacon are golden and crisp and the mozzarella is nice and gooey. While this is grilling make sure you keep an eye on it, as it can turn into a charred kebab very quickly. To make the dressing, chop up the olives and mix with the chilli, 5 tablespoons of the lemon juice and the same of olive oil. Season to taste.

To serve the kebabs, dress the herbs with half of the olive dressing right at the last minute so the leaves stay nice and fresh, then use the other half of the dressing drizzled over the kebabs.

Try this: Do exactly the same as above but swap the mozzarella for cubes of fresh white fish such as haddock, cod or monkfish.

SERVES 4

1 loaf of ciabatta bread

8 rashers of thinly sliced dry-cured smoky bacon, or pancetta

zest of 2 lemons

4 large buffalo mozzarella cheeses

8 sticks of fresh rosemary

1 clove of garlic

extra virgin olive oil

3 handfuls of mixed fresh herbs (chives, chervil, mint, basil, parsley)

for the dressing

1 good handful of nice black olives, stones removed

1 fresh red chilli, deseeded and finely chopped

5 tablespoons lemon juice

5 tablespoons extra virgin olive oil

sea salt and freshly ground black pepper

best chargrilled steak

If you love your weekly steak, here's a great way to take it up a few notches. The combination of thyme, beef and mushrooms with the salsa verde is so so good and can't be beaten.

First of all, make your salsa verde.

Tie up the stalk end of your bunch of thyme, place the leafy end in a pestle and mortar and give it a good bash. This will remove the tasty leaves and leave you with what looks like a miniature broom. Put this to one side. Add your garlic, anchovy fillet and lemon zest to the mortar. Bash to a paste and stir in your olive oil.

Your fillet steaks should be about 2.5cm/1 inch thick. Wrap a piece of bacon around each steak (this gives it a really good flavour) and secure loosely with a piece of string. Peel the mushroom skins off, which only takes a second and helps them absorb the marinade. Brush the steaks and mushrooms with some of your flavoured thyme oil, keeping the rest for the cooking.

Try to become instinctive about cooking basic things like steaks and to understand heat, sizes and cuts of meat. Chefs test their meat by the way it looks and the resistance it gives when squeezed. Preheat your griddle pan or barbecue until really hot. I don't want to give you a specific time to cook them, as your steaks may be thicker or thinner than the ones I'm using. Whether using fillets or sirloins, I cook mine for roughly 3 or 4 minutes each side and let them rest for a couple of minutes to give me a medium cooked steak – you can do them for a little more or less time to your preference.

Season the meat on both sides and place on the griddle pan with your mushrooms. Turn every minute, and brush each time with your thyme oil brush. The mushrooms will be cooked after about 6 minutes and should be soft to the touch – cooking them this way means they don't go all soggy but they do have an intense meaty flavour. Once the beef is cooked to your liking, remove the string, divide the steaks between 4 warmed plates with your mushrooms, allow to rest for 2 minutes and put a big dollop of salsa verde over the top.

SERVES 4

1 x salsa verde recipe (see page 263)

1 large bunch of fresh lemon thyme or thyme

1 clove of garlic

1 anchovy fillet

zest of 1 lemon

10 tablespoons extra virgin olive oil

4 x 225g/8oz fillet steaks or sirloins

4 rashers of smoked streaky bacon

8 medium large Portobello or other flat-gilled mushrooms

sea salt and freshly ground black pepper

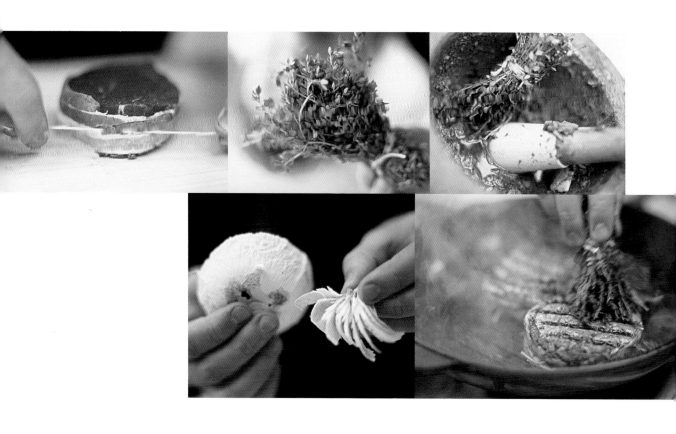

1. Secure a slice of bacon to each steak with a piece of string.

2. Bunch of thyme tied at the stalk end.

3. Make a marinade by bashing up the leafy end of the thyme bunch.

4. Peel the mushroom skins off.

5. Use the thyme stalk ends to brush the marinade on to each steak.

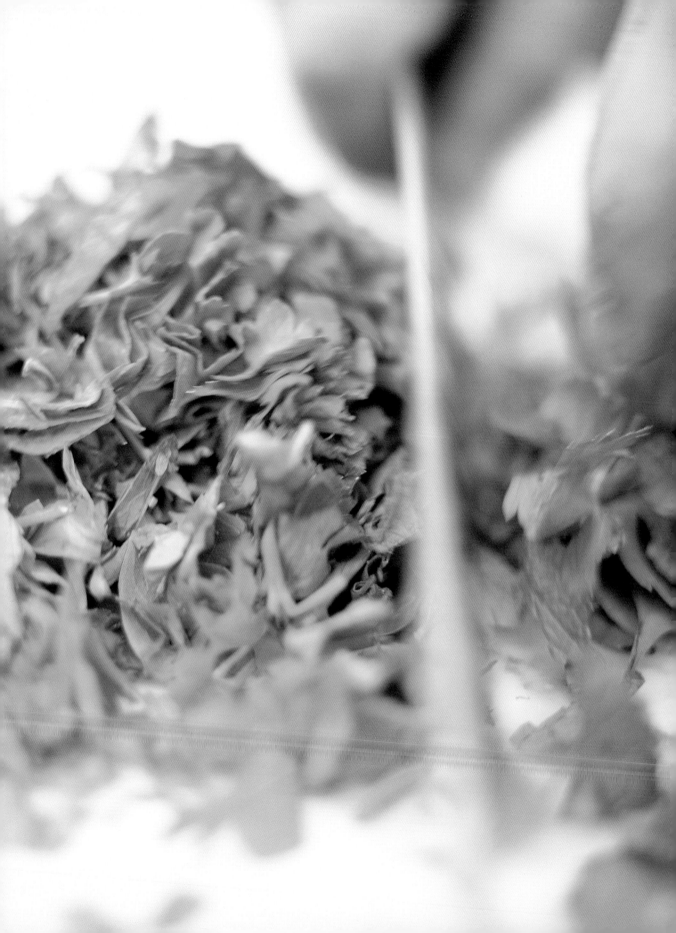

salsa verde

The best way to make salsa verde is to chop all the ingredients very finely by hand. It's great served with grilled or roasted meat and fish.

Finely chop the garlic, capers, gherkins, anchovies and herbs and put them into a bowl. Add the mustard and vinegar, then slowly stir in the olive oil until you achieve the right consistency. Balance the flavours with freshly ground black pepper, a bit of salt and maybe a little more vinegar.

SERVES 8

1½–2 cloves of garlic, peeled

1 small handful of capers

1 small handful of gherkins pickled in sweet vinegar

6 anchovy fillets

2 large handfuls of flat-leaf parsley, leaves picked

1 bunch of fresh basil, leaves picked

1 handful of fresh mint, leaves picked

1 tablespoon Dijon mustard

3 tablespoons red wine vinegar

8 tablespoons really good extra virgin olive oil

sea salt and freshly ground black pepper

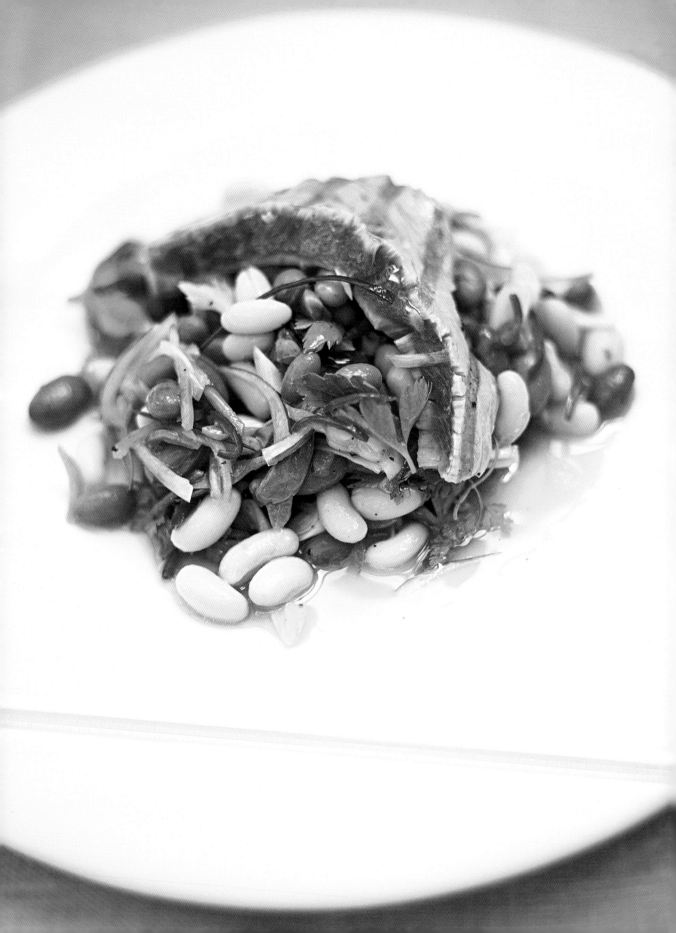

chargrilled tuna with dressed beans and loadsa herbs

This is a really beautiful summer dish that takes hardly any time at all to prepare – and of course you can use different kinds of beans, such as black-eyed beans, flageolets, butter beans or even lentils. It's a terrific hot snack or main dish – and with the tuna all torn up it makes a great salad. I like to griddle the tuna for a minute on each side so it has colour on the outside but still remains a little pink in the middle. A lot of people still want to cook tuna all the way through (which I think is madness!), but you must do it how you like best. It's worth seeing if you prefer it pink in the middle though. I'm really going heavy on the herbs in this recipe – 4 or 5 years ago this might have been a bit OTT, but it's really easy to get hold of a good selection of herbs now, so the more the merrier.

Feel free to use a couple of tins of beans if it's more convenient. Tinned beans aren't bad these days – they have got much better for some reason. But if you're using dried, which still taste better, soak them overnight in water. They'll double in size. You then just need to drain them and put them into a pan with fresh water to cover. Bring to the boil, then simmer them for around 40 minutes or until tender – sometimes I put a squashed tomato and a potato in the water with them, as it helps to soften the skins. When done, drain them, discarding the tomato and potato, and put them into a large bowl with 8 tablespoons of peppery olive oil, the red onion, anchovies and chillies. Season with salt and pepper and the lemon juice – for a bit of a twang.

Preheat your griddle pan until really hot. Season the tuna steaks with salt and pepper, sprinkle over the lemon zest and pat a little olive oil on both sides. Sear the steaks for a minute on each side. While the fish is searing, get your guests round the table. Throw the herbs into the dressed beans, mix up and divide between the plates. Take the tuna off the heat, tear it up and place on top of the warm beans. Nice with some cold white wine.

SERVES 4

100g/3 1/2oz dried cannellini beans

100g/3 1/2oz dried borlotti beans

optional: 1 tomato

optional: 1 potato

extra virgin olive oil

1 red onion, peeled and finely sliced

4 anchovy fillets, finely chopped

1–2 fresh red chillies, deseeded and finely sliced

sea salt and freshly ground black pepper

1 x 225g/8oz bluefin or really good dark yellowfin tuna steaks, about 1cm/1/2 inch thick

zest and juice of 2 lemons

3 handfuls of mixed fresh herbs (chives, chervil, basil, parsley, mint), roughly chopped

KNIFE TECHNIQUES

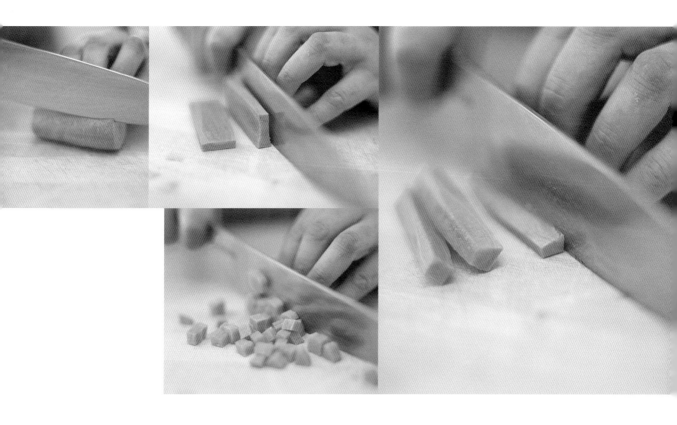

1. To stop the carrot moving about, simply slice down the length of one side and then roll it on to its flat edge.

2. Slice the carrots to your required thickness – very thin or a bit thicker. If the carrot feels at all unstable at any point then make sure you roll it on to its flattest edge. Be careful.

3. You can slice the carrots into lengths to make batons, which can be handy for stews and veg dishes.

4. Or gather up the batons and slice across to give you diced vegetables.

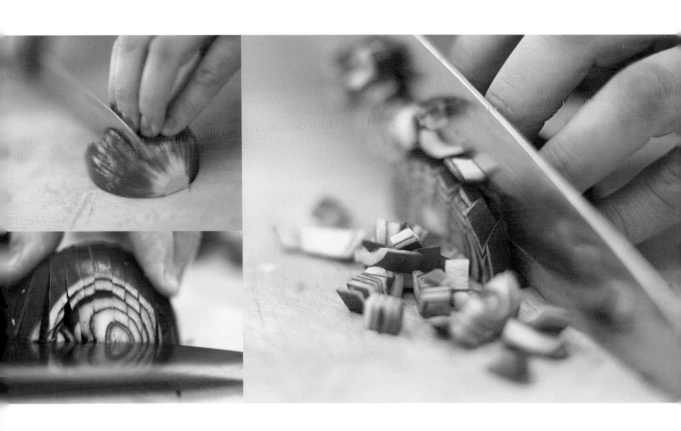

1. To chop an onion, peel, cut it in half and, with the core facing away from you, slice through but not quite to the core end, as this will hold the onion together.

2. Slice horizontally through the onion, but again, not quite to the core end.

3. Slice across your slices to give you chopped onion. You can do this fine or coarse depending on what you need. P.S. If you cry easily, wear swimming goggles!

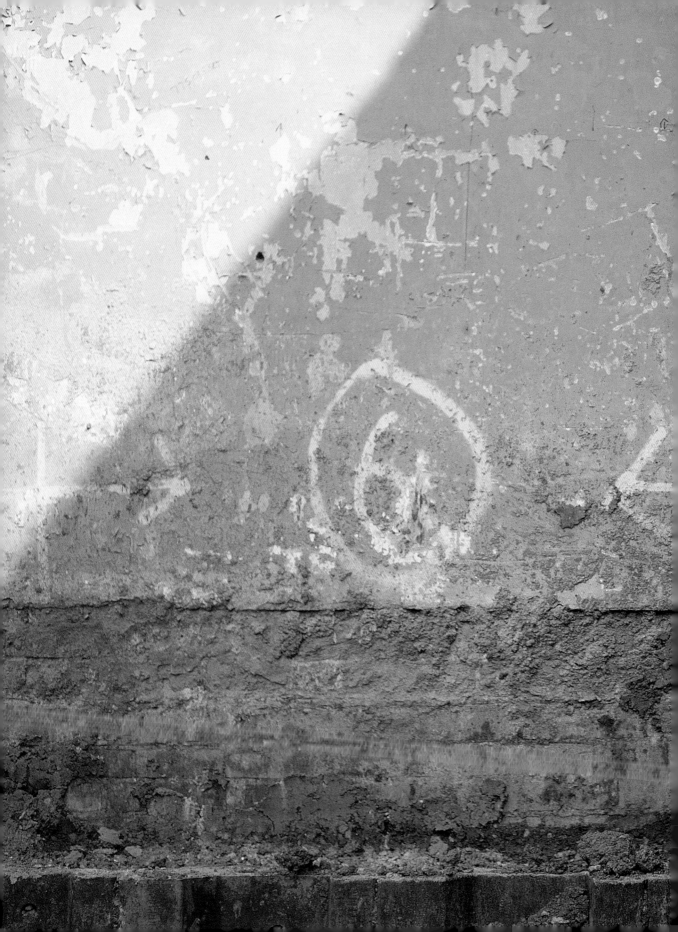

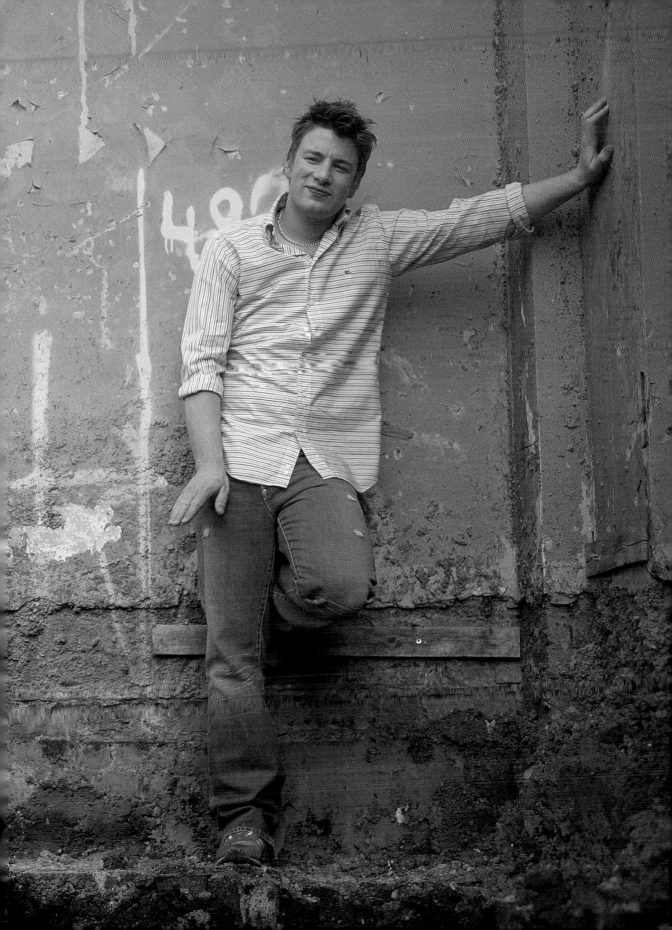

chargrilled pork leg with asparagus

This is a really good way to turn a cheap cut of meat into something special. In this recipe we're going to get nice thin escalopes of pork from the leg, flavour them and prepare them so they cook quickly. You could also use chicken or even veal in the same way if you fancy.

Rub the goat's cheese with a little olive oil and cook on a hot griddle on both sides until nicely coloured. Remove and put to one side. Bash up the garlic and lemon thyme in a pestle and mortar (or use a metal bowl and the end of a rolling pin). Add a couple of splashes of olive oil, stir, and rub the mixture all over the pork escalopes. Season the pork then put the escalopes one by one between 2 large pieces of clingfilm and hit them with something heavy and flat until they're about 0.5cm/¼ inch thick. This will make them really tender. Do this to all 4 escalopes.

Check that your griddle pan is hot, and chargrill your asparagus, then your courgettes, on both sides. Mark them nicely to give a bit of flavour and character to them. Put them into a salad bowl with the vinegar, 8 tablespoons of olive oil and half the fresh mint. Using the griddle pan again, chargrill your pork escalopes on both sides until nicely marked – about 4 minutes. Tear each escalope in half and scatter these into the salad bowl with the rest of the mint (for a lovely fresh burst of flavour) and the crumbled goat's cheese. Toss well, then place the bowl in the middle of the table and let everyone tuck in.

SERVES 4

150g/5½oz hard goat's cheese

8 tablespoons extra virgin olive oil plus a little extra

1 clove of garlic

1 small bunch of fresh lemon thyme, leaves picked

4 x 225g/8oz pork escalopes, about 1cm/½ inch thick

sea salt and freshly ground black pepper

500g/1lb 2oz asparagus, finely sliced lengthways

250g/9oz green and yellow courgettes, finely sliced lengthways

4 tablespoons cider vinegar or white wine vinegar

1 bunch of fresh mint, leaves picked

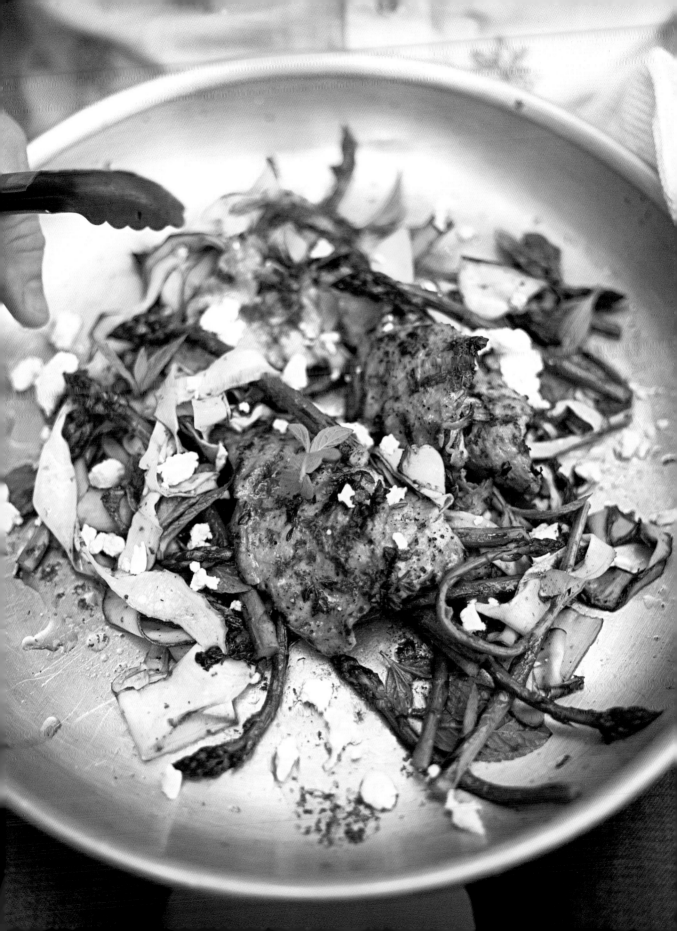

BAKING AND
SWEET THINGS

This is about the only time you'll ever hear Mr Oliver being very specific about measurements and weights and cooking times and sizes of tins and moulds, so please excuse me. But this is baking and I suppose it's a little like chemistry to get it right. It covers bread, cakes, tarts and all sorts of different desserts. I'll give you a nice selection of things to try which I bake at home all the time. The method of baking is similar to roasting, in that you've got dry heat from above and below in an oven, sometimes with a convection fan, but the cooking process doesn't rely on fat being on the surface of the food (though it may well be present within it). The actual cooking method is very simple – but because baking usually involves cakes and puddings that have to rise and cook within a certain amount of time, you have to stick to the recipes to get them just right.

pears in amarone

When I went to Italy this year with my mate David Gleave from Liberty Wines, he took me to a wine estate near Verona called Allegrini. All their wines are fantastic, but especially their Amarone, which is perfect for drinking and cooking with. After serving us a fantastic lunch they gave us these pears poached in Amarone. I've tweaked the recipe slightly to my own taste. It is so simple and delicious – if you can get some nice pears and a really good bottle of Amarone-style red you'll be laughing. If you use rubbish wine and manky old pears, the finished dish will be horrible, so don't try and do it half-heartedly.

Preheat the oven to 190°C/375°F/gas 5. Split the vanilla pods and remove the seeds (see page 304). Put the seeds and pods into an appropriately sized casserole-type pan that will hold all your pears snugly, and add the wine, sugar, cinnamon, and orange juice and zest. Throw in your thyme, secured together in a little bunch with string. Bring to the boil, turn down to a simmer, and add your pears, sitting upright. Put the lid on the pan and bake in the preheated oven for around 1 hour until the pears are soft and tender but not falling apart. They should be soft all the way through but retain their shape. (Sometimes they can take less or more time depending on the ripeness of the pears.) When they're ready they will have taken on the flavour and colour of the wine and should smell delicious.

By now the wine and the sugar will have thickened and the flavour will have intensified. Remove the pears to a dish, turn up the heat under the pan, and reduce the wine by about half. Remove from the heat and add the butter – agitate the pan but don't give it any more heat. This will give you a really intense, tasty sauce which is to die for. Put the pears back in the pan and leave until ready to serve. Warm is the best temperature to serve this dish, and it's best with some nice whipped sour cream or crème fraîche – a lovely contrast to the richness of the sauce.

SERVES 8

2 vanilla pods

1 bottle of Amarone or Barolo red wine

225g/8oz sugar

a small cinnamon stick

zest and juice of 1 orange

a small bunch of fresh thyme

8 Comice pears, peeled and base removed

250g/9oz butter

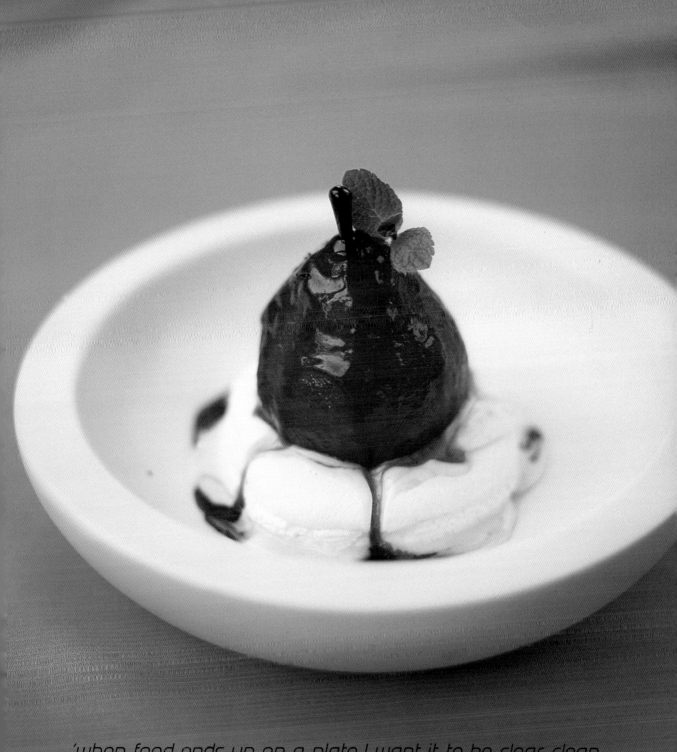

'when food ends up on a plate I want it to be clear, clean
and fresh, but most of all unfussy'

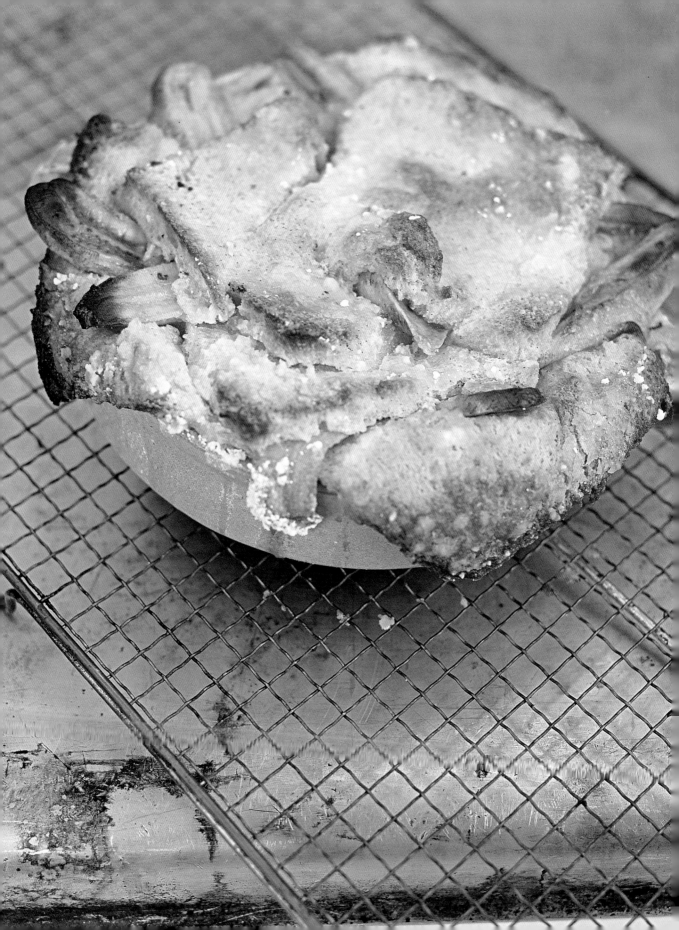

baileys and banana bread and butter pudding

Having grown up in a pub, two of the alcoholic drinks I tried and got a taste for at a very early age were Baileys and a cocktail called a Snowball. Now I'm older I detest the taste of both of them! Jools has a little drop of Baileys every now and again, so there's usually a bottle hanging about, and one day I had some bananas and it was as simple as that – I tried this recipe out and it was fantastic, one of the best possible twists on a bread and butter pudding.

Preheat the oven to 180°C/350°F/gas 4. Flatten each slice of bread down as flat as possible. Butter each piece thinly but thoroughly with the softened butter, then cut the slices of bread in half and put to one side.

In a bowl whisk together the sugar, vanilla seeds and eggs till pale and fluffy, then add the cream, the milk and the Baileys and whisk until smooth. Slice up your peeled bananas and lightly toast your almonds in the preheated oven. Take an appropriately sized baking dish (or you could do individual ones) and rub the sides with a little butter. Dip each piece of bread in the egg mixture then begin to layer the bread, the sliced banana and the almonds in the baking dish. Repeat until everything has been used up, ending with a top layer of bread. Pour over the rest of your egg mixture, using your fingers to pat down the bread to make sure it soaks up all the lovely flavours.

Generously dust the top of the pudding with icing sugar and bake in the oven for around 35 minutes or until the custard has set around the outside but is just slightly wobbly in the centre. Allow it to cool and firm up slightly. Some people like to serve it with ice cream or double cream, but if you get it gooey enough in the middle then it is nice just on its own. Feel free to take this recipe in any direction you like – using raisins or dried apricots or different types of bread like brioche or pannetone.

SERVES ABOUT 6

½ a loaf of pre-sliced white bread, crusts removed

55g/2oz or ¼ pack of butter, softened

140g/5oz caster sugar

seeds from 1 vanilla pod (see page 304)

8 free-range eggs

500ml/18fl oz double cream

565ml/1 pint milk

4 shots of Baileys

5 bananas

4 tablespoons flaked almonds, toasted until golden

icing sugar to dust

surprise pudding

When I was little, a gym opened around our way and it had a juice bar where they served this amazing carrot cake with a twangy sour cream topping. This is one of my efforts at making boring old carrot cake remotely credible. My mate Peter Begg, the friendly Scotsman, suggested I swap carrot for beetroot, which I did, and the result was marvellous. Thanks Pete!

Boil the beetroots until soft, then drain and allow to cool a little. Rub the skins off then mash in a food processor or with a masher till smooth. Preheat the oven to 180°C/350°F/gas 4. Put the beetroot purée, ginger, egg yolks, honey and olive oil in a bowl and add the seeds from 1 vanilla pod. Whisk together, then add the baking powder, polenta, orange zest and juice, salt, allspice, cinnamon and flour. In a separate bowl beat the egg whites until stiff and fold them into the beetroot mixture. Get yourself a 25cm/10 inch cake tin or cheesecake mould. Rub with butter and dust with a little flour to stop the cake sticking. You could also line it with greaseproof paper (see page 174 for how to make a cartouche) to be really sure. Pour in the mixture then bake in the preheated oven for around 35 minutes until spongy. Test whether it's ready by poking a cocktail stick into it – if it's clean when it comes out you know the cake's done. Allow to cool. Whisk the crème fraîche with the vin santo, sugar and the seeds from the remaining vanilla pod. Taste and adjust to your liking with a bit more sugar and vin santo. Serve the cake in wedges with a big dollop of the vin santo and vanilla cream.

SERVES 8

500g/1lb 2oz raw beetroots, preferably organic

2 thumb-sized pieces of fresh ginger, finely chopped

3 large organic eggs, separated

150ml/5 1/2fl oz honey

170ml/6fl oz olive oil

seeds from 2 vanilla pods (see page 304)

2 heaped teaspoons baking powder

100g/3 1/2oz polenta

zest and juice of 1 orange

a good pinch of salt

a good pinch of allspice

a good pinch of cinnamon

150g/5 1/2oz plain flour

200g/7oz crème fraîche

1 wineglass of vin santo, Marsala or sherry

2 heaped tablespoons caster sugar

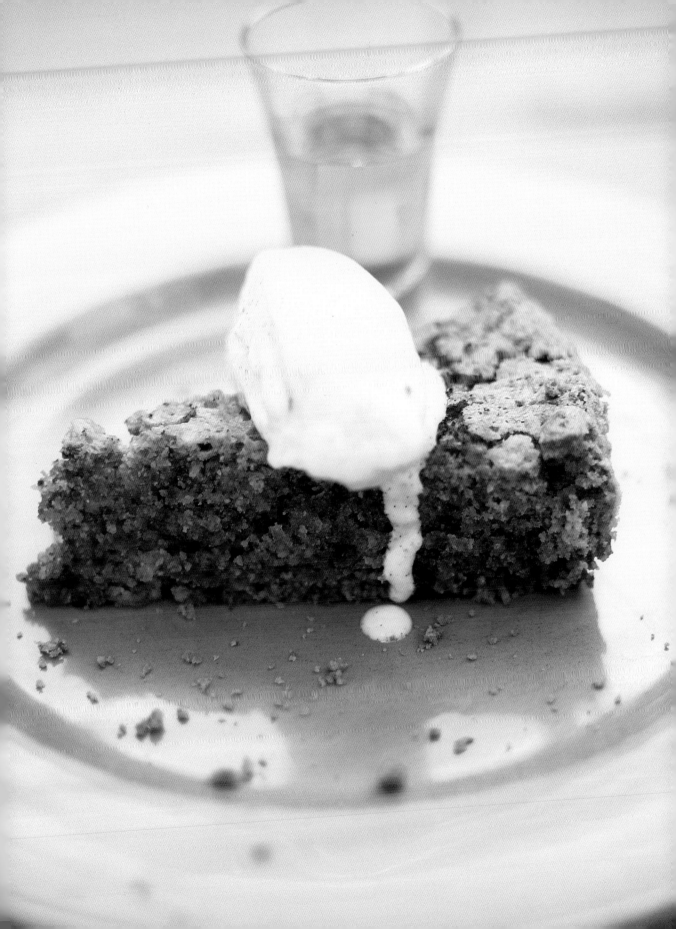

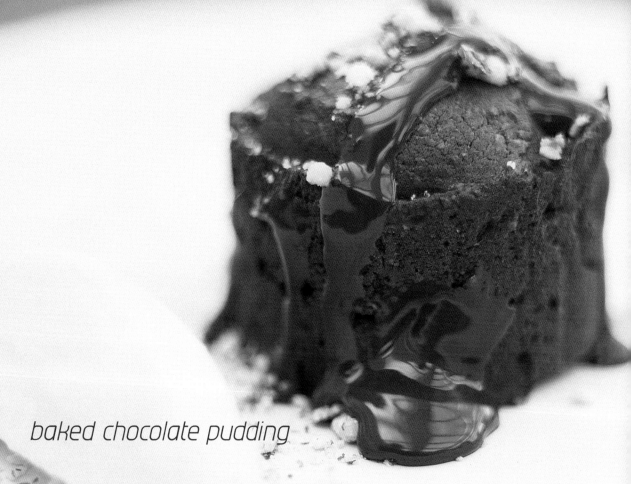

baked chocolate pudding

This pudding is chocolate heaven! The original recipe idea for it came from my mate Ben, the head chef at Monte's. I've changed it round a bit to make it easier to make at home.

Melt 125g/4¹/₂oz chocolate with the coffee, then pour into small ice-cube moulds and freeze until hard. Take 6 small 7.5cm/3 inch pastry rings, dariole moulds or cappuccino cups and grease well with some butter. Place in the fridge while you make your sponge mixture. Melt the remaining chocolate with the butter in a bowl over a pan of boiling water, then in a separate bowl whisk the egg whites with the sugar until firm. Fold the yolks into the cooled chocolate and butter mixture, then add the almonds and flour. Finish by carefully folding in the egg white mixture. Preheat the oven to 190°C/375°F/gas 5. Take your moulds out of the fridge and spoon a little mixture into each one, then push in a cube of the frozen coffee and chocolate mixture. Cover with the rest of the sponge mixture so each ice cube is completely enveloped. Bake in the preheated oven for about 18–20 minutes, then remove carefully from the moulds while hot. Serve immediately sprinkled with hazelnuts.

SERVES 6

455g/1lb best-quality cooking chocolate (70% cocoa solids)

50ml/2fl oz hot espresso or good strong instant coffee

125g/4¹/₂oz butter, plus extra for greasing

6 eggs, separated

200g/7oz caster sugar

100g/3¹/₂oz ground almonds

100g/3¹/₂oz rice flour

1 small handful chopped hazelnuts, toasted

rice pudding

Sometimes the golden oldies are the best! This rice pudding is dead easy, very comforting and can be varied with all types of different flavours.

Put the butter, sugar, milk, vanilla seeds, salt and rice in a pan and bring to a gentle simmer. Cover and leave to simmer until the milk has been absorbed and the rice is soft but not too stodgy. Serve in bowls while hot.

Try this: For a nice surprise, drop a spoonful of jam into the middle of each pudding, or melt about 200g of best-quality cooking chocolate (70% cocoa solids) in a bowl over some simmering water and stir this into your rice pudding before serving.

SERVES 4

100g/3½oz butter

115g/4oz caster sugar

1.3 litres/2 pints milk

seeds from 2 vanilla pods (see page 304)

a pinch of salt

140g/5oz pudding rice

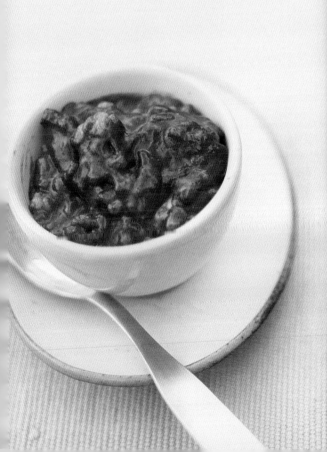

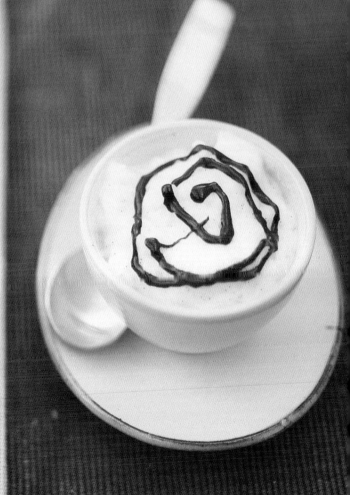

perfect sweet pastry

You can make this pastry by hand or in a food processor. I never make less than this quantity, so when I say 'l x basic pastry recipe' in the recipes which follow it's always a good idea to freeze the extra tart shell for use another day. Turn the page for some great step by step pictures showing how to make the pastry and then bake it 'blind'.

Stage 1: Cream together the butter, icing sugar and salt, then rub or pulse in the flour, vanilla seeds, lemon zest and egg yolks. When this mixture has come together, looking like coarse breadcrumbs, add the cold milk or water. Pat together to form a ball of dough. Lightly flour and then squeeze it into shape. The idea is to get your ingredients to a dough form with the minimum amount of movement, i.e. keeping your pastry flaky and short (the more you work it the more elastic it will get, causing it to shrink in the oven and be chewy, and you don't want that to happen).

Stage 2: Roll the pastry into a really large, short and fat sausage shape, wrap it in clingfilm and put it in the fridge to rest for at least 1 hour.

Stage 3: Carefully slice off very thin slivers of your pastry lengthways. You can make the slices thicker if you like, but remember that the tart will take longer to cook. Place the slivers all around your tart mould, fitting them together like a jigsaw. Push the pieces together and tidy up the sides by cleaning any excess pastry from the rim of the mould. Place in the freezer for at least 1 hour.

Stage 4: If I'm going to fill my tart shells with an uncooked filling I usually bake them 'blind' (i.e. with no filling) for around 15 minutes at 180°C/350°F/gas 4 – this will cook them all the way through, colouring them slightly. Once completely cooled, the shells can be filled. With baked fillings the tart shell has to be baked blind for around 12 minutes at 180°C/350°F/gas 4 before being filled and then baked once more.

Try this: Once your tart shell has been baked blind, brush the inside of it with a little egg white and then put it back in the oven for 30 seconds – no longer. This will give it a nice waterproof layer which will protect it from a moist filling. The pastry will stay crumbly and crisp for longer instead of going all soggy.

TO MAKE 2 x 28CM/ 11 INCH TART SHELLS

250g/9oz butter

200g/7oz icing sugar

a medium pinch of salt

500g/just over 1lb flour

seeds from 1 vanilla pod

zest of 1 lemon

4 egg yolks

2–4 tablespoons cold milk or water

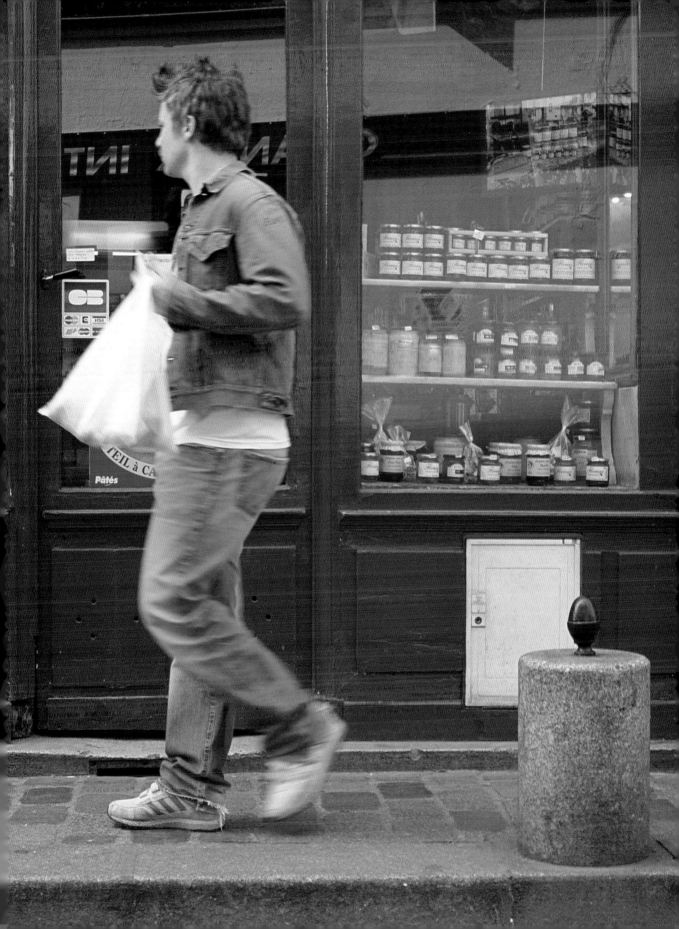

MAKING THE PERFECT SWEET PASTRY

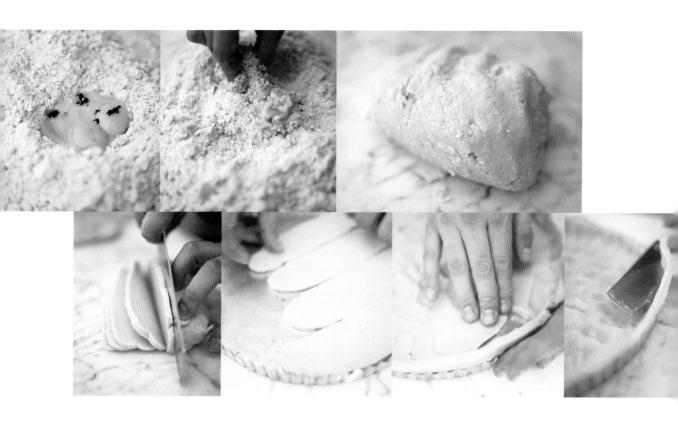

1. Add the egg yolk, lemon zest and vanilla seeds to the flour mix.

2. Rub together until the mixture is like coarse breadcrumbs.

3. Pat together to form a ball of dough.

4. Slice off in slivers.

5. Place the slivers in your tart mould.

6. Push the pieces together.

7. Tidy up the sides by trimming off any excess pastry.

BAKING 'BLIND'

I find that if you freeze your pastry case you can bake it blind straight from the freezer without it shrinking. If you haven't got time to freeze it, then simply line the case with clingfilm (yes, it's absolutely fine) or greaseproof paper, fill it with dried beans and bake it, as shown below.

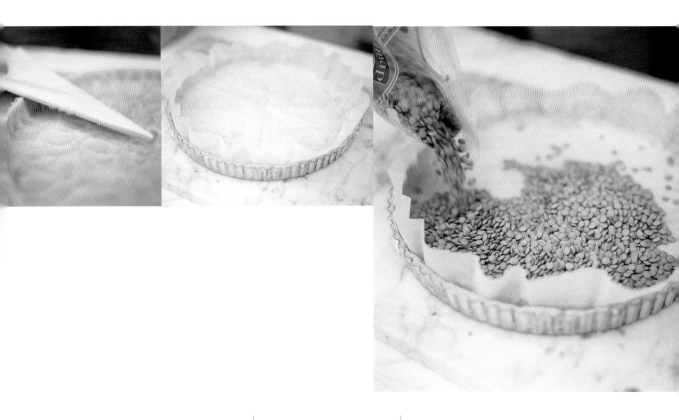

1. Measure a folded piece of greaseproof paper against the pastry case and tear off to give you a cartouche (see page 174).

2. Line the pastry case with the cartouche.

3. Fill the pastry case with dried beans and then bake for 12–15 minutes at 180°C/350°F/gas 4 until lightly golden.

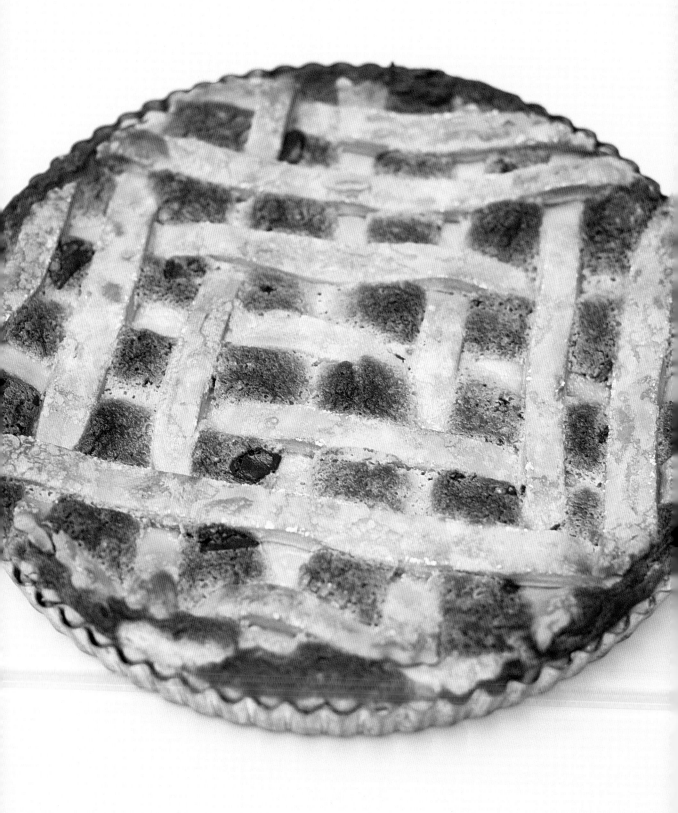

baked ricotta and mascarpone tart with chocolate and orange

When I used to work at the Neal Street Restaurant with Gennaro Contaldo (a superb chef who taught me such a lot), he used to make 4 or 5 things similar to this every morning using just ricotta and candied fruit. This is a really fantastic tart – great with a cup of tea in the afternoon. Terrific with a little crème fraîche and segmented oranges. For this version I used half ricotta and half mascarpone and put my own flavour combination together.

Make the pastry and line a loose-bottomed 28cm/11 inch flan tin. Bake blind (see page 285) and allow to cool. Roll the extra pastry out to the same thickness in a long rectangular shape, dusting as you go, and divide into 14 strips 2.5 cm/1 inch wide. Set these aside – you will need them to finish off the tart.

Turn the oven down to 170°C/325°F/gas 3. Whip together the ricotta, mascarpone, icing sugar, orange zest, vanilla seeds and egg yolks until smooth and shiny. In a separate bowl whip up your egg whites until stiff – you can test if they're done by holding the bowl upside down over your head. Obviously the mixture should stick to the bowl and not fall on your head! Gently fold the egg whites into the mixture. Pour into your cooled tart mould and sprinkle the chocolate over the top. Lay 7 strips of pastry across the tart, equally spaced, and then place the other 7 the other way on top of them like a lattice. Use your thumbs to trim any excess pastry off the side of the mould – this will stick it to the pastry below. Brush the pastry with a little of the beaten egg and then dust with a little icing sugar. Bake in the preheated oven for 40–45 minutes.

This tart can be served hot or cold with some ice cream, crème fraîche or cream.

SERVES 8

1 x basic pastry recipe
(see page 282)

250g/9oz ricotta cheese

250g/9oz mascarpone

125g/4½oz icing sugar

zest of 3 oranges

seeds from 2 vanilla pods
(see page 304)

2 eggs, separated

100g/3½oz best-quality cooking chocolate (70% cocoa solids), roughly chopped

1 egg, beaten

icing sugar, for dusting

hazelnut torte

I must have made this torte hundreds of times when I first moved to London – it was one of the first classic Italian dessert recipes that I learned to make and it's great!

Preheat the oven to 190°C/375°F/gas 5. Butter a 28cm/11 inch loose-bottomed flan tin or cheesecake mould, line it with greaseproof paper and place it in the fridge. Put the hazelnuts on to a baking tray and roast in the oven for about 5 minutes until lightly golden. Allow to cool, then whizz up in a food processor until you have a fine powder – be careful not to over-whizz. You can bash the nuts up in a tea towel using a rolling pin if you don't have a food processor.

Beat the butter and sugar together either in the food processor, or in a bowl with a whisk, until pale. Add the egg yolks one by one, and the orange zest. Sieve in the flour, crumble in the ricotta and stir in the powdered hazelnuts and the poppy seeds. In a separate bowl, beat the egg whites with a pinch of salt until they are really stiff, then fold them slowly into the hazelnut mixture. Pour the mixture into the cake tin and bake in the preheated oven for around 25–30 minutes until there is a little colour on the top of the torte. You can check to see that it's ready by sticking a cocktail stick into the centre of the torte. It should come out clean and not sticky. Remove from the oven and allow to cool. While it's cooling, place the jam in a little pan with 4 tablespoons of water and bring this slowly up to the boil. Brush this over the top of the torte and, when cool, sprinkle with the grated chocolate. Serve with some crème fraîche or fromage frais.

SERVES 8

115g/4oz butter, softened to room temperature, plus extra for tin

125g/4¹/₂oz hazelnuts

125g/4¹/₂oz sugar

4 large organic eggs, separated

zest of 1 orange

30g/1oz plain flour

125g/4¹/₂oz ricotta cheese

2 tablespoons poppy seeds

a pinch of salt

3 heaped tablespoons jam, preferably apricot

50g/1³/₄oz best-quality cooking chocolate (70% cocoa solids), finely grated

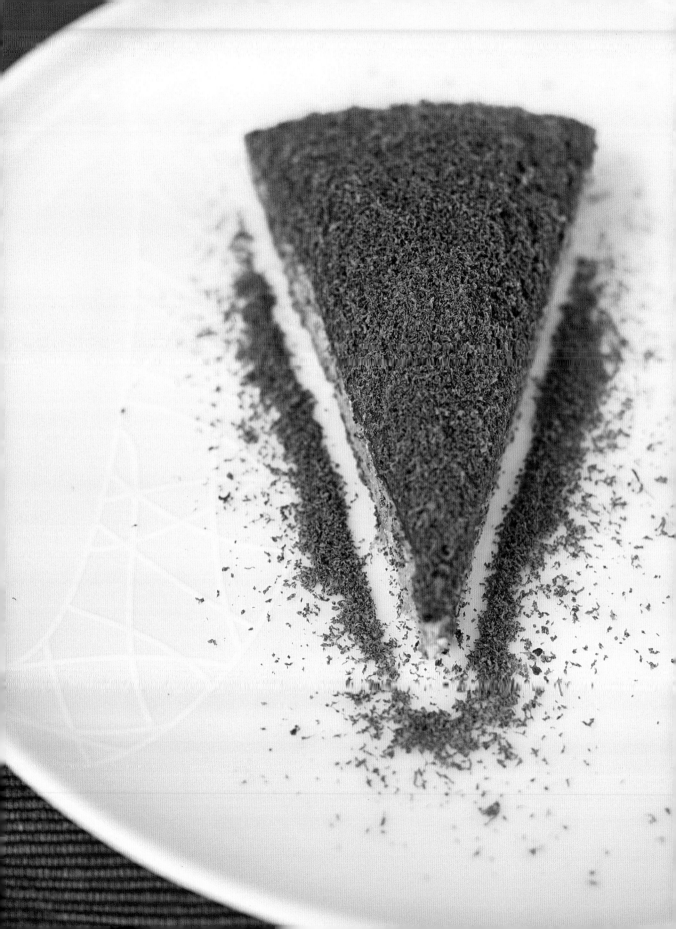

nectarine meringue pie

A really lovely dessert with a gorgeous peachy flavour. It can be made with any fruit combination you fancy. Try using apricots, peaches or plums.

Preheat the oven to 180ºC/350ºF/gas 4. Make the pastry, then line a 28cm/11 inch loose-bottomed flan tin with it. Place in the freezer to stop the pastry from shrinking. Wash the nectarines then run your knife round each one and twist to remove the stone. Slice up and put into a small baking dish or tray with the 115g/4oz sugar, butter and cornflour. Stir well and cover with tin foil.

Take the pastry case out of the freezer. Place in the oven with the dish of nectarines on a shelf below, and bake for around 15 minutes until the pastry is lightly golden and the nectarines have softened.

Beat the egg whites to peaks – you can tell if they're done by holding the bowl upside down over your head. If the meringue is stiff enough it should stay in the bowl! Add the 125g/4½oz sugar and whisk in.

When the pastry case and nectarines are ready, remove them from the oven. Pour the nectarines and all their lovely juices into the pastry case. Dollop the meringue on top and peak it with a fork so it's not all smooth and flat. Put the tart back into the oven for around 8 minutes until the meringue is lightly golden. Serve this either hot or cold.

SERVES 8

1 x basic pastry recipe (see page 282)

1.2kg/2½lb ripe nectarines or peaches

115g/4oz vanilla sugar or caster sugar

a little butter

1 level tablespoon cornflour

5 large egg whites

125g/4½oz caster sugar or vanilla sugar

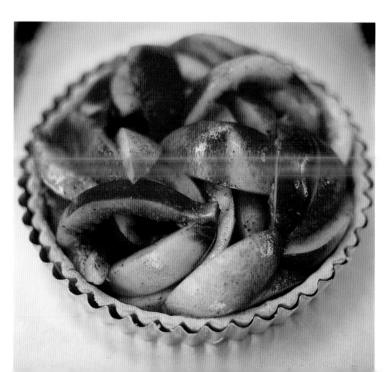

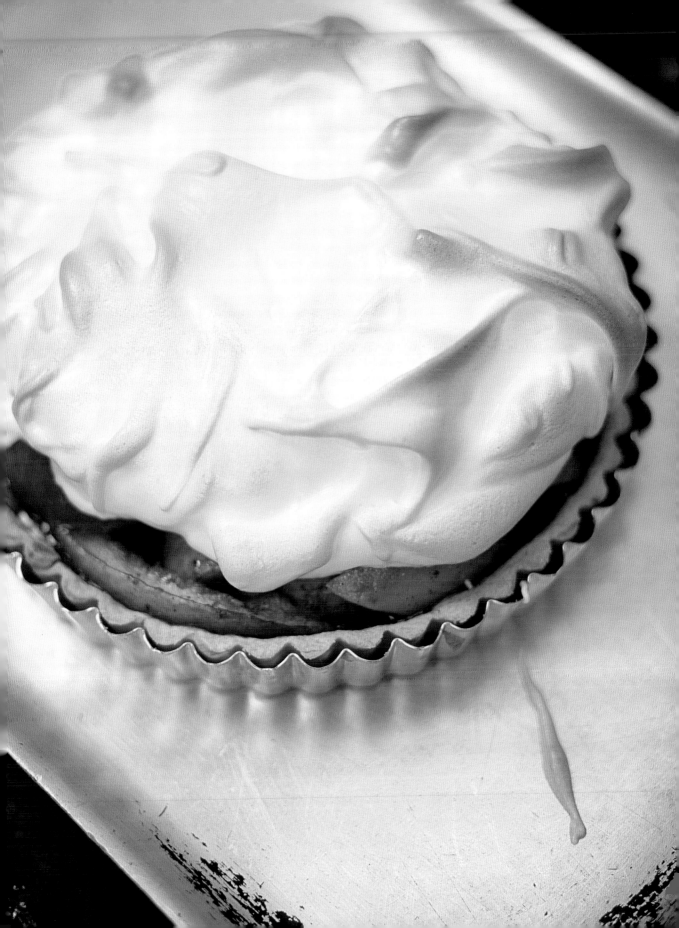

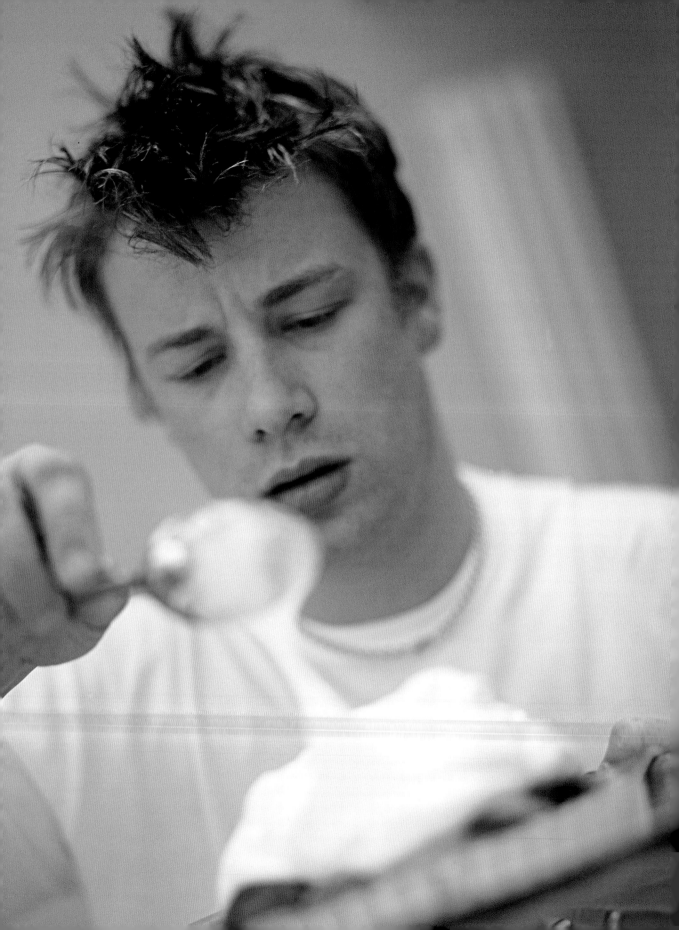

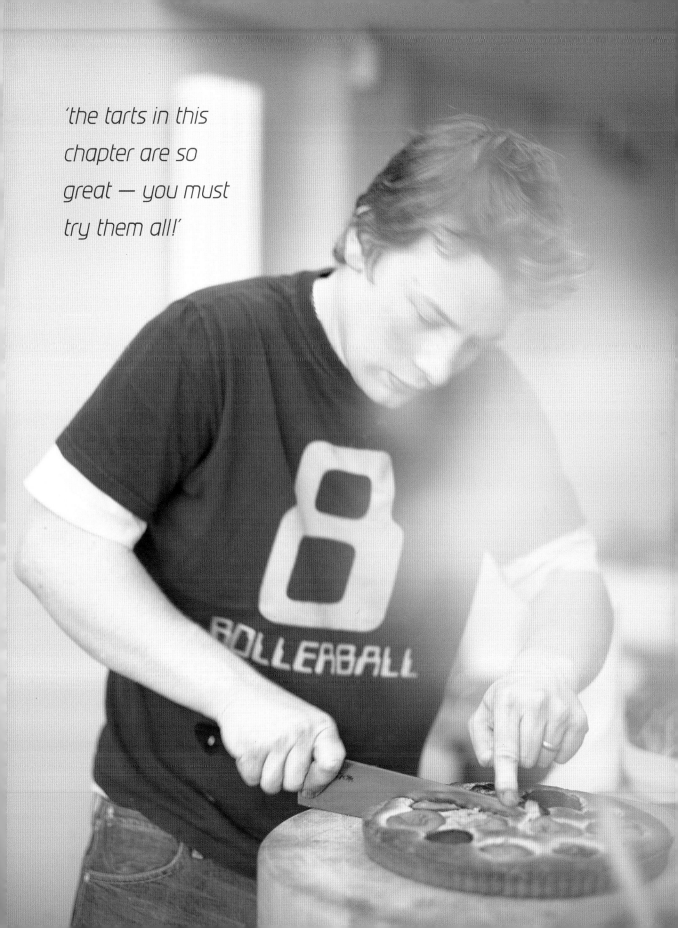

'the tarts in this chapter are so great — you must try them all!'

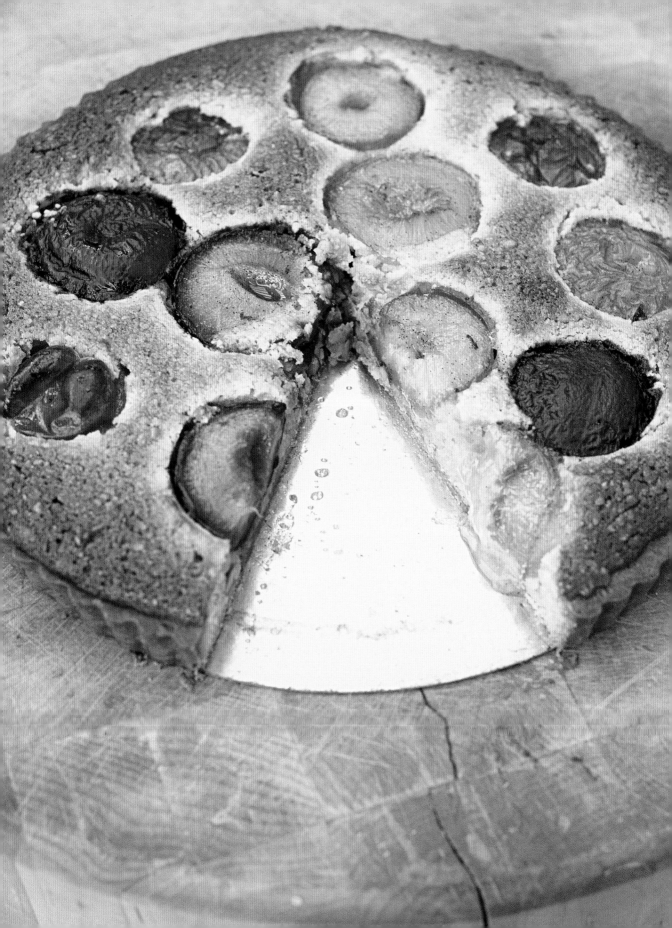

plum and almond tart

This is a great filling for a tart. It gives you a lovely frangipane mixture, with the delicate taste of almonds, and the lovely texture of baked plums.

Make the pastry then line a 28cm/11 inch loose-bottomed flan tin with it and bake it blind (see page 285).

In a food processor, blitz the whole almonds to a fine powder and put into a bowl. Then blitz the butter and sugar until light and creamy. Add this to the almonds with the lightly beaten eggs and fold in until completely mixed and nice and smooth. Stir in the pistachio nuts, then place in the fridge to firm up slightly. Once the mixture has chilled, pour it into your tart case about three-quarters full. You don't want to over fill it otherwise it will spill over the edge when you add the plums.

Toss the plums in the vanilla sugar, let them sit for 10 minutes, then push them into the tart mixture. Bake the tart on a tray at 180°C/350°F/gas 4 for about 1 hour, or until the almond mix has become firm and golden on the outside but is still soft in the middle. Allow to cool for about ½ an hour and serve with ice cream or crème fraîche.

SERVES 8

350g/12oz blanched whole almonds

300g/10½oz unsalted butter

300g/10½oz caster sugar

3 whole free-range eggs

1 handful whole pistachio nuts, shelled

1 x basic pastry recipe (see page 282)

6–7 plums, halved and destoned

3 tablespoons vanilla sugar

citrus curd tart — my favourite ways

The great thing about this recipe is the way in which it can be varied. The classic lemon curd tart is still my favourite but sometimes it makes a nice change to blend some lime or orange juice with the lemon. Or try a straight orange tart. Just make sure your juice amount is always 320ml/11fl oz.

Make the pastry and line a 28cm/11 inch loose-bottomed flan tin. Bake blind (see page 285). To make the filling, put the yolks, whole eggs, sugar, citrus juice and zest into a thick-bottomed pan and whisk over a very low heat. Keep whisking for around 4 minutes until the mixture slowly begins to thicken, then you can change from a whisk to a wooden spoon. Add the butter and continue stirring. Make sure you stir up every bit of curd mixture from the bottom of the pan. As soon as it nicely coats the back of the spoon like really thick custard, you can remove it from the heat and allow it to cool down a little bit. Give it one final whisk so that it's nice and smooth. At this point pass the mixture through a sieve to get rid of the little pieces of lemon zest. Using a spatula, scrape every last bit of lemon curd mixture into the tart mould while it's still lukewarm and shake gently so the mixture goes nice and flat. Allow to set and cool for 30 minutes and then you can serve it as it is, or try one of my favourite ways below.

Try this: I love dusting the tart with a good layer of icing sugar then caramelizing it with a blowtorch to give a thin snappy layer of caramel. Or try chilling it and then topping it with meringue using the 7 egg whites left over from the ingredients above and whisking them with 200g/7oz sugar.

Or this: This tart is fantastic served with any seasonal fruit, especially raspberries and strawberries.

SERVES 8

1 x basic pastry recipe (see page 282)

7 large egg yolks

7 whole eggs

375g/13oz caster sugar

320ml/11fl oz citrus juice, plus zest from the fruit

320g/11½oz unsalted butter, room temperature

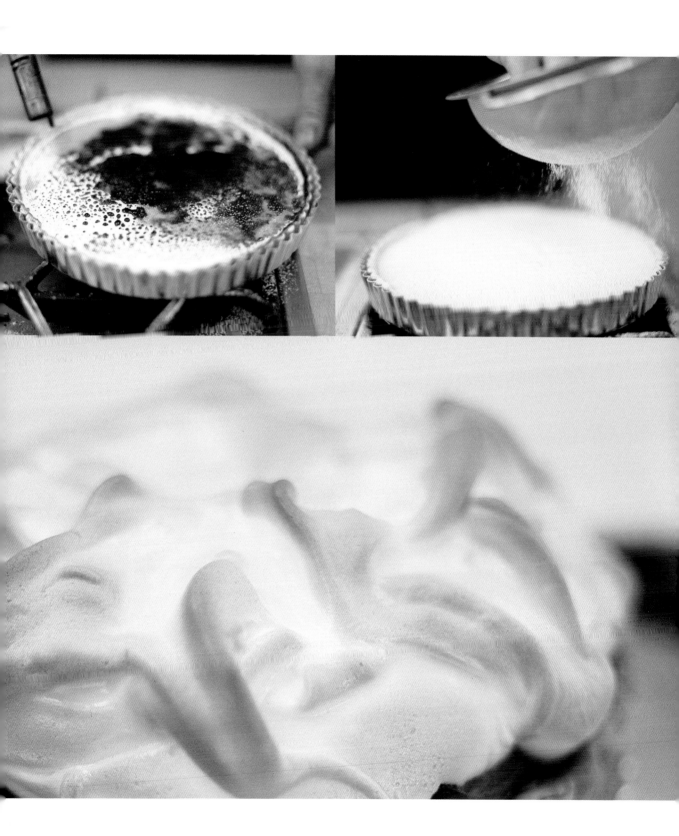

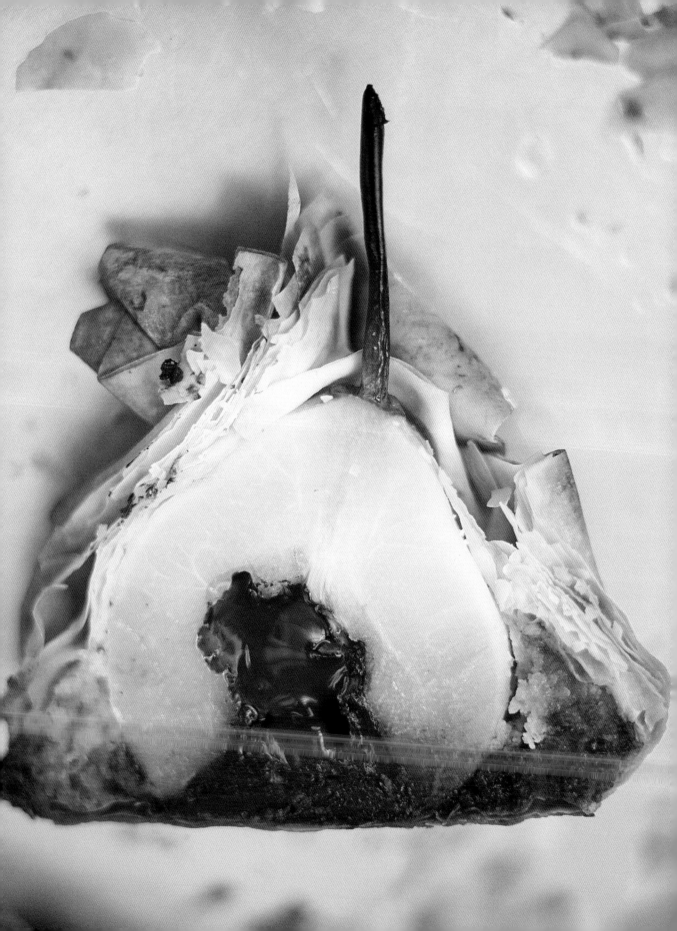

baked pears stuffed with almonds, orange and chocolate in flaky pastry

I've been mucking about with filo pastry quite a lot at home recently, because you can buy it frozen, it's dead cheap, and just by brushing a couple of sheets of filo with some melted butter you can wrap or line things to give you a fantastic texture and crunch. I'm cooking whole pears in this recipe, but you can try it with poached apples or nectarines as well. I chisel out each core (with nectarines, remove the stones as carefully as possible), then stuff them with my kind of frangipane, cover them with filo and bake them. Absolutely amazing and dead simple

Preheat the oven to 170°C/325°F/gas 3. Carefully peel the pears and remove out the core from the bottom. This will give you a hole about 4cm/1½ inches deep. Put the pears to one side.

Put your blanched almonds into a food processor and whizz up until really fine. (You could always do this by placing them in a tea towel and bashing them with a rolling pin.) Put them in a bowl with 70g/2½oz of the butter, the sugar and the zest and juice of the orange. Add the vanilla seeds to the bowl, then mix everything up until nice and smooth. Bash up the chocolate into small pieces, adding these to the mixture as well. Divide into 4 balls and put to one side.

Melt the rest of the butter in a little pan for brushing on to the filo pastry. Dampen a clean tea towel and wring it out – use this to cover the unused filo pastry so it doesn't dry out and become too brittle. Working with one piece of filo at a time – they are normally about A4 size – spread it out in front of you and brush the sheet with melted butter. Lay the next sheet of pastry on top and repeat until you have 4 brushed layers of filo pastry. Cut the layered pastry down to a 20cm x 20cm/8 inch x 8 inch square.

Take a pear and one ball of almond mix and fill the hole in the base, packing the excess filling around the base of the pear. Place in the middle of the filo square then gather up the pastry around the stalk and pinch tight. You can leave it looking nice and rustic and flopping all over the place, as this will look really good when it's cooked. Repeat this process with the other 3 pears. Brush the outside of the pastry with any remaining melted butter then cook in the preheated oven for 25–30 minutes until the pastry is golden and crisp. Serve with fromage frais, crème fraîche or vanilla ice cream.

SERVES 4

4 perfectly ripe pears

40g/1½oz blanched almonds

150g/5½oz butter

50g/1¾oz sugar

zest and juice of 1 orange

seeds from 1 vanilla pod (see page 304)

70g/2½oz best-quality cooking chocolate (70% cocoa solids)

16 sheets of filo pastry, defrosted if frozen

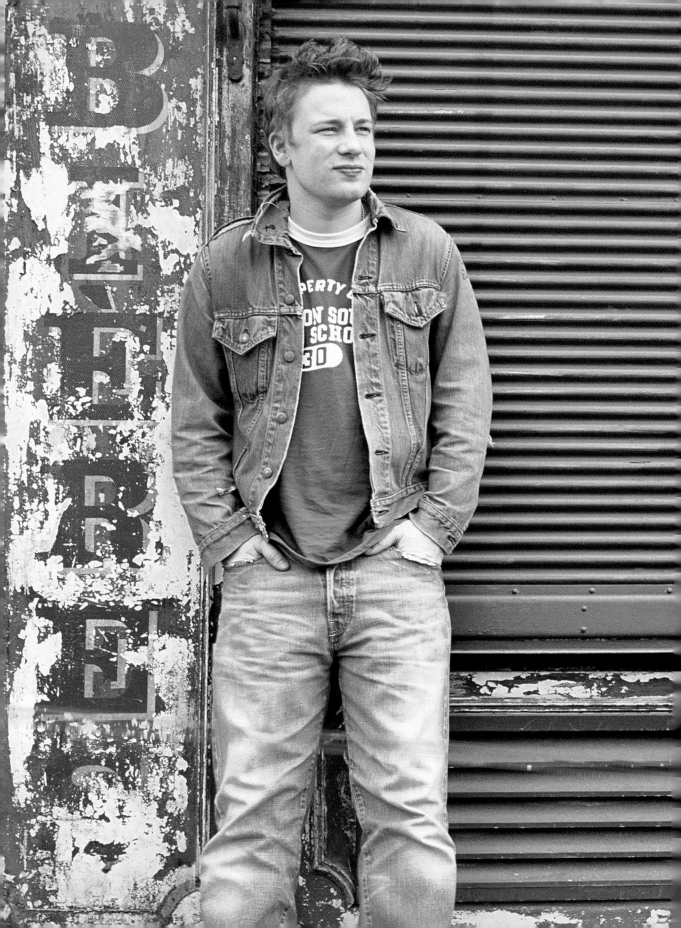

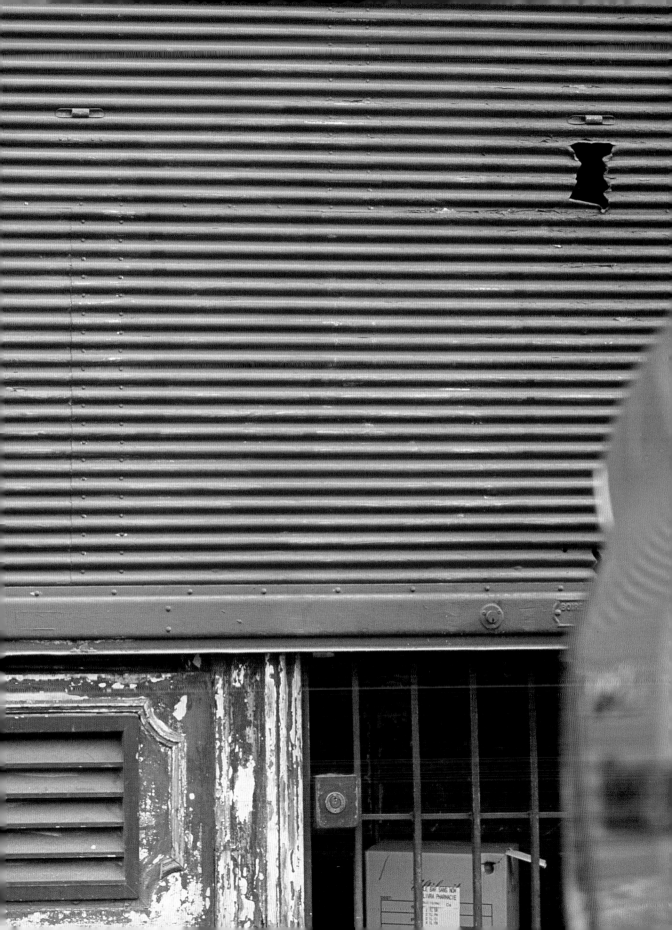

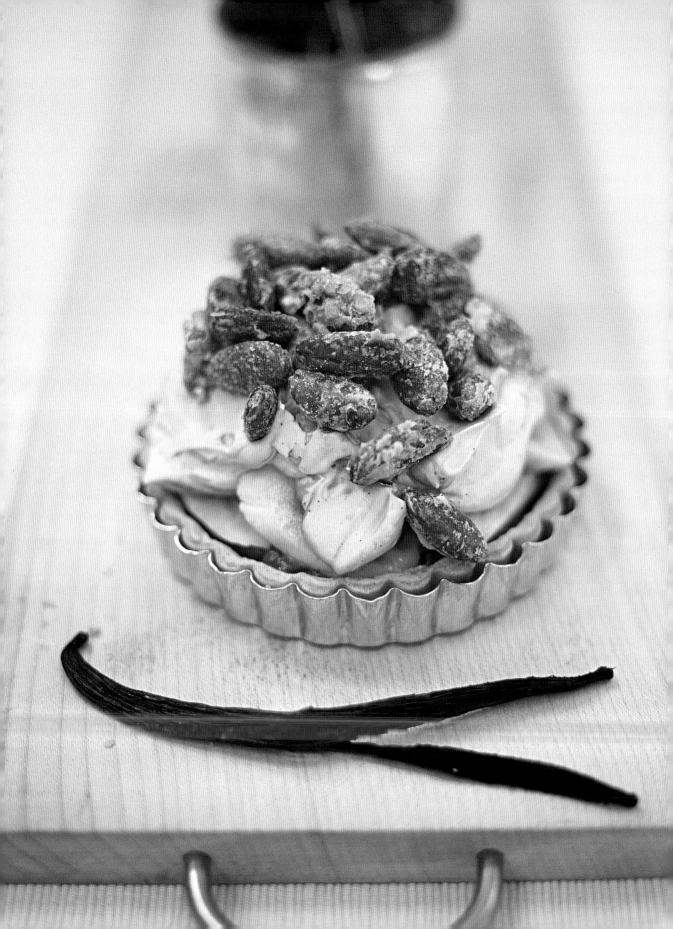

banoffee pie

When I was little we used to make banoffee pies at the pub which everyone loved. To make a big batch the trick was to boil up loads of unopened tins of condensed milk in one big pan for about 4 hours. I suggest that at home you boil a couple of tins up, because when you've made this banoffee pie once, you'll definitely want to make it again. It's really important to keep the water topped up though, so make sure you keep checking it – if the pan boils dry the tins will explode and you'll have toffee all over your ceiling – not only dangerous, but a bugger to clean up! When the tins are boiled and left unopened, they keep for months in the larder and even longer in the freezer. It is also important to let the tins cool down on their own and make sure they have cooled completely before you open them. However, jars of pre-made toffee are now sold in the supermarkets, so I've used one in this recipe, but feel free to boil your own if you want to live life on the edge!

Preheat the oven to 180°C/350°F/gas 4. Give the almonds a rinse in water, drain them a little and mix them quickly with the icing sugar in a bowl until they are really sticky. Place on a baking tray and toast for 15 minutes in the oven until they are golden and crispy, turning them every couple of minutes. Don't let them turn black or they will taste bitter. Remove from the oven and allow to cool. Make the pastry, line a loose-bottomed, buttered 28cm/11 inch flan tin (or you could try making smaller individual ones) and bake it blind for 15 minutes until lightly golden (see page 285). Remove from the oven and let it cool.

Spread the toffee as thick as you like across the base of the pastry. Slice the bananas and place on top of the toffee, then whip the cream. Add the Camp coffee – add a little less if you'd like a more subtle coffee flavour – and the vanilla seeds. Then dollop the cream on top of the bananas, as high and as rough as you like.

Sprinkle the almonds over the top of the banoffee pie and serve immediately.

SERVES 8

200g/7oz blanched, whole almonds

280g/10oz icing sugar

1 x basic pastry recipe (see page 282)

1 jar of Merchant Gourmet Dulce de Leche toffee or 2 x 397g/14oz tins of condensed milk, boiled

6 bananas

565ml/1 pint double cream

1 tablespoon Camp coffee

seeds from 1 vanilla pod (see page 304)

clementine chocolate salad

I love the idea of having a refreshing salad for dessert. You can have some real fun with this sprinkling different nuts, herbs and chocolate over the top.

Peel the clementines, slice across thinly and remove the pips. Arrange on 4 plates and sprinkle over the almonds and mint. Bring the sugar and water to the boil, add the vanilla seeds and allow to simmer until the liquid becomes a light golden syrup. Try not to touch it too much at this stage. Drizzle the syrup over the clementines and top with the shaved chocolate before serving.

SERVES 4

8 clementines

1 large handful of flaked almonds

10 fresh mint leaves, finely sliced (see page 112)

6 tablespoons caster sugar

4 tablespoons water

seeds from 1 vanilla pod (see below)

100g/3 ½oz best-quality cooking chocolate (70% cocoa solids), shaved

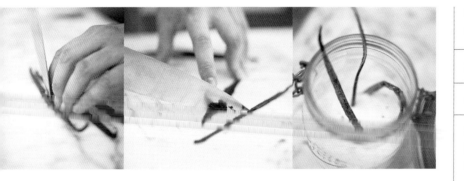

REMOVING SEEDS FROM VANILLA PODS

1. Score the pods.

2. Scrape the seeds out.

3. Put the unwanted pods in a jar of sugar for delicious flavoured vanilla sugar.

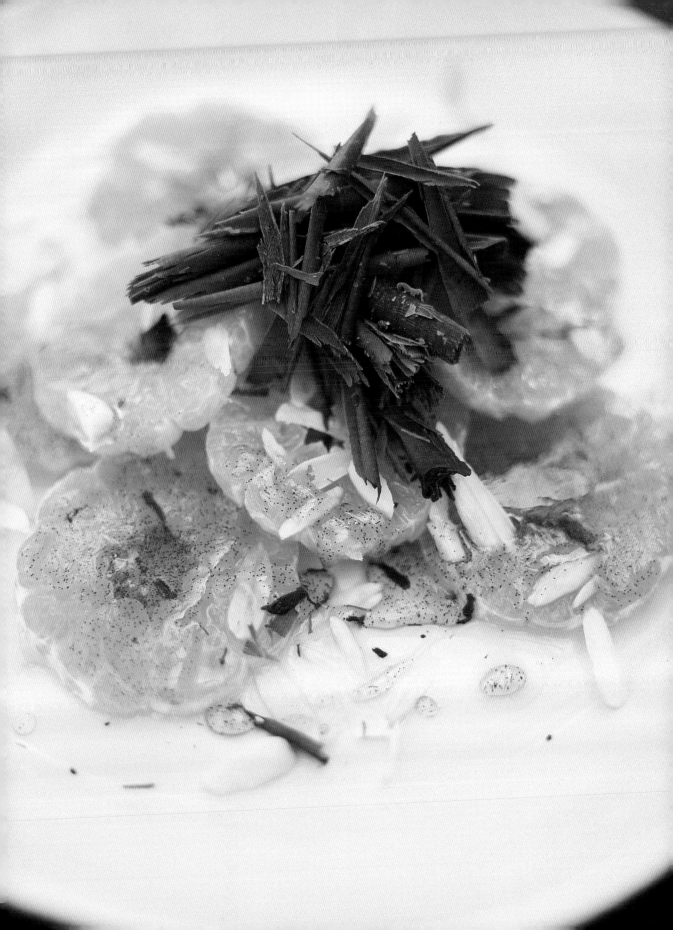

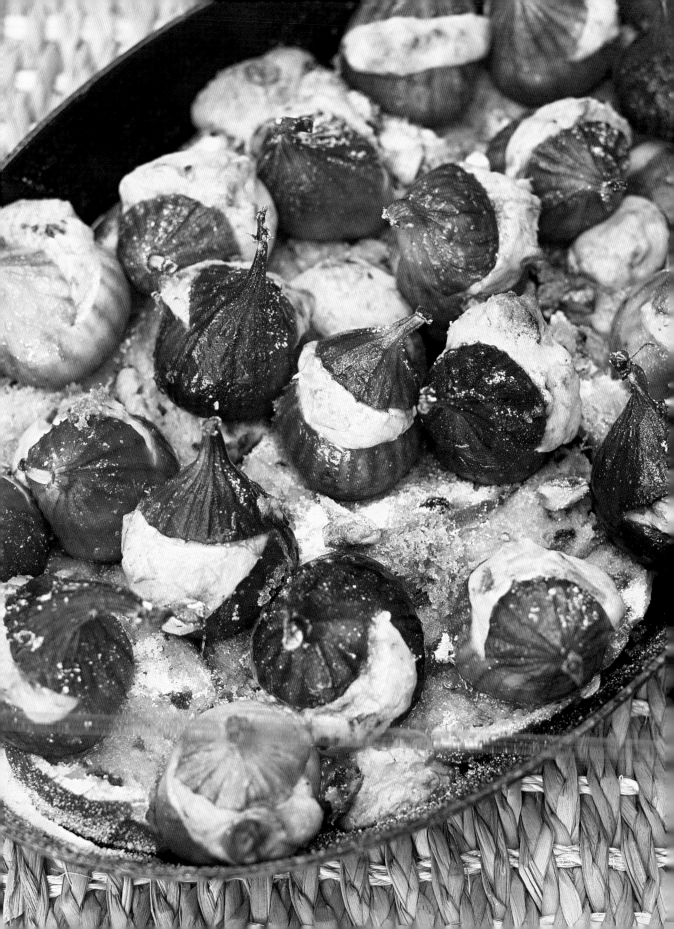

scrumptious baked figs with mascarpone, orange, pistachios and hot cross buns

This is a really quick and tasty little dish which always makes me feel good.

Preheat the oven to 180°C/350°F/gas 4. Put your mascarpone in a bowl. Chop up half of the pistachios and add to the mascarpone, along with half the honey, half the orange zest and the orange juice. If you like you can also add the bashed-up chocolate at this point. Mix everything together and taste for sweetness – you may need a little more honey.

Butter an appropriately sized earthenware dish. Slice your hot cross buns any way you like into 4 or 5 pieces and lay these in the dish. With a sharp knife, carefully cut across the top of each fig, but not quite all the way through – you want to leave a sort of hinged lid. Poke your finger into each fig to make a little extra room, then spoon some of the mascarpone mix into the gap so it almost oozes out. Keep any leftover filling to one side. Place the figs in, around and on top of the buns. Drizzle with the remaining honey and sprinkle with the extra pistachios and orange zest. Dab any leftover mascarpone mix around the buns in the baking dish then dust the whole lot with some icing sugar. Bake in the preheated oven for around 35 minutes until the bread is golden and crisp and the figs look yummy. Serve with some really cold crème fraîche or ice cream.

Try this: Hot cross buns, or currant buns, are great, but you can also try using some lovely brioche bread or croissants.

SERVES 6

250g/9oz mascarpone cheese

1 handful of unsalted shelled pistachio nuts

4 tablespoons honey

zest of 2 oranges and juice of 1

optional: 100g/3½oz dark chocolate, bashed up

1 knob of butter

4 hot cross buns, or currant buns

12 nice ripe figs (green or black)

2 tablespoons icing sugar

funky coke float

This is a ridiculous dessert which brings back a lot of old memories of when I lived in my parents' pub. I used to make coke floats for all my mates – we would all creep into the pub between lunch and dinner service and take the home-made ice cream cartons out of the freezer. If I was in luck there would be some melted chocolate in the pastry section – I'd pour this over 2 scoops of ice cream in a glass and top it off with Coca-Cola and a sprinkle of sugar-encrusted pecans and almonds. These are dead easy to make – just dip the nuts in water, shake off any excess, then mix with plenty of icing sugar until they are sticky. Place them on a baking tray and toast in the oven for 15 minutes at 180°C/350°C/gas 4 until golden. You can serve this as a dessert or a drink, and it's obviously OTT, but to this day it always seems like a bit of a treat – although now I'm a big boy I've replaced Coca-Cola with a double shot of espresso which works just as well!

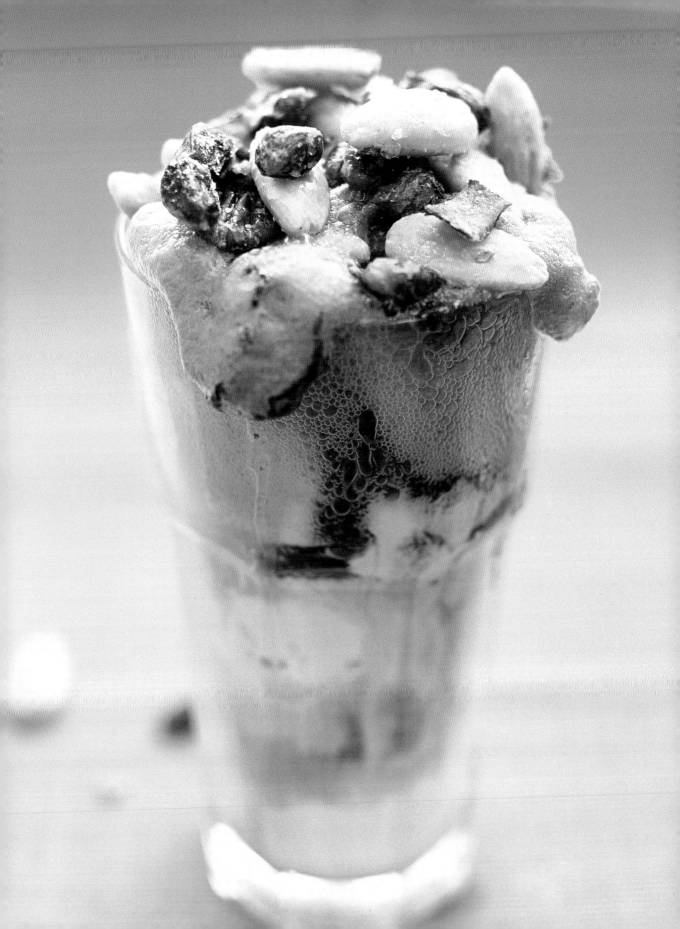

my perfect cheese plate

I really want to get you lot into cheese. I know I'm lucky as I've got the lovely Patricia from La Fromagerie down the road, but if you love your food, you'll manage to find somewhere near you that does good cheese. And with farmers' markets and family-run delis becoming more prominent, you're bound to find some half-decent stuff somewhere local.

The other day I asked Patricia to do a cheese-tasting with the fifteen Jamie's Kitchen kids – a brave woman! I was being quite forceful, to make sure that every one of them tried every cheese – even the ones that they thought smelt horrible. You've got to remember that a lot of these guys have not had an enormous repertoire of food throughout their lives, so most of the shapes, sizes and smells were completely new to them. I knew just how they felt, because I knew bugger all about cheese until about six years ago, when Patricia did a similar tasting at the River Café, where I was working. But the great thing was watching their faces light up when they realized they'd never tasted a Brie or a Cheddar like that before. Or seeing them really tucking into some of the more unusual ones, like goat's cheese with truffles or rolled in ash, going back for seconds of the humming Taleggio and Torta Gorgonzola. Or watching their total amazement when they tasted the difference between buffalo mozzarella and rubbery cow's mozzarella. And, yes, some of them did say that they still preferred the more predictable Bries and Cheddars they'd grown up with, but it was a real pleasure hearing some of the others say their favourite was one of the more obscure cheeses, which shocked even them.

To me the perfect cheese plate encapsulates as many sensations as possible – fresh, mild, strong, hard, soft, crumbly, smelly or fragrant, tangy, oozy, grainy ones rolled or rubbed in this, that or the other – and ones made from different milks – goat's, cow's, buffalo and sheep. My perfect cheese plate would be a mixture of all these things, depending on what I could get hold of at the time. Always eat the milder, fresher cheeses on the board first and then build up to the climax of the strongest blue and gorgonzolas. I'd be really excited if I was given a cheese plate like this at a dinner party or a restaurant.

With regard to what you eat with cheese, some lovely fresh bread or lightly grilled sourdough is my favourite. I've never been a fan of biscuits or crackers to be honest but if it makes you happy, go for it. Sometimes you can really complement a cheese by eating little dried fruits with it. It's hard to say what's right and wrong here. All I would suggest is that you try things, and if they don't suit you then there's your answer.

I was really interested to find out that grapes and celery are used between cheese to clean the palate, so that you can taste the full potential of the next cheese. At home I serve bread, 6 or 7 cheeses ranging from a mild fresh goat's cheese to a strong blue, some nice organic apples from the farmers' market, grapes, celery and, even better, some peeled baby carrots, fresh peas and, around early summer, beautiful thin-skinned cherry tomatoes. I love the way you can leave the board in the middle of the table and as the conversation flows you can return to your favourite cheese after you've tasted them all.

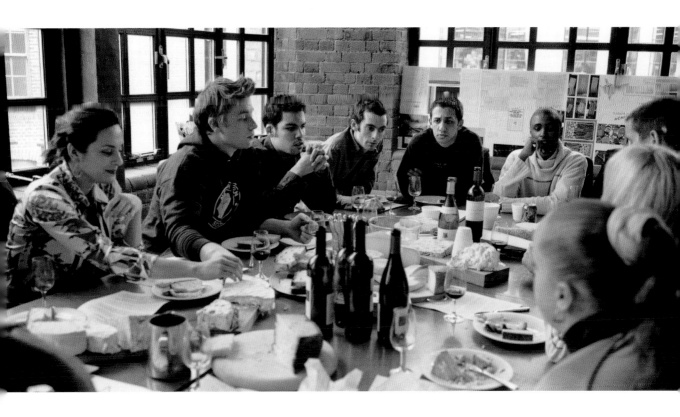

'it may only be a cheese plate, but it could be the highlight of the evening'

the perfect basic bread recipe

Stage 1: Dissolve the yeast and honey (or sugar) in half the tepid water.

Stage 2: On a clean surface or in a large bowl, make a pile of the flour and salt. Make a well in the centre and pour in all the dissolved yeast mixture. With 4 fingers of one hand, make circular movements from the centre moving outwards, slowly bringing in more and more of the flour until all the yeast mixture is soaked up. Then pour the other half of the tepid water into the centre and gradually incorporate all the flour to make a moist dough. (Certain flours may need a little more water, so don't be afraid to adjust the quantities.)

Stage 3: Kneading! This is the best bit, just rolling, pushing and folding the dough over and over for 5 minutes. This develops the gluten and the structure of the dough. If any of the dough sticks to your hands, just rub them together with a little extra flour.

Stage 4: Flour both your hands well, and lightly flour the top of the dough. Make it into a roundish shape and place it on a baking tray. Score it deeply with a knife allowing it to relax and prove with ease until it's doubled in size. Ideally you want a warm, moist, draught-free place for the quickest prove, for example near a warm cooker or in the airing cupboard, and you could cover it with clingfilm if you want to speed things up. This proving process improves the flavour and texture of the dough and should take around 40 minutes, depending on the conditions.

Stage 5: When the dough has doubled in size you need to knock the air out of it by bashing it around for a minute. Now you can shape it into whatever shape is required — round, flat, filled, trayed up, tinned up or whatever — and leave it to prove for a second time until it doubles in size again. The important thing is not to lose your confidence now. Don't feel a need to rush through this, because the second proving time will give you the lovely, delicate soft texture that we all love in fresh bread.

Stage 6: Now it's time to cook your loaf. You want to keep all the air inside it, so gently place it in the preheated oven and don't knock it or slam the door. Bake according to the time and temperature given in the recipe variations which follow. You can tell if your bread is cooked by tapping its bottom (if it's in a tin you'll have to take it out). If it sounds hollow it's cooked, if it doesn't then pop it back in for a little longer. Put it on a rack to cool before tucking in!

30g/1oz fresh yeast or 3 x 7g sachets of dried yeast

30g/1oz honey (or sugar)

625ml/just over 1 pint tepid water

1kg/just over 2lb strong bread flour

30g/1oz salt

some extra flour for dusting

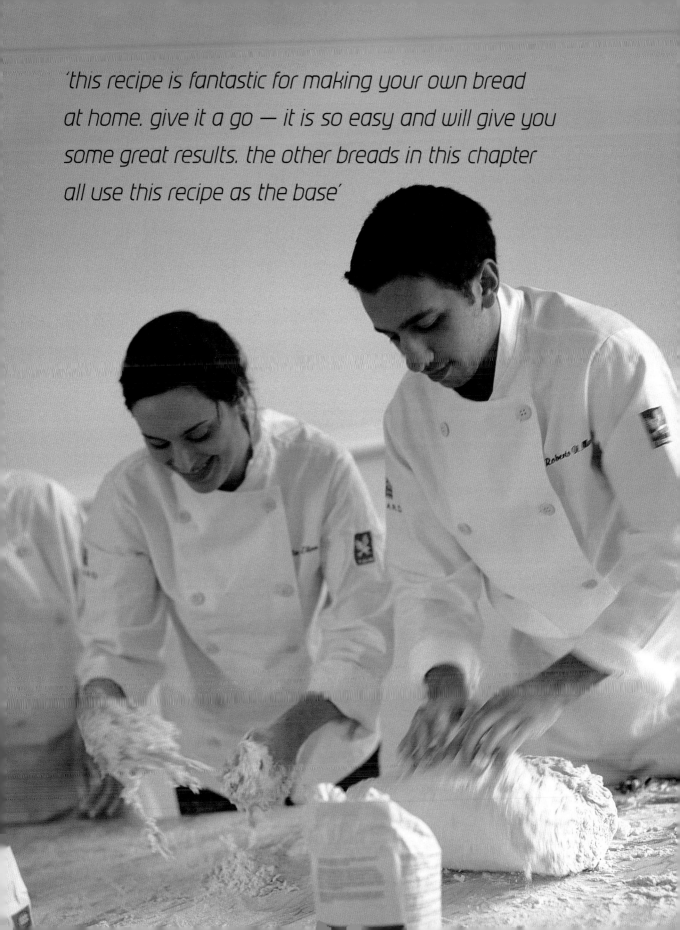

'this recipe is fantastic for making your own bread
at home. give it a go — it is so easy and will give you
some great results. the other breads in this chapter
all use this recipe as the base'

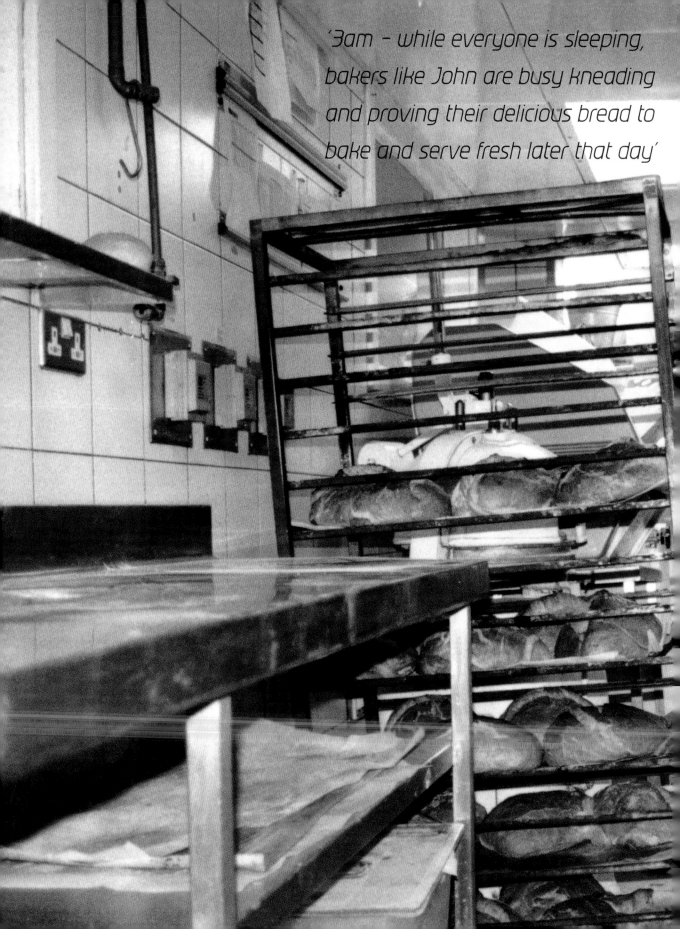

'3am – while everyone is sleeping, bakers like John are busy kneading and proving their delicious bread to bake and serve fresh later that day'

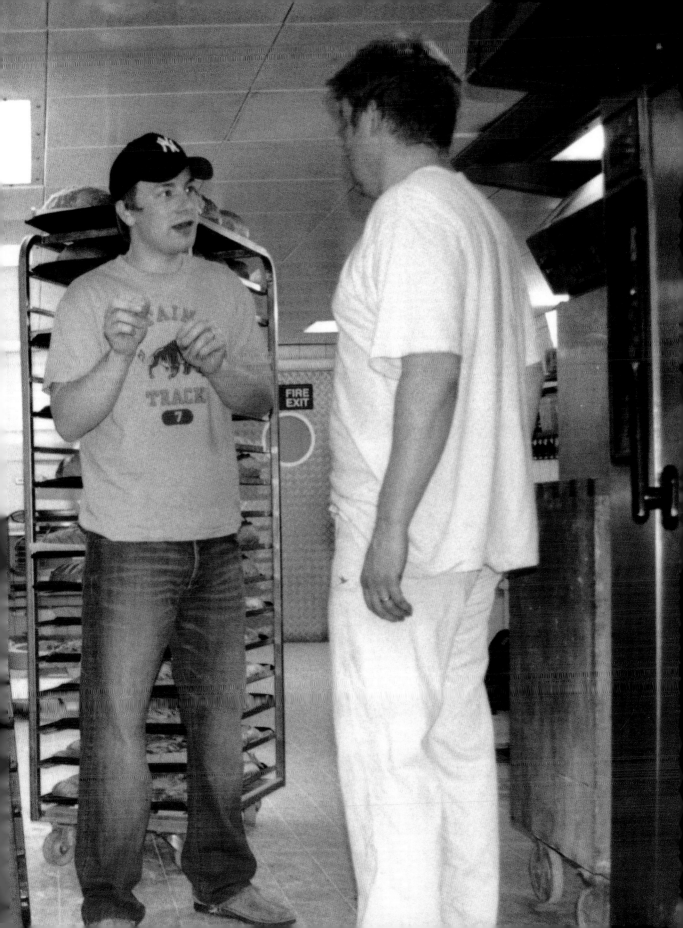

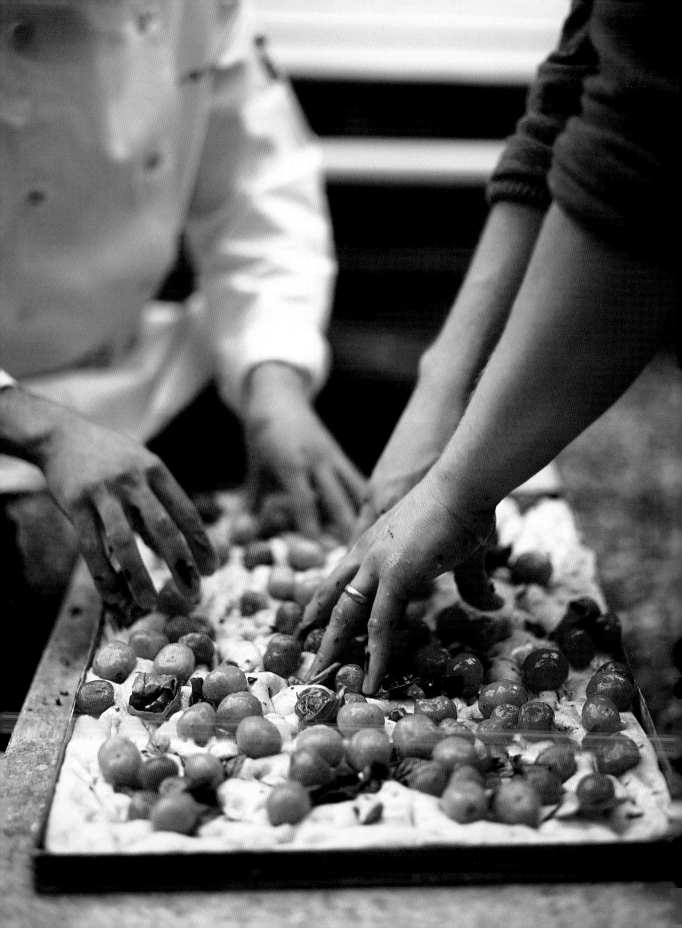

tomato focaccia

I've been a big fan of focaccia bread for a long time, and this is my favourite this year, using fantastic little cherry tomatoes – green, red and yellow – and of course their best mate, basil. It makes a fantastic picnic sandwich or main course bread which everyone seems to love.

Make up your basic bread recipe and allow to prove for 40 minutes. While it's proving, prick your tomatoes with a knife and drop them into boiling water for around 30 seconds (see page 110). Drain, cool them under cold water, and remove the skins, keeping them whole if possible as they're nice and small. Put the tomatoes in a bowl, cover with the olive oil and put to one side. I usually make one large focaccia but you can make 2 smaller ones if you like.

Take your proved dough and bash the air out, then put it on a floured surface and roll it out about 2.5cm/1 inch thick. Transfer it to a floured baking tray and push the dough to fill the tray. Pour over the olive oil and tomatoes and sprinkle over the basil. Push your fingers to the bottom of the tray across the whole dough, using them like a poker, pushing them through the dough and then flattening them out when you hit the tin. This gives the bread its classic shape and makes indentations so you get little pools of oil while it's cooking. Leave to prove until it has doubled in size again then sprinkle with salt and pepper and carefully place into a preheated oven at 220°C/425°F/gas 7. Cook for around 20 minutes, until the bread is crisp and golden on top and soft in the middle. Drizzle with more extra virgin olive oil when you take it out of the oven.

MAKES 1 LARGE OR 2 SMALLER FOCACCIAS

1 x basic bread recipe (see page 312)

600g/1lb 6oz cherry tomatoes

10 tablespoons extra virgin olive oil

flour

1 good handful of fresh basil, leaves picked

sea salt and freshly ground black pepper

rosemary and raisin bread

This is such a fantastic combination – and really works well as a table bread served with anything. It's especially good with a little ploughman's lunch and even better in a Cheddar cheese sandwich with Branston pickle. The sweetness of the raisins makes it absolutely fantastic, so give it a go.

Start making your basic bread dough, adding the rosemary and raisins at the start of Stage 3. You may want to add a little more flour if the dough is too sticky. Continue with the basic recipe until the dough is nice and elastic, then allow it to prove for about 30–60 minutes. Divide the dough in half and knead it with a little extra flour – you can shape it any way you like, but I like to make 2 long sausage-shaped loaves. Place on a tray, dust with flour, and leave to prove again until doubled in size. Score down the length of the bread with a really sharp knife (sometimes I poke a stick of rosemary into each loaf) and bake in the preheated oven at 180°C/350°F/gas 4 for around 25 minutes, until golden and crisp. Leave to cool before eating.

MAKES 2 MEDIUM-SIZED LOAVES

1 x basic bread recipe (see page 312)

1 large bunch of fresh rosemary, leaves picked

500g/1lb 2oz raisins, chopped

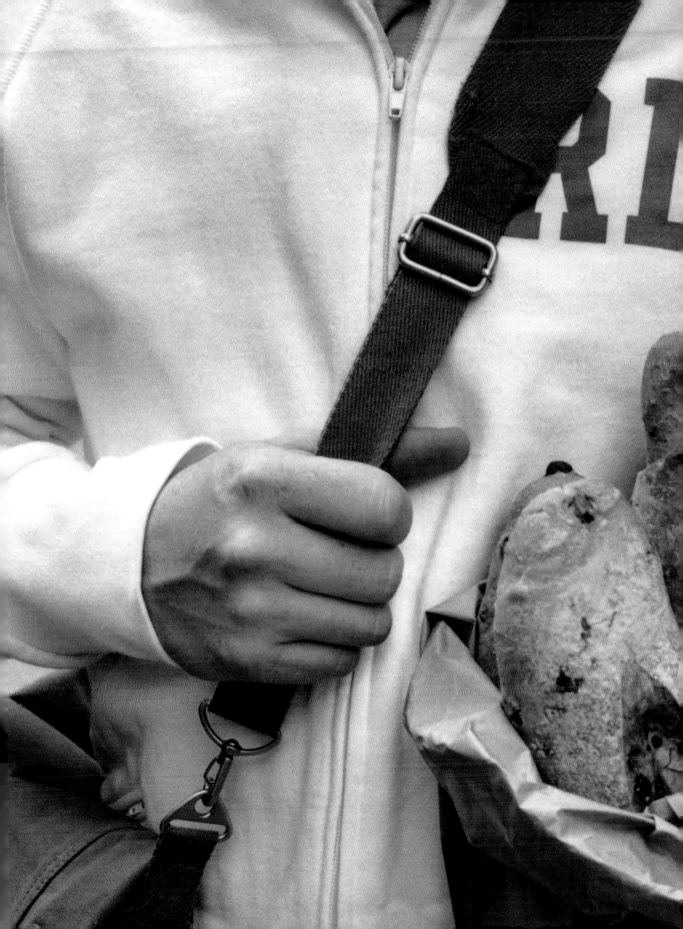

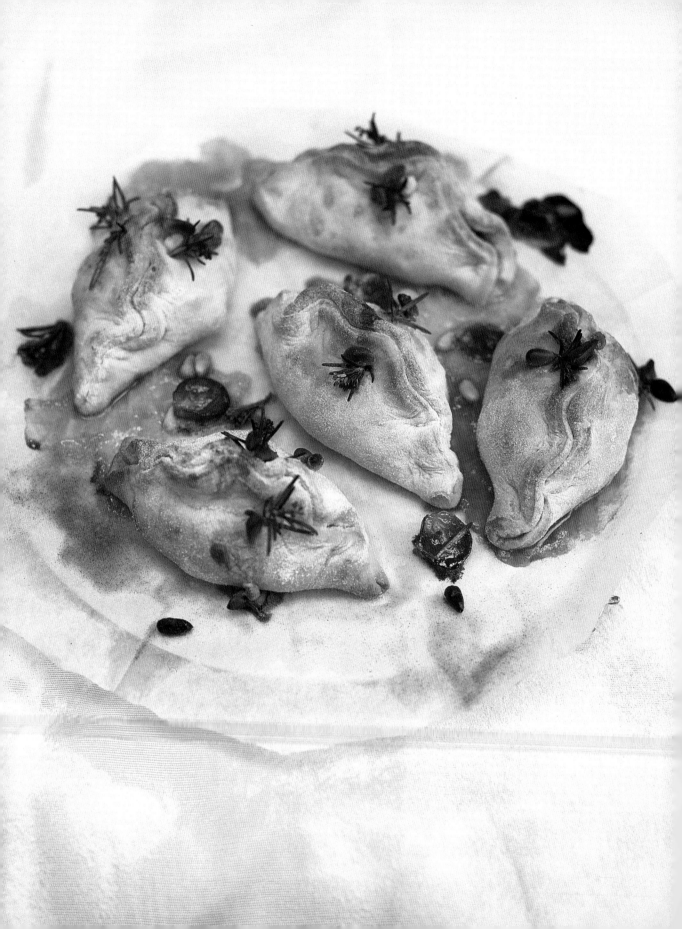

little sweet grape and rosemary calzones

Calzones are little stuffed folded breads. I've made them really small and I've made them really large, and I've served them on the menu at Monte's as a dessert with some nice vanilla and rosemary ice cream. These small ones would be just as at home with a nice cheese plate (see page 310).

Start your basic bread dough and work through the recipe until the first prove. While the dough is proving, mix your grapes, cinnamon, rosemary, vin santo, sugar and pinenuts in a bowl. The sugar will draw all the lovely syrupy juice out of the grapes. Allow your grapes to marinate until the dough has doubled in size.

Divide the dough into 2 pieces, roll each of these out 1cm/½ inch thick, and dust with flour to stop it sticking. Using a 15cm/6 inch pastry cutter or a saucer as a template, cut out circles. Of course you can do any size you like, but small ones are quite cute for desserts. Put a dessertspoon of filling in the middle of each circle, fold in half, then crimp the edges together (see the pictures below). You don't want any cracks, so just pinch them together if you see any appearing. Drizzle the calzones with a little olive oil and spike them with some rosemary leaves if you like. Bake in a preheated oven at 180°C/350°F/gas 4 for 20 minutes until golden.

Try this: Add 100g/3½oz of crumbly ricotta to the grapes. This is nice and makes it a bit more cakey.

MAKES 10–14 SMALL CALZONES

1 x basic bread recipe (see page 312)

500g/1lb 2oz seedless green or red grapes, washed, picked and halved

½ teaspoon cinnamon

3 sprigs of fresh rosemary, leaves picked

1 small wineglass of vin santo or sweet white wine

150g/5½oz sugar

1 handful of pinenuts, lightly toasted

flour

extra virgin olive oil

optional: sticks of rosemary

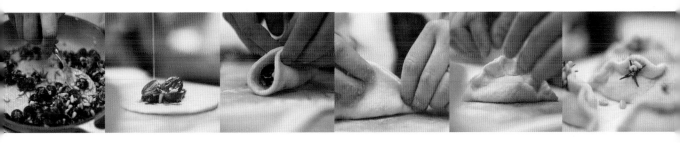

sweet roasted red onion and garlic bread

This is a genius little bread and, to be honest, served warm it's almost like a meal in itself. Great in lunchboxes or for picnics or barbecues.

Make up the basic bread recipe. While it's proving preheat the oven to 190°C/375°F/gas 5. Put all the other ingredients apart from the flour in a small roasting tray and bake in the preheated oven for half an hour. Allow to cool, then finely chop. Bash the air out of your proved dough and roll out in a roundish shape to about 1cm/½ inch thick on a flour-dusted surface. Smear the sweet onion and garlic mixture over the bread, then roll the bread up, folding in the sides and pushing it roughly into the shape that you want. Place it on an oiled baking tray, dust with flour, and score with a sharp knife. Leave to prove until doubled in size, then bake in a preheated oven at 220°C/425°F/gas 7 for about 35 minutes until the bread is crisp and golden and sounds hollow when tapped.

MAKES 1 LARGE LOAF

1 x basic bread recipe (see page 312)

4 red onions, peeled and sliced

2 bulbs of garlic, cloves peeled and sliced

10 tablespoons balsamic vinegar

4 tablespoons olive oil

1 small handful fresh thyme, leaves picked and bashed up

flour

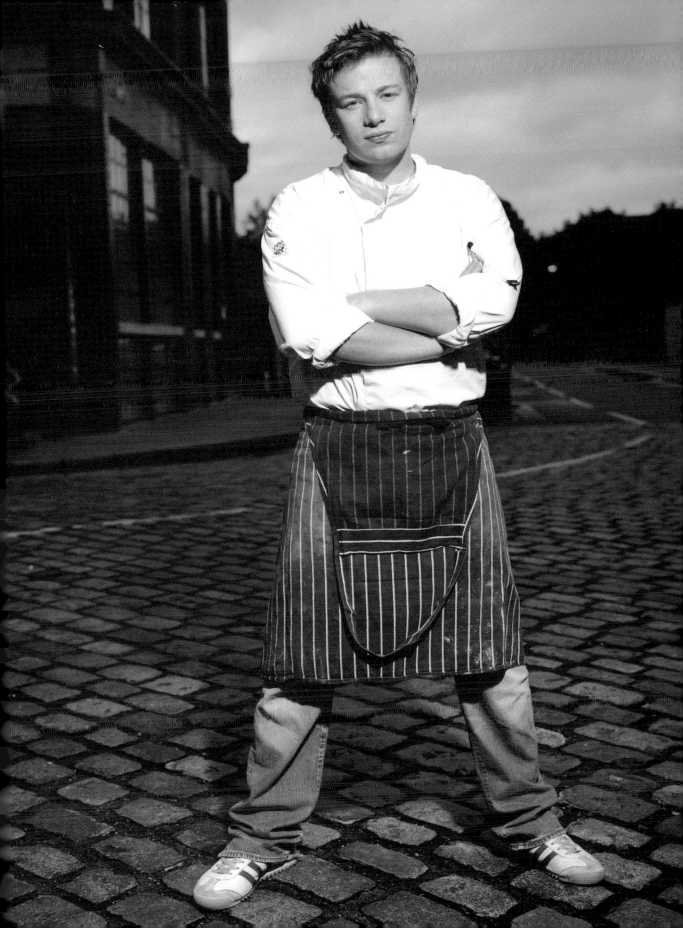

slow-roasted tomato bread

This is a lovely intense sweet bread. It's brilliant for lunch, toasted with some mozzarella cheese and a little basil, or served simply with dinner. You can make a large loaf or smaller ones as I have here, using some old tomato tins which I have washed out and lined with greaseproof paper.

Preheat the oven to 150°C/300°F/gas 2. Prick the tomatoes with a knife – you can leave them on the vine. Toss them into an appropriately sized roasting tray with the garlic – you want the tomatoes to fit nice and snugly so you only have one layer. Rip in your basil, season well with salt and pepper and even a little chilli crumbled over if you like, and add 2 or 3 lugs of extra virgin olive oil. Place the tray in the preheated oven and roast for about 1 hour.

When the tomatoes are done, remove and allow to cool. Squeeze the sweet garlic out of its skin and throw the skins away. Choose 6–8 really nice tomatoes and put them aside to use on top of your bread. Remove all the stalks from the remaining tomatoes, then mash them up with the garlic, scraping up all the lovely, sticky goodness from the bottom of the tray. Start making your basic bread dough, and when it comes to adding the water, at Stage 2, pour your mushed tomatoes into a measuring jug and just top up with water to give you the same amount of liquid as in the basic recipe. Carry on with the rest of the recipe, adjusting the amount of flour so you end up with a non-sticky, elastic, shiny bread dough. Allow it to prove for half an hour.

Shape the dough into a large loaf or smaller rolls. If you're using tins, like I have, oil them well with olive oil and divide the dough between them and then push the remaining tomatoes into each one. Leave to prove again until doubled in size (about 15 minutes). Bake at 180°C/350°F/ gas 4 for around 20 minutes until golden and crisp. A larger loaf will need an extra 10–15 minutes. To check if the bread is ready, tap the bottom of it. A dull thud means it's done.

Try this: As a quick alternative, you could work through the basic bread recipe and simply add sun-dried tomatoes. Just tear them up and squeeze them into the dough at Stage 5.

And this: Push some pieces of mozzarella into the bread with the tomatoes before baking.

MAKES 6–8 'TIN' BREADS

1kg/2¼lb cherry vine tomatoes (or plum tomatoes)

1 bulb of garlic, cut in half crosswise

1 handful of fresh basil, leaves picked

sea salt and freshly ground black pepper

optional: 1–2 dried red chillies

extra virgin olive oil

1 x basic bread recipe (see page 312)

optional: 6–8 empty tomato tins, or equivalent, to cook the bread in

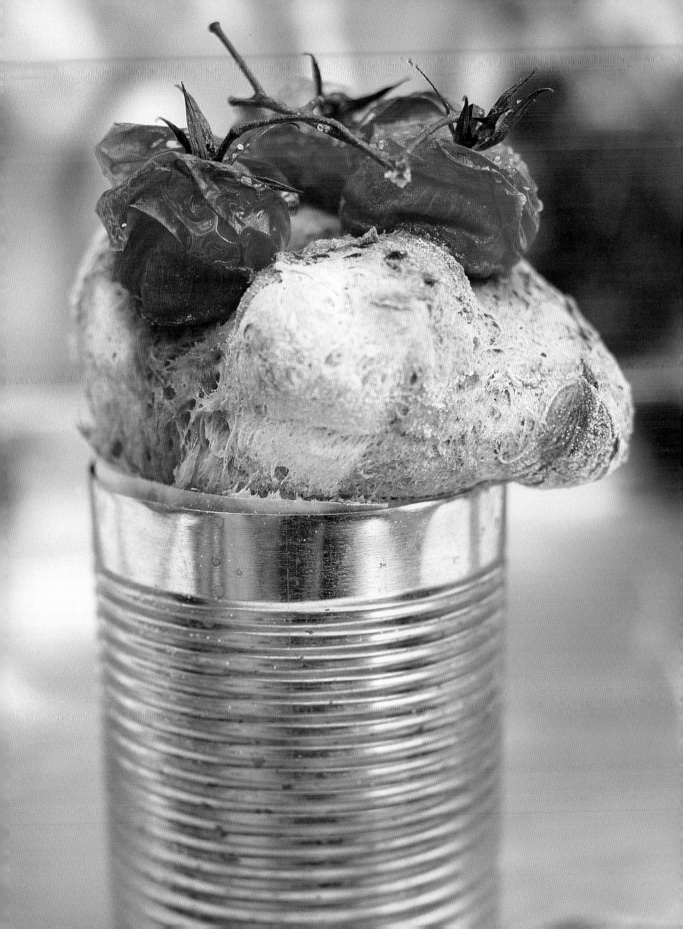

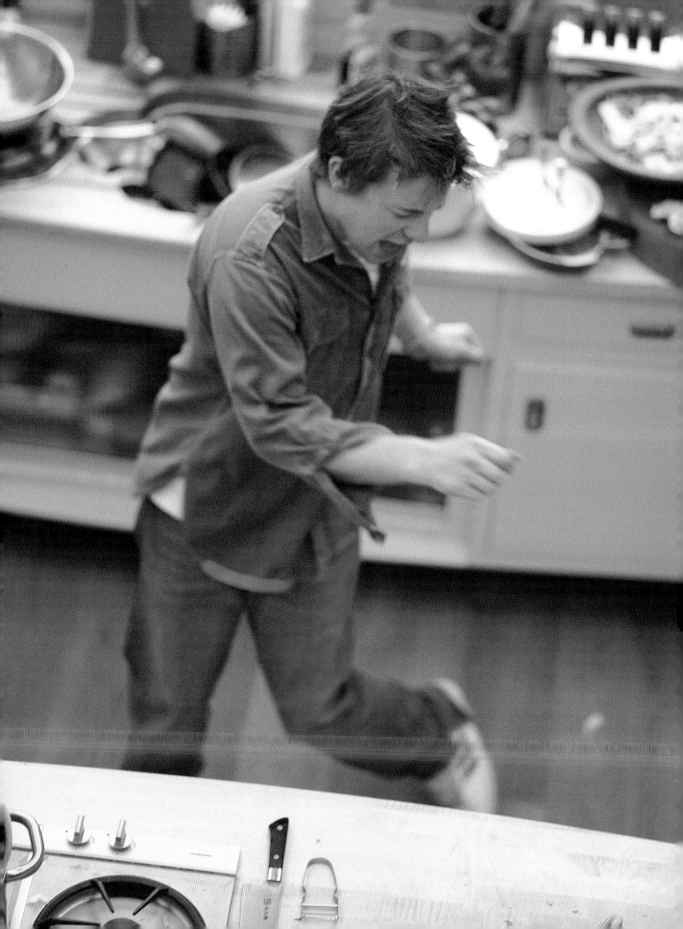

index

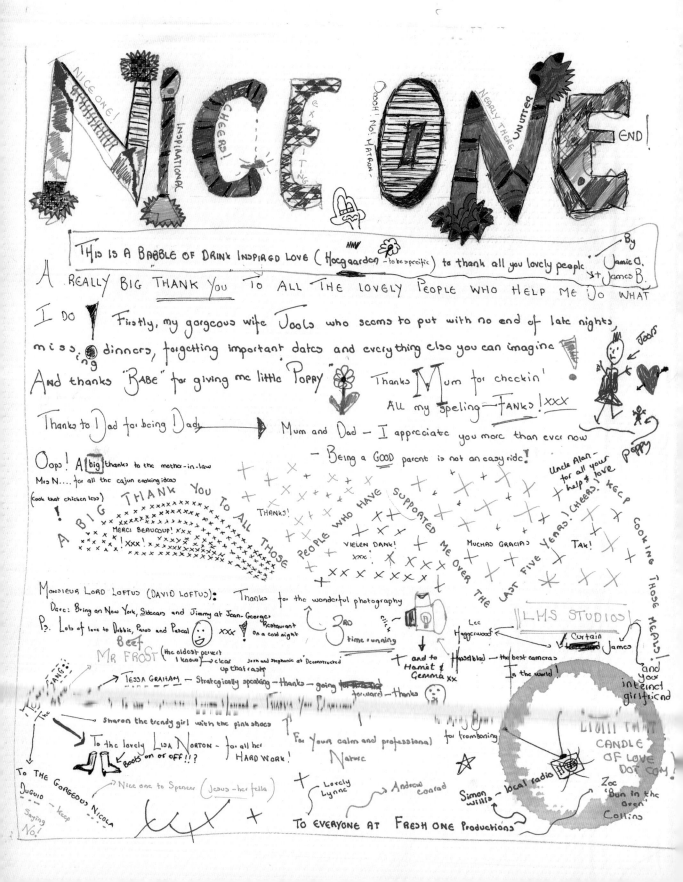

NICE ONE

Nice one! Aaaahhhhh! Cheers! Inspirational! Exciting! Oooh! No! Matron. Nearly there. Utter. End!

THIS IS A BABBLE OF DRINK INSPIRED LOVE (Hoegaarden - to be specific) to thank all you lovely people. By Jamie O. & James B.

A REALLY BIG THANK YOU TO ALL THE LOVELY PEOPLE WHO HELP ME DO WHAT I DO! Firstly, my gorgeous wife Jools who seems to put with no end of late nights, missing dinners, forgetting important dates and everything else you can imagine. And thanks "BABE" for giving me little Poppy. Thanks Mum for checkin' all my speling - FANKS! xxx

Thanks to Dad for being Dad → Mum and Dad - I appreciate you more than ever now - Being a GOOD parent is not an easy ride!

Oops! A big thanks to the mother-in-law Mrs N.... for all the cajun cooking ideas (cook that chicken less)

A BIG THANK YOU TO ALL THOSE PEOPLE WHO HAVE SUPPORTED ME OVER THE LAST FIVE YEARS! CHEERS. KEEP COOKING THOSE MEALS!

Uncle Alan - for all your help & love

THANKS! MERCI BEAUCOUP! xxx !xxx! VIELEN DANK! xxx! MUCHAS GRACIAS! TAK!

Monsieur Lord Loftus (DAVID LOFTUS): Thanks for the wonderful photography - 3RD time running - click

Dave: Bring on New York, Sidecars and Jimmy at Jean-George's Restaurant on a cold night

P.S. Lots of love to Debbie, Paros and Pascal xxx! Beef

and to Hamet & Gemma xx

LHS STUDIOS

Lee Haggerwood → Hasselblad - the best cameras in the world! - and your internet girlfriend

Mr FROST (the oldest pervert I know) - clear up that rash! Josh and Stephanie at Deconstructed

Curtain James

TESSA GRAHAM - Strategically speaking - thanks - going forward - thanks

Sharon the trendy girl with the pink shoes

To the lovely LISA NORTON - for all her HARD WORK! Boots on or off!!?

For your calm and professional Nature for tromboning

Nice one to Spencer (Jesus - her fella)

To THE GORGEOUS NICOLA DUGUID - keep saying No!

Lovely Lynne Andrew Conrad Simon Willis - local radio

TO EVERYONE AT FRESH ONE Productions

LIGHT THAT CANDLE OF LOVE DOT COM!

Zoe "Bun in the oven" Collins

To JEKKA (the best organic herb lady in the world) — GET YOUR WINDOW BOXES DONE

www.jekkasherbfarm.com

Completely legal promotion

mean girl

(psycho olive)

GIVE ELVIS Hair

To Gennaro and Liz — Passione Restaurant

Thank you for being a constant inspiration and friend

(10 Charlotte Street)

Stronzo!

Book a table if you want to try some great food

020 7636 2833

Dan Dimbleby (unflexible object)

WE LOVE JOOLS + HER!

To Jamie Scouser — The Restaurant Manager

Sandy
+ Store Directors

TALKBACK You have done me proud Mate

STICKY TOFFEE PUDDING

(thanks to Ginny and John Pratt)

endone was not to posh to posh — oi oi!!

Give Baby

World's Best mother xxx!!

I give up!! AHHHH

(this is meat)

Joat Golborne Fishing Peter Rincham

Lovely Daisy Goodwin

Frenchman Peter Moore Rushton's

Rushton's Cynic Boob

Come and See

WWW.JAMIEOLIVER.COM

Harvey Nichols

to lunch at Allens

Gary at M. Moen and Sons

John / Claire / Sadie + Hamilton

GUILD BOOKS

Thanks to Cockerton Thanks for all the fruit and veg

Hany Mate

Sheila Keating — Dad + Liam
Love + Embraces

HASSELBLAD
you make the best cameras everything.

Peter Bowron

and all the rest of the PENGUIN sales team

Mr Boss Man
Tom

To my publisher John Hamilton

Have not heard any complaints from you this time! You must trust me — Thanks for everything. JUMxxxxx

To my Editor: LINDSEY JORDAN

Ok you're getting on at your job but don't get cocky! I can tell that you are married because you are better at chewing my ear off.

Luv u and Gary — Bless!

Nicky Barneby Your the Best

Annie Lee (copy editor)
Love You J xxx

VERY GOOD DRAWING By JOliver

Sophie Brewer

Mr Richards - thanks for all your dedication to the kids at catering college.

WINES

To David Gleave
ON: 020 7720 5350

For the best Italian wines / helping me source the best Olive Oil

The handsome PETE BEGG... the Sean Connory of the kitchen! Cheers mate. And to little Tommy too.

POULET LA GHOTTE

Chaise Ric—a

You're tasty Mark Gautier

Everyone at Borough Market — Peter Gott, Sharpy, Les the Shrimp man, Mr Turnip and the Game + everyone else

Keith Taylor (sorry about the deadline)

Tara Ont — Poulett You're Gorgeous

Marie Cassidy Do it!!

To My AGENT: Borra / Aden / Michelle

Alex @ The Roost

Jimmy — the

THANKS TO EURODST FOR A COUPLE OF FREE TICKETS

To Peter and Alex at the Outside digivation

Nature boy

where it is!!

Thanks 4 David Beckhams Boots I've used them well

To Ben, Guy + the Gang at Moving Brands

Sorry again about the fad

Cheese on toast coming TO

To Andy the Gasman

VILLAGE IDIOT — get a girlfriend it's been 13 year. I am starting to think you are turning

2 Neighbour James B thanks 4 the small writing... get your Boy out xxx

British Gas — (Servicing all your needs)!!

Patrick + Don
from LA FROMAGERIE

Shut up Jools

Jamie Oliver Jamie

YOUR THE best SORRY!!

MAKING LIFE TASTE BETTER

To Sir Peter Davis
Sarah Weller and all the gang at SAINSBURYS

This thanks page or won't... I CANT

I love you Jamie... but will u just come home now and stop getting legless with James... I'm hungry

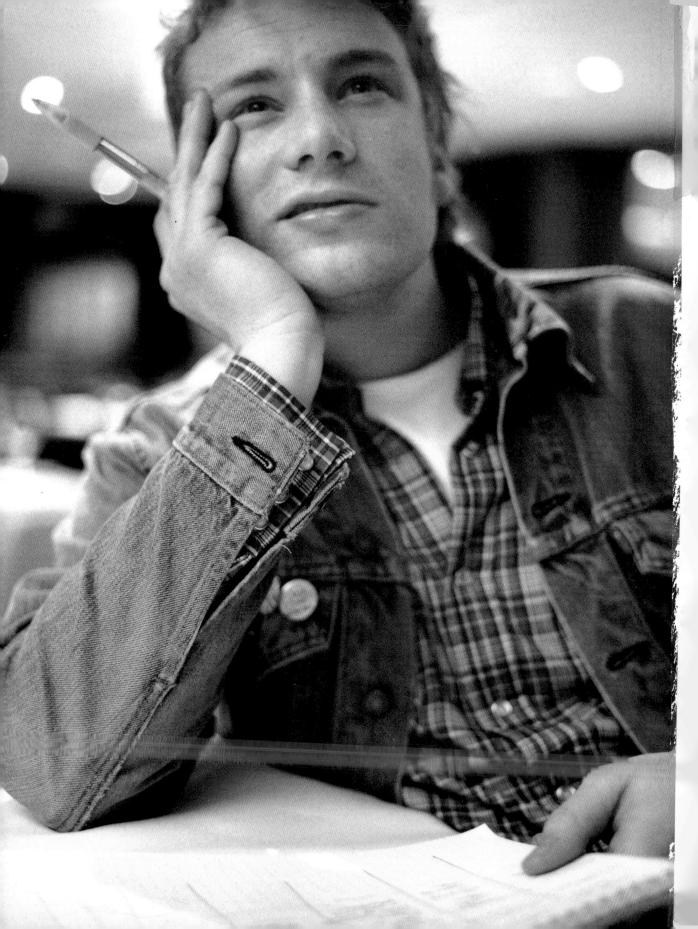